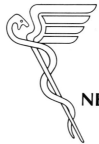

1979
YEAR BOOK OF

NEUROLOGY
AND
NEUROSURGERY

THE 1979 YEAR BOOKS

The YEAR BOOK series provides in condensed form the essence of the best of the recent international medical literature. The material is selected by distinguished editors who critically review more than 500,000 journal articles each year.

Anesthesia
Drs. Eckenhoff, Bart, Brunner, Holley and Linde.

Cancer
Drs. Clark, Cumley and Hickey.

Cardiology
Drs. Harvey, Kirkendall, Kirklin, Nadas, Paul and Sonnenblick.

Dentistry
Drs. Hale, Hazen, Moyers, Redig, Robinson and Silverman.

Dermatology
Dr. Dobson.

Diagnostic Radiology
Drs. Whitehouse, Bookstein, Gabrielsen, Holt, Martel, Silver and Thornbury.

Drug Therapy
Drs. Azarnoff, Hollister and Shand.

Endocrinology
Drs. Schwartz and Ryan.

Family Practice
Dr. Rakel.

Medicine
Drs. Rogers, Des Prez, Cline, Braunwald, Greenberger, Bondy and Epstein.

Neurology and Neurosurgery
Drs. De Jong and Sugar.

Nuclear Medicine
Drs. Quinn and Spies.

Obstetrics and Gynecology
Drs. Pitkin and Zlatnik.

Ophthalmology
Dr. Hughes.

Orthopedics and Traumatic Surgery
Dr. Coventry.

Otolaryngology
Drs. Strong and Paparella.

Pathology and Clinical Pathology
Drs. Carone and Conn.

Pediatrics
Drs. Oski and Stockman.

Plastic and Reconstructive Surgery
Drs. McCoy, Brauer, Dingman, Hanna, Haynes and Hoehn.

Psychiatry and Applied Mental Health
Drs. Romano, Freedman, Friedhoff, Kolb, Lourie and Nemiah.

Surgery
Drs. Schwartz, Najarian, Peacock, Shires, Silen and Spencer.

Urology
Dr. Gillenwater.

The YEAR BOOK of

Neurology and Neurosurgery

1979

NEUROLOGY

Edited by

RUSSELL N. DE JONG, M.D.

Professor Emeritus of Neurology,
The University of Michigan Medical School

NEUROSURGERY

Edited by

OSCAR SUGAR, M.D.

Professor and Head of the Department of
Neurosurgery, University of Illinois
Abraham Lincoln School of Medicine

YEAR BOOK MEDICAL PUBLISHERS, INC.
CHICAGO • LONDON

Printed in U.S.A.

Library of Congress Catalog Card Number: CD38-24

International Standard Book Number: 0-8151-2419-8

Table of Contents

The material covered in this volume represents literature reviewed up to April, 1979.

Current Literature Quiz

The significant advances described in this YEAR BOOK introduce new diagnostic and therapeutic procedures useful for treating conditions seen frequently in your practice. The following questionnaire will test your familiarity with the current literature. References to the articles on which the questions are based are given in the back of the book.

1. What parts of the spinal cord are most apt to be affected by hypoxia or anoxia?
2. What are the major causes of transverse myelopathy?
3. What pathologic changes are found in studies of cerebellar biopsies performed on patients with intractable epilepsy?
4. Need one be concerned about possible sequelae of febrile convulsions?
5. Is the absence of pulsation of the retinal veins a reliable index of increased intracranial pressure?
6. What is a probable mechanism for the development of drusen of the optic nerve?
7. Are all aspects of neurologic function affected by aging?
8. What are some of the causes of recurrent hypersomnia?
9. Does one run any risk of untoward effects by using glucocorticoid hormones in the perinatal period?
10. What is meant by basilar migraine and in what group of patients does it usually occur?
11. What readily available stimulant can sometimes be used instead of closely regulated prescription drugs in the treatment of hyperactive children?
12. How does juvenile Huntington's chorea differ from Huntington's chorea which occurs in adults?
13. What is prolonged twilight state and what is its usual etiology?
14. What types of lesions produce delta waves in the EEG?
15. What is the Lennox or Lennox-Gastaut syndrome?
16. Levels of anticonvulsant drugs in what body fluid, other

than the blood, may be used for accurate calculations of the body concentration of these drugs?

17. In the control of what types of seizures is clonazepam particularly valuable?

18. It is accepted that carbamazepine is an effective anticonvulsant drug. What advantages does it have over other anticonvulsant drugs in the treatment of epilepsy?

19. Why is it important to monitor all anticonvulsant drugs in patients receiving sodium valproate?

20. How does the action of levodopa differ from that of bromocriptine and lergotrile in bringing about relief of symptoms in Parkinson's disease?

21. What brings on attacks of familial paroxysmal dystonic choreoathetosis?

22. How do cluster headaches and migraine differ from each other?

23. The inactivated poliomyelitis vaccine should be reserved for use of what groups of patients?

24. What diagnostic procedure should be carried out prior to instituting treatment of herpes simplex encephalitis with adenine arabinoside?

25. What approaches to therapy other than the parenteral administration of antibiotics are indicated in neonatal meningitis?

26. What special precautions should be used in the handling of materials from and the medical care of patients with Creuztfeldt-Jakob disease?

27. Are the peripheral nerves ever affected in multiple sclerosis?

28. If it is true that there is an association between household pets and multiple sclerosis, what specific pets are involved and by what means are they carriers of the disease?

29. What is the mode of action of corticosteroids in myasthenia gravis?

30. Is it possible to make the diagnosis of Duchenne's muscular dystrophy during the prenatal period?

31. What are the dangers of cervical myelopathy in patients with rheumatoid arthritis?

32. What is the mechanism of cardiopulmonary arrest in patients with diabetic autonomic neuropathy?

33. Why is it important to make the diagnosis of giant cell arteritis as early as possible?
34. What are the factors that influence stroke recurrence in patients with transient ischemic attacks?
35. Why is Holter monitoring essential in many patients having periodic cerebral symptoms?
36. Is an EEG helpful in predicting anoxic brain damage after resuscitation of patients who have had a cardiac arrest?
37. What clinical manifestations indicate a poor prognosis after cardiopulmonary arrest?
38. What is alpha-pattern coma?
39. What cerebrospinal fluid changes are found in 90% of patients with clinically definite multiple sclerosis?
40. What is the mode of action of baclofen in the relief of spasticity?
41. How can recordings of brain stem auditory responses be used to reveal lesions of the posterior fossa that are not clinically apparent?
42. What are three effective measures to reduce intracranial hypertension?
43. What are the benefits of ventriculosubgaleal shunts?
44. Is section of the dentate ligaments of the spinal cord worth the trouble?
45. Which end of the central canal of the spinal cord should be opened for syringomyelia?
46. Pantopaque and radioactive materials can be used to detect, grossly, the general location of cerebrospinal fluid leaks. What materials can be used for more precise localization?
47. In cranial defect surgery, what determines the choice of available materials for replacement of the skull?
48. When are radiologic techniques other than computerized tomography scans necessary in diagnosis of cerebellopontine angle lesions?
49. What can be done to aid computerized tomography diagnosis when subdural hematomas are isodense with brain?
50. How can nuclide injections be used to confirm brain death?
51. What types of arachnoiditis can be diagnosed by myelography?

52. Should computerized tomography scanning be required in all patients with head injuries?
53. What variations exist in frequency of postoperative neurologic infections, causative organisms and prophylactic antibiotics?
54. How much of the calvarium can be removed for neonatal craniosynostosis?
55. Is early urinary diversion the best way of dealing with bladder control in open myelomeningocele?
56. Henk Verbiest believes that most acquired lumbar canal stenosis is superimposed on preexisting developmental stenosis. What treatment does he use, and with what results?
57. Do intrathecal steroids reduce or promote adhesive arachnoiditis?
58. What is the dilemma concerning treatment of childhood optic gliomas?
59. Is biopsy an essential prelude to radiation therapy of tumors of the posterior 3d ventricle and pineal region?
60. What is the rationale for use of high doses of methylprednisolone in patients with inoperable brain tumors?
61. Is radiation therapy of brain tumors worthwhile?
62. What is the best way of dealing with spinal cord compression due to metastatic breast cancer?
63. What should be done about unruptured asymptomatic intracranial aneurysms?
64. When should one consider anastomosis of the occipital to the posterior inferior cerebellar artery?
65. What are the relative merits of radiofrequency lesions versus posterior fossa decompression of the trigeminal nerve for trigeminal neuralgia?
66. What are the indications for operating on the brachial plexus?

NEUROLOGY

RUSSELL N. DE JONG, M.D.

Introduction

During recent years there have been many advances in clinical neurology and the neurologic sciences. Concepts of neurologic disease have been altered by our expanding knowledge of brain chemistry, functions and pathology, of the biology and pathology of the peripheral nervous and autonomic nervous systems, and of the neuromuscular junction and the muscle tissue itself and their abnormalities in pathologic states. New information about neurotransmitters and neuromodulators has changed our concepts of the pathophysiology of important neurologic and psychiatric diseases. Advances in neuroanatomy, neuropathology and neuropsychology have expanded our knowledge of the details of cerebral function. Developments in virology and immunology have thrown light on the etiology of many neurologic diseases, several of them belonging to the category of illnesses once referred to as "degenerative." Studies on the enzyme systems, metabolic functions and genetics have even further clarified the underlying causes of important diseases. Finally, neuroradiology and related disciplines have improved our diagnostic methods, especially in developing that diagnostic technique of major importance, computerized axial tomography.

Although research into factors underlying multiple sclerosis continues on a large scale, the specific etiology of this disease has not yet been demonstrated. Evidence continues to accumulate, however, to suggest that the disease is virus related, probably to a virus to which the patient was exposed early in life. Most investigators believe, however, that the virus is not the direct cause of the disease, but the neurologic changes are the result of an immune response to the virus. Various specific viruses have been suggested as causes of multiple sclerosis, including those of measles and other common childhood infections, as well as paramyxoviruses, but none has been specifically proved to be responsible. Interestingly viral and antibody investigations similar to those carried out in multiple sclerosis are now being conducted in amyotrophic lateral sclerosis also. Further studies in this disease are being awaited with interest. It is too early to make any statement about a possible relationship between multiple sclerosis and contact with household pets and a distemper virus that might be carried by them.

At the same time that research is being conducted into solving the etiology of multiple sclerosis and other diseases of the nervous system, investigations are being pursued into diagnosis and treatment. It is now possible, by analysis of the cerebrospinal fluid by techniques using newly introduced commercial reagents and apparatus, to demonstrate diagnostic abnormalities in more than 90% of patients with clinically definite multiple sclerosis. The major changes noted are an elevation of immunoglobulin G expressed as percentage of total protein, elevation of the immunoglobulin G-albumin ratio and the presence of oligoclonal immunoglobulin G bands.

Among the most dramatically significant advances in knowledge about the functions of the brain has been the demonstration of the presence of neurotransmitters and neuromodulators in the nervous system. Of particular significance was the finding that a specific neurotransmitter, dopamine, is normally present in large amounts in the caudate nucleus, putamen and globus pallidus and that in patients with Parkinson's disease it is selectively depleted in these structures. This depletion seems to be correlated with the degree of degeneration of the pigmented cells in the substantia nigra. One of the major therapeutic advances of the past 2 decades was the demonstration that levodopa, a precursor of dopamine, increases the concentration of the latter in the basal ganglia and brings about improvement in the symptoms of Parkinson's disease. Unfortunately, such improvement does not occur in all patients, levodopa often causes distressing side effects, only some of which can be eliminated by the simultaneous administration of a decarboxylase inhibitor, and the therapeutic effects seem to lessen with time. It has now been demonstrated that certain ergot alkaloid derivatives, bromocriptine and lergotrile, are dopamine agonists that have pharmacologic properties attributable to direct stimulation of dopamine receptors.

These, when available for general use, will be added to the drugs that bring about relief from parkinsonian manifestations.

Traditionally, death has been defined as the cessation of vital functions (e.g., heartbeat and respiration). Brain function usually ceases at approximately the same time. Using the criterion of cessation of circulation of the blood and breathing, it is relatively simple, under most circumstances, to determine the exact time of death. During recent years, however, the development of modern technology has made it possible to resuscitate patients after cessation of heartbeat and respiration and to provide life-support methods for them. As a result, there is need for reevaluation of the formerly accepted criterion. Accurate determination of the exact time of death has become increasingly important to physicians and the general public since organ transplantation has become refined and often lifesaving. If the classic concept of cessation of heartbeat and respiration continues to be used as the sole criterion for death, delay in the removal of the organs to be transplanted may cause them to be irreparably damaged and the success of the transplantation operation seriously jeopardized. During approximately the same period during which organ transplantation surgery has been developed, significantly increased information about normal and abnormal cerebral function has been obtained, and the concept of *brain death* has evolved. During a relatively short time, rather voluminous literature has appeared dealing not only with the clinical and electrophysiologic aspects of this subject, but also its ethical, moral, sociologic, religious and philosophic aspects. A summation of this may be found in the chapter entitled "Cerebral Death" by A. E. Walker, published in *The Nervous System*, Volume 2, edited by D. B. Tower and Y. N. Chase (New York: Raven Press, 1975), pages 75 – 87.

For a number of years the United States Food and Drug Administration failed to release any new anticonvulsant drugs for sale and general use. During the past 2 years, however, three new anticonvulsant drugs have become available. Carbamazepine, which had been available in Europe for both the treatment of trigeminal neuralgia and related painful states and as an anticonvulsant, was available in the United States until recently only for the treatment of neuralgic conditions. It has now been made available for use also as an anticonvulsant. It is especially helpful in the treatment of focal or partial seizures with complex symptomatology (including psychomotor seizures) and for major motor seizures. Clonazepam is especially helpful in the treatment of epilepsy associated with myoclonus, petit mal and petit mal varian attacks and akinetic seizures. It is also of use in the control of photosensitive epilepsy. Sodium valproate is most helpful in the treatment of petit mal and tonic-clonic seizures, but seems to be of some value in the control of all varieties of epileptic attacks.

Computerized axial tomography has been rapidly accepted and is now widely used in neurologic diagnosis. Recently a group of British physicists have developed a new technique of medical imaging that is termed "nuclear magnetic resonance" or "zeugmatography." (Lauterbur, P. C.: Nature 242:190, 1973). This gives diagnostic information comparable to that provided by computerized tomography. For a number of reasons it may even replace tomography. Magnetic fields and radiofrequency energy utilized in the technique are harmless. Malignant cells have been shown to have abnormal relaxation times and it is possible that abnormal metabolic states are also measurable (e.g., ischemia and edema). The impact of nuclear magnetic resonance on medicine is awaited with interest (Larrick, J. W.: N. Engl. J. Med. 298:634, 1978).

RUSSELL N. DE JONG, M.D.

Neuroanatomy, Neurophysiology and Neuropathology

Localization of Pyramidal Tract in Internal Capsule of Man. Localization of the pyramidal tract in the anterior half of the posterior limb of the internal capsule has long been accepted, but recently this view has been challenged. J. Hanaway (Washington Univ.) and R. R. Young[1] (Harvard Med. School) present evidence supporting the thesis that the pyramidal motor fibers are located posteriorly in the posterior limb of the internal capsule.

Man, 72, was admitted with sudden severe right leg weakness after 6 months of stiffness and weakness of the legs. Blood pressure on admission was 220/100 mm Hg. Mild right-sided hemiparesis was present. The patient walked with aid and without ataxia. A right-sided facial palsy was noticed about 12 hours after the ictus, with increased tone in all limbs, especially on the right side, and extensor plantar responses. The right arm and then the leg became totally paralyzed over the next 12 hours. The face moved bilaterally during grimacing but speech became dysarthric. Strength then increased in the right leg, but extensor spasticity increased and the patient could walk only with aid. When he was last seen, 8½ months after the ictus, tone was increased in the right upper limb, and leg strength was fairly well preserved. Severe dysarthria and a right central facial weakness were present. The patient died of aspiration pneumonia.

A necrotic lesion confined to the posterior half of the posterior limb of the internal capsule was found at autopsy. A 3-mm old infarct was present in the right basis pontis at the level of the trigeminal nerve. The internal capsule infarct was old. Wallerian degeneration was evident down to the level of the cerebral peduncles.

Motor paralysis and spastic dystonia on the right side were associated with ischemic infarction of the posterior half of the posterior limb of the left internal capsule in this patient. This case supports localization of the pyramidal

---

(1)   J. Neurol. Sci. 34:63–70, October, 1977.

tract fibers to a compact region in the posterior half of the
posterior limb of the internal capsule.

▶ [The traditional view suggested by Dejerine (1901) that the descending
pyramidal fibers lie in the anterior half of the posterior limb of the internal
capsule is refuted by this report. New evidence strongly suggests that they
are confined to a compact region in the posterior half of the posterior
limb. It is obvious that a time-honored concept cannot be changed on the
basis of a single observation. Further studies are certainly necessary.
—Ed.] ◀

What Hope for Repair of the Brain? Geoffrey Raisman[2]
(London) points out that the consequences of axonal injuries
in the adult nervous system depend on the location of the
axons. It has long been believed that the adult mammalian
central nervous system has a rigid structural arrangement,
and that the only anatomical changes possible are those
caused by advancing age, trauma or disease. In contrast to
peripheral nerve lesions, the treatment of brain and spinal
cord injuries is usually undertaken with the tacit assumption that anatomical repair is not possible. This apparently
static situation contrasts markedly with the process of em-
bryologic development. One would expect the most effective
repair process to be that in which developmental events
could be reenacted. Data from studies on axonal injuries in
adult rats have shed light on this problem. Studies on animals having transection of the fimbria on one side showed
that fimbrial axons can efficiently form new synapses in
adult rat brain and that those postsynaptic targets that
were originally innervated by fimbrial axons remain in
some way selective for fimbrial axons.

Experimental manipulations have unmasked the presence in the adult neuropil of growth potential and growth-
regulating factors that would not be suspected from simple
observation of the normal situation. The defect appears to
lie in the glial cells. It may prove possible by surgical reap-
proximation or grafting to bring presynaptic and postsynaptic elements into suitable apposition, permitting correct
synaptic corrections to form. Brain and spinal cord injuries
may not always be irreparable.

▶ [Because the observations indicate that the neutropil of the central
nervous system is capable of highly efficient synapse formation after injury, the repair of central nervous system damage might be possible if

---

(2)   Ann. Neurol. 3:101–106, February, 1978.

methods could be devised to regulate the direction of growth of the axon sprouts. — Ed.] ◄

Anterograde Transneuronal Degeneration in the Limbic System: Clinical-Anatomical Correlation. Little has appeared in the clinical neurologic literature on trans-synaptic or transneuronal degeneration except for reports associated with visual or olivary-dentatorubral lesions. William C. Torch, Asao Hirano and Seymour Solomon[3] (New York) report a case representing an experiment of nature that demonstrated the synaptic organization of the human limbic system. Anterograde transneuronal degeneration delineated the chain of neurons between the hippocampus and anterior thalamus in this case.

Man, 64, with a 1-year history of well-controlled hypertension, was admitted with arteriovascular disease in the legs, present for 10 years. He had become increasingly irritable, childlike, paranoid and depressed starting 8 years before. Sexual potency had declined and personal hygiene was neglected. Daytime somnolence and anorexia had occurred in the 6 months before admission, with a 40-lb weight loss. The patient was cachectic and had a blood pressure of 150/100 mm Hg. Retinal arteriosclerotic changes were noted and peripheral pulses were absent in the legs. He was alert but disoriented to time and place. Judgment and recent and short-term memory were impaired. The gait was ataxic and shuffling. Hyperreflexia was noted at the knees and ankles. An EEG showed diffuse disorganization with intermittent 2- to 3-Hz medium-voltage activity in the left temporal region. After discharge his personality deteriorated and the dementia worsened in the next month. The day-night sleep pattern reversed. Bladder and bowel incontinence developed. The patient was readmitted in delirium that progressed rapidly to coma, with no focal neurologic signs, and died shortly afterward.

Autopsy showed mild bronchopneumonia, generalized arteriosclerosis and gangrenous cystitis. Arteries at the base of the brain showed segmental narrowing from atherosclerosis. A large old cystic infarct was present in the inferior part of the left temporal lobe that destroyed the fusiform gyrus, posterior part of the hippocampal gyrus and underlying white matter. The left fornix and mamillary body were severely atrophic and gliotic, as were the left mammillothalamic tract, hypothalamus and anterior thalamus. No cerebral atrophy or degenerative disease was noted. The brain stem and cord were unremarkable.

---

(3)   Neurology (Minneap.) 27:1157–1163, December, 1977.

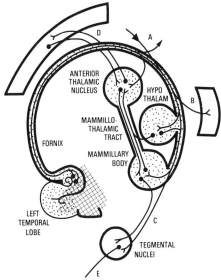

Fig 1.—Schematic diagram of the rhinencephalic-limbic circuit and sites of pathology. The cross-hatched area represents the old temporal lobe infarct. The stippled area represents the sites of severe atrophy. The fornix projects mainly from the hippocampus to the mamillary body, hypothalamus and anterior thalamic nucleus, in addition to the commissure of the fornix (*A*), the septal, preoptic and paraolfactory areas (*B*) and the brain stem tegmental nuclei (*C*). Shown also is the mammillothalamic tract, the thalamocortical and corticothalamic fibers between anterior thalamus and cingulate gyrus (*D*) and the tegmentospinal tract and dorsal longitudinal fasciculus (*E*). (Courtesy of Torch, W. C., et al.: Neurology (Minneap.) 27:1157–1163, December, 1977.)

The rhinencephalic-limbic circuit is illustrated in Figure 1. Transneuronal degeneration depends on relatively complete deafferentiation and typically occurs in "closed neuronal systems," those with limited connections to other parts of the central nervous system. Bilateral limbic involvement appears not to be necessary for limbic symptomatology. Transneuronal degeneration may be a cause of hitherto unsuspected progressive clinical deterioration in other areas of the central nervous system as well.

► [Such extensive retrograde transneuronal degeneration has rarely been described in man. The development of changes such as these may be a mechanism underlying the cognitive, behavioral and autonomic dysfunctions that are part of many different pathologic conditions. — Ed.] ◄

Cerebral Atrophy: Immunologic˙ Disorder? Cerebral atrophy of unknown origin is a psychiatric enigma. Branislav D. Janković, Slobodan Jakulić and Jozef Horvat[4] (Belgrade) investigated a possible relationship between cerebral atrophy and delayed skin hypersensitivity to human brain protein (HBP). Both HBP and human liver protein (HLP) fractions of fresh human tissues were utilized. A total of 594 subjects, 187 of them with cerebral atrophy, received injections intradermally of 100 μg HBP and HLP in the forearm. Reactions were read 24 hours later. Intellectual deterioration was the chief symptom. Neurologic examinations showed a variety of disinhibition signs. About 30% of the patients had had a head injury 1–5 years before the onset, and about 25% consumed alcohol regularly without showing signs of intoxication. The patients were treated with neuroleptic drugs. Patients with nuclear forms of schizophrenia as well as a combined group of neurotic and normal subjects served as controls.

Allergic encephalomyelitis did not develop in guinea pigs and rats immunized with HBP. Animals immunized with HLP showed delayed skin hypersensitivity but no histologic lesions in the liver. The frequency of delayed skin hypersensitivity reactions to HBP was significantly higher in patients with cerebral atrophy (69%) than in the control groups (35% and 2.5%). Exclusion of proved cases of head trauma increased the rate of positive skin reactions to 76.8%. The test was found to be reproducible when repeated after 3–14 months in 47 patients with cerebral atrophy and positive skin reactions and 14 normal subjects with negative reactions. Test results were not related to age or duration of illness in patients with cerebral atrophy. No aggravation of the disease was apparent in the 8 months after the skin testing. About a fifth of the study patients acquired local reactions to HLP, and 18% had antibrain antibodies in their serums.

These findings suggest a relationship between cerebral atrophy and cellular immunity, but it is not clear that the antigens cause the brain damage. Whether or not cerebral atrophy is a direct result of an autoimmune process remains to be seen. Senile and presenile psychoses caused by or asso-

---

(4) Lancet 2:219–220, July 30, 1977.

ciated with brain damage and dementias of unknown origin may have a common immune denominator. Cell-mediated immunity, as well as the proposed activity of a unique anti-brain antibody, may be involved in the development of schizophrenia.

► [This study suggests that both schizophrenia and cerebral atrophy have a correlation with cell-mediated immunity. Cerebral atrophy is not a psychiatric enigma; it is a neuropathologic one. The resulting dementia is a psychiatric (and also neurologic) enigma. – Ed.] ◄

Ataxic Hemiparesis: Pathologic Study. Fisher and Cole, in 1965, described a stroke syndrome characterized by weakness and ataxia of the ipsilateral extremities, believed to be due to ischemia rather than hemorrhage. C. Miller Fisher[5] (Harvard Med. School) report the finding in 3 pathologically studied cases of this syndrome.

Man, 82, with hypertension, had transient left arm weakness with gait unsteadiness a week before admission. The left side was almost totally paralyzed on the day of admission and the patient felt dizzy and vomited once. Return of power began within 4 hours. Examination showed horizontal nystagmus on gaze to each side

Fig 2. – Section of pons showing small tandem infarcts. (Courtesy of Fisher, C. M.: Arch Neurol. 35:126 – 128, March, 1978; copyright 1978, American Medical Association.)

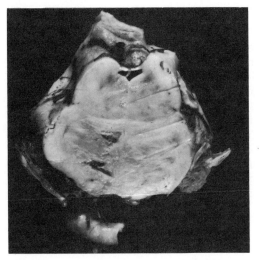

and a coarse vertical nystagmus on upward gaze. There was slight weakness of the left side of the face, slight dysarthria and deviation of the tongue to the left. Strength was reduced in the left extremities, and a left Babinski sign was present. Dysmetria was also present on the left side. The cerebrospinal fluid was normal. The patient was discharged after 6 weeks; he died 3½ years later of pneumonia complicating senile dementia.

The brain showed advanced cortical atrophy. The large cerebral arteries were moderately atherosclerotic but patent. Cavitation was noted in the right upper basis pontis (Fig 2). A small basilar branch artery running to the region of the infarct exhibited a thick plaque of atherosclerosis at its junction with the basilar artery.

The main features of this stroke syndrome were weakness of one side, increased tendon reflexes, a Babinski sign, dysmetria, slow alternating movements, slight dysarthria and nystagmus. The lesions lay approximately at the junction of the upper third and lower two thirds of the basis pontis on the side opposite the pyramidal and cerebellar signs. All patients were hypertensive and had a patent basilar artery. The prognosis for recovery is excellent. The hemiparesis is variable in distribution and severity in these cases. The term "ataxic hemiparesis" is proposed for this syndrome.

► [As he has done on so many other occasions, Doctor Fisher has identified a specific syndrome and has demonstrated its etiology. He has shown that a lesion of the pons may be associated with a contralateral hemiparesis that is cerebellar in character. The designated term "ataxic hemiparesis" is appropriate. — Ed.] ◄

Diffuse "Anoxic" Myelopathy. B. Azzarelli and U. Roessmann[6] (Case Western Reserve Univ.) report the neuropathologic findings in the spinal cord in 16 patients having hypoxia or circulatory arrest. "Anoxic" lesions of the central nervous system were found in 44 of 544 autopsies done over a 16-month period and 16 of these showed evidence of anoxic damage in the spinal cord. The sexes were equally represented. Eleven patients were adults, 2 were infants and 3 were neonates. Episodes of cardiorespiratory arrest or ventricular fibrillation were documented in 12 patients; 4 patients had severe hypoxic episodes due to pulmonary disease. All patients remained comatose and died 1 – 21 days after the anoxic episodes, without neurologic recovery occurring.

(6) Neurology (Minneap.) 27:1049 – 1052, November, 1977.

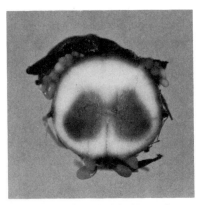

Fig 3. — Lumbar spinal cord with marked duskiness of gray matter. (Courtesy of Azzarelli, B., and Roessmann, U.: Neurology (Minneap.) 27:1049–1052, November, 1977.)

Four patients with respirator brain had complete transverse necrosis of the upper cervical segments. Marked duskiness of the gray matter in the lumbosacral region was noted in 1 cord (Fig 3). Twelve patients had severe anoxic changes in the brain and 2, slight changes. Symmetric anoxic lesions were confined to the gray matter of the cord. The age of the cord lesions corresponded to that in the brain and to the timing of the clinical anoxic episode. The lumbosacral segments were affected in all patients, the lower thoracic and lumbosacral regions in 2 and the cervical and lumbosacral areas in 1. Nine patients had lesions throughout the cord. In the thoracic region, the posterior horn was most consistently involved. Both anterior and posterior horns were damaged in most patients in the lumbosacral segments. The substantia gelatinosa was relatively severely damaged. The cord was most severely damaged in patients with severe brain anoxia, hypotensive brain stem necrosis and "central necrosis" of the spinal cord nuclei.

Selective involvement of the gray matter in these patients with anoxic damage may explain the neurologic deficit after aortic surgery. The frequent involvement of the substantia gelatinosa may explain the selective deficit for temperature and pain sensations. The possibility of diffuse anoxic damage must be considered as an alternative to the anterior spinal artery syndrome.

► [Changes in the brain caused by hypoxia and anoxia have been studied extensively, but little attention has been given to the spinal cord. This study shows that the spinal cord, too, especially the gray matter, may be damaged by anoxia. – Ed.] ◄

Autoimmune Features of Acute Transverse Myelopathy. The pathogenesis of acute nonmechanical transverse myelopathy (ATM) is largely unknown, but some evidence implicates the involvement of an immune mechanism in idiopathic ATM. Oded Abramsky and Dvora Teitelbaum[7] examined the possibility that idiopathic ATM might be the result of a cell-mediated autoimmune response to a component of nervous system tissue.

Five men and five women aged 14–61 years with acute idiopathic transverse or ascending myelitis were studied. Three had had a virus-like illness before the onset of the myelopathy. No patient had objective evidence of peripheral nerve involvement. The duration of neurologic symptoms to maximal deficit ranged from less than an hour to 10 days. Myelography, done in 6 cases, gave negative results. Six patients who were recovering from an acute neurologic insult were also evaluated.

Seven of 10 study patients showed definite lymphocyte transformation with the central nervous system myelin basic encephalitogenic (BE) protein. The 3 with negative results were receiving steroids; 1 steroid-treated patient had a positive response. Three of 8 patients showed significant stimulation to the peripheral nerve basic protein P_2. The degree of lymphocyte responsiveness was not related to the severity of disease. Virtually no stimulation was seen with peripheral nerve basic protein P_{1L} or acetylcholine receptor. Four initially positive patients showed essentially no response to BE or P_2 a few months after the acute stage of disease. Responses to BE were also seen in patients with acute disseminated encephalomyelitis, acute myeloradiculitis and multiple sclerosis. Essentially no response to BE or P_2 was found in patients with multiple sclerosis who were not receiving steroids.

It would seem that ATM and ADE are related disorders, or possibly variants of the same condition. Apparently, several distinct types of acute autoimmune, probably postinfectious demyelinating disorders can be defined in the nervous

(7) Ann. Neurol. 2:36–40, July, 1977.

system. Specific sensitization to BE and P_2 occurs in ATM, ADE and acute myeloradiculitis. Sensitization to the neuritogenic P_{1L} occurs in pure peripheral nerve syndromes such as Bell's palsy and Guillain-Barré syndrome. Other demyelinating disorders such as chronic relapsing polyneuropathy and multiple sclerosis may also involve cell-mediated immunity to myelin antigens.

▶ [Not infrequently, the etiology of acute transverse myelopathy cannot be determined. In some of these enigmatic cases a postinfectious autoimmune mechanism may be an important factor in the pathogenesis. — Ed.]

Gustatory Phenomena after Upper Dorsal Sympathectomy. Reports of pathologic gustatory phenomena have increased in recent years, but most refer to Frey's syndrome. Alexander Kurchin, Raphael Adar, Amikam Zweig and Mark Mozes[8] analyzed postoperative gustatory phenomena in 100 patients who underwent bilateral upper dorsal sympathectomy for palmar hyperhidrosis in 1971 – 75. About half were of each sex; average age was 23 years. A supraclavicular approach was used to remove the T2 and T3 ganglia. Follow-up was completed on 93 patients 4 – 50 months after operation (average, 18 months).

Fifteen (18%) of 85 patients questioned reported having gustatory phenomena before operation. After operation 68 (73%) of 93 patients had such phenomena. Only 3 patients had preoperative gustatory phenomena from anything other than spicy food. Eight patients noticed a definite change in the intensity or nature of the phenomena postoperatively. Mean time of onset of postoperative gustatory phenomena was 5.1 months. Hot and spicy foods were the most common stimuli, but other stimuli were implicated in about half the cases. The face and scalp were the main sites, but in one fourth of cases the phenomena also affected a wide variety of other locations. Sweating was the most common phenomenon, but most patients had other phenomena also. Sweating alone was present in 13 patients. Most patients did not consider the phenomena to be a problem. Gustatory phenomena were more frequent in patients without severe Horner's syndrome. There was no correlation between return of moisture to the hands and gustatory phenomena. Complete dryness of the face after surgery was unrelated to gustatory phenomena.

(8)   Arch. Neurol. 34:619 – 623, October, 1977.

This is the highest rate of gustatory phenomena yet reported after upper dorsal sympathectomy. The phenomena may be related to regeneration per se or to collateral sprouting. The gustatory phenomena are usually mild, and they should not be considered to be a significant complication of the operation.

► [Gustatory sweating and other phenomena (flushing, tingling, paresthesias) that occur with gustatory stimulation occasionally follow upper dorsal or cervicodorsal sympathectomy as the result of either preganglionic sympathetic regeneration or collateral sprouting with aberrant synapses in the superior cervical ganglion. – Ed.] ◄

Neuropathologic Changes in Cerebellar Biopsies of Epileptic Patients. Michael Salcman, Richard Defendini, James Correll and Sid Gilman[9] (Columbia Univ.) examined cerebellar cortical biopsy specimens from 5 male patients with pharmacologically intractable epilepsy, which were obtained at surface electrode implantation for therapeutic stimulation. The patients had had incapacitating seizures for 4–37 years. The findings were compared with autopsy

Fig 4.–Cerebellar biopsy specimen, showing degeneration of all three cortical layers. Besides complete loss of Purkinje's cells, there is atrophy of molecular layer, moderately severe depletion of granule neurons and rarefaction and astrocytosis of folial white matter. Hematoxylin-eosin; reduced from ×110. (Courtesy of Salcman, M., et al.: Ann. Neurol. 3:10–19, January, 1978.)

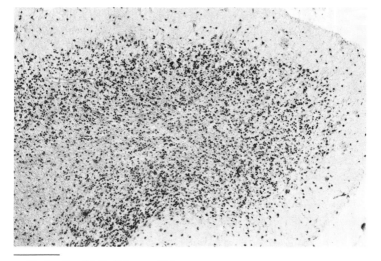

(9)   Ann. Neurol. 3:10–19, January, 1978.

findings in 5 young children who died of status epilepticus of uncertain cause and 5 adults with seizures secondary to cerebral oligodendroglioma. A thin wedge of cerebellar cortex was taken from the posterior edge of the superior semilunar lobule. Three patients had bilateral biopsies. All 5 patients had received high doses of phenytoin and combinations of other anticonvulsants.

The eight specimens from the study patients showed severe degeneration of the Purkinje cell layer. The findings in 1 case are shown in Figure 4. Two patients had never had a generalized convulsion, but all had marked Purkinje cell degeneration.

Similar findings have been obtained in two other series of similar cases, but the incidence of permanent nerve cell damage in epilepsy is unknown. It has been suggested that certain anticonvulsants may function by activating Purkinje cell inhibition, and that enhanced Purkinje cell activity in the course of an epileptic attack may provide a mechanism of seizure control through suppression of activity in a cerebellothalamocortical circuit. Progressive damage to the Purkinje cells may result in progressive loss of an important system controlling epileptic attacks and lead to increasingly intractable epilepsy.

► [These observations suggest that permanent neuronal damage in epilepsy is related to the cumulative effects of the frequency and chronicity of the disorder. – Ed.] ◄

Neurologic Sequelae of Experimental Febrile Convulsions. Febrile seizures occur in about 5% of children in the United States. Whether such seizures damage the central nervous system is uncertain. James G. T. Nealis, N. Paul Rosman, Theslee J. De Piero and Eileen M. Ouellette[1] (Boston Univ.) conducted a laboratory study to investigate the effect of experimental hyperthermic seizures on the developing rat brain. Radiant heat was produced in a hyperthermia chamber. About 3 minutes was needed to produce a seizure after the subcutaneous temperature reached 41.5 C in a rat aged 5 days and $3\frac{1}{2}$ minutes at 42.5 C in a rat aged 15 days. The rats were exposed at age 5 days, when mitotic activity is high in the rat brain, and at 15 days, equivalent to the 1st year of human life. Some groups of rats were ex-

(1) Neurology (Minneap.) 28:246–250, March, 1978.

posed to hyperthermia but were not permitted to have convulsions.

No significant group differences in ages of acquisition of developmental reflexes were found. No rats lost acquired reflexes after exposure to hyperthermia, with or without seizures. Differences in numbers of training sessions needed to master maze-solving ability were insignificant, but error scores in the maze test were significantly greater in convulsed than in control rats.

The findings suggest that experimentally induced hyperthermic seizures occurring early in life may damage the developing brain and result in impaired problem-solving ability at a later age. The findings may be relevant to febrile convulsions in childhood.

▶ [These studies suggest that febrile seizures in the extremely young may damage the developing brain. — Ed.] ◀

Neuro-ophthalmology

Clinical Significance of Spontaneous Pulsations of the Retinal Vein. Spontaneous retinal vein pulsations are noted at ophthalmoscopy in 15 – 90% of normal subjects and are abolished by elevated intracranial pressure. Barry E. Levin[2] (New Jersey Med. School) evaluated the usefulness of this sign in 146 unselected subjects: 76 men and 70 women aged 20 – 90 years as controls, 9 patients with elevated intracranial pressure, 24 with elevated intracranial pressure from mass lesions without papilledema, 10 with papilledema of varying origin and 29 patients with spontaneous pulsations who required lumbar puncture.

Spontaneous venous pulsations occurred in 87.6% of control subjects. Bilateral absence of pulsations was more frequent in men of most ages, especially in the 5th and 6th decades. No significant correlations with blood pressure or with various medical illnesses were found. Lumbar-puncture patients variably had spontaneous venous pulsations when the cerebrospinal fluid pressure fell below 190 mm water. Pulsations were useful in judging intracranial pressure elevations. None of the patients with elevated intracranial pressure without papilledema had spontaneous venous pulsations and no patient with papilledema exhibited spontaneous pulsations. None of the patients studied serially at lumbar puncture had a cerebrospinal fluid pressure above 180 mm water; all had spontaneous pulsations present before lumbar puncture.

This study shows the usefulness of spontaneous venous pulsations as a clinical sign of normal intracranial pressure and in predicting intracranial pressure. The presence of venous pulsations makes it very unlikely that intracranial pressures above 190 – 195 mm water are present; the presence of transtentorial or tonsillar herniation, or both, is

---

(2) Arch. Neurol. 35:37 – 40, January, 1978.

usually clinically apparent. Loss of spontaneous venous pulsations precedes frank papilledema.

▶ [Retinal vein pulsations may be absent in patients with normal intracranial pressure. Consequently, their absence is not a reliable indication of elevated intracranial pressure. — Ed.] ◀

Pathogenesis of Optic Nerve Drusen: Hypothesis. Joel G. Sacks, Richard B. O'Grady, Earl Choromokos and Jan Leestma[3] (Northwestern Univ.) conducted a histologic examination of the eyes of a patient with optic nerve drusen and concluded that drusen are not static in size, but grow from microscopic, subclinical particles.

Youth, 19, with sudden onset of vertigo, impaired speech and inability to walk that lasted less than 2 weeks, showed hypesthesia and minimal weakness in the right arm and a flattened right nasolabial fold. The optic discs were elevated and had blurred margins. A fluorescein retinal angiogram showed no late stain. After a sudden, marked exacerbation of the symptoms, a cerebrospinal fluid pressure of 270 mm water was found, and angiography suggested a cerebrovascular accident in the left opercular area. Subsequent vertebral angiography showed two aneurysms. The patient's condition deteriorated rapidly after rupture of the aneurysm and he died.

A massive subarachnoid hemorrhage was seen at autopsy, with a hematoma about the base of the brain and brain stem. The larger basilar artery aneurysm had thrombosed and ruptured laterally into the pons. The patient had been ventilated after death until his donor kidneys could be removed. Basophilic, acellular, laminated bodies distorted the optic nerves anterior to the lamina cribrosa without extending to the disc surface. Small basophilic granules were grouped about dilated vascular channels adjacent to the large laminated bodies. In one section a blood vessel was outlined by perivascular granules.

A review of 53 fluorescein retinal angiograms of patients with optic nerve drusen showed a frequent abnormal branching pattern on the disc (Fig 5), relatively large vessels connecting the superficial and deep disc circulations, and increased disc capillarity.

The findings in the present case cannot be reasonably attributed to chronic disc swelling from elevated intracranial pressure. It is proposed that drusen originate from leakage of unformed elements of the blood, such as plasma proteins, which serve as the nidus for the deposit of other materials

(3)   Arch. Ophthalmol. 95:425 – 428, March, 1977.

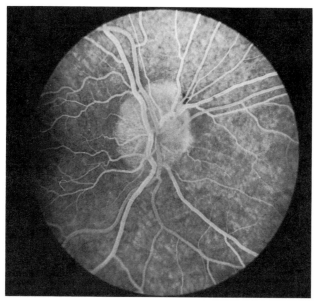

Fig 5. – Typical early branching pattern of retinal vessels. Capillaries on temporal side of this right disc are unusually prominent. (Courtesy of Sacks, J. G., et al.: Arch. Ophthalmol. 95:425–428, March, 1977; copyright 1977, American Medical Association.)

within the perivascular space. The dysoria hypothesis could explain the formation of drusen-like bodies in chronic papilledema. Abnormal pressure relations within the microvasculature of the optic nerve head may contribute to the dysoria.

▶ [Although optic nerve drusen are well known to ophthalmologists (and may cause neurologists to have diagnostic problems), little is known about their pathogenesis. This article suggests that they result from an inherited abnormal disc vascular pattern that allows transudation of plasma proteins that in turn serve as a nidus for the deposition of extracellular materials. – Ed.] ◀

Subclinical Eye Movement Disorders in Patients with Multiple Sclerosis. Early neurologic signs of multiple sclerosis (MS) may be focal, with no clear history of fluctuation, and the finding of other signs of disseminated disease could shorten the workup of affected patients. Leda Datz Solingen, Robert W. Baloh, Lawrence Myers and George

Ellison[4] (Univ. of California, Los Angeles) assessed eye movements quantitatively in 16 patients with well-documented MS who lacked clinically apparent extraoculomotor impairment. Patients with gaze nystagmus were included. Mean age was 39 years, and duration of disease ranged from 2 to 38 years. Six patients had gaze nystagmus, 5 on horizontal gaze only. Induced saccade and pursuit eye movements were recorded by direct-current electro-oculography; special amplifiers were used to minimize drift and noise interference.

Seven patients (44%) had fixation instability. One patient showed saccade overshoot dysmetria, and 2 patients had cogwheel pursuit apparent at the lowest target velocity. Four patients had gaze nystagmus at 30 degrees of eye deviation. Four had vestibular nystagmus only with the eyes closed; it was unidirectional and increased with gaze in the direction of the fast component. Thirteen patients in all had significantly impaired saccades, smooth pursuit or both, compared with 25 normal subjects. Eight patients showed saccade dysmetria, 5 had delayed saccade reaction time and 4 had bilateral saccade slowing. Nine patients exhibited two or more abnormalities on the test battery.

Quantitative assessment of eye movements in patients with suspected MS can help in identifying the important "second lesion." Routine clinical assessment of extraocular motor function misses abnormalities that are found on electro-oculographic recording. By careful reexamination of the patients after the tracings are reviewed, some of the abnormalities may be appreciated.

▶ [These data suggest that quantitative assessment of eye movements in patients with suspected multiple sclerosis can help in identifying multiplicity of lesions. — Ed.] ◀

Amaurosis Fugax from Disease of the External Carotid Artery. Recognition of the source of emboli causing amaurosis fugax is important in prevention of transient ischemic attacks, cerebral infarction or retinal infarction. Atheromatous emboli often originate in the extracranial carotid system. Atheromatous disease of the external carotid artery is not well documented as a source of retinal emboli. Mitchell D. Burnbaum, John B. Selhorst, John W. Har-

(4) Neurology (Minneap.) 27:614–619, July, 1977.

bison and John J. Brush[5] (Med. College of Virginia) describe 3 patients with proved internal carotid occlusion and a diseased external or common carotid artery who had amaurosis fugax.

Man, 58, with angina for 16 years, within 1 week had 4 attacks of loss of vision in the right eye for 10 minutes, with right-sided headache, diaphoresis, vertigo and numbness in the left fingers. A bruit was heard over the right carotid artery, and right temporal artery pulsation was reduced. Right carotid angiography showed occlusion of the internal carotid artery at its origin.

Multiple attacks of amaurosis fugax occurred for 3 weeks, during one of which a white plug was seen in the central retinal artery of the right eye and its proximal branches. Right carotid compression caused severe right hemicranial pain, and several additional cholesterol emboli were seen in the fundus of the right eye (Fig 6, A).

A week later, the right external and common carotid arteries were clamped and divided, the bifurcation was resected, and the arteries were reanastomosed. The removed segment contained a large ulcerated plaque. Postoperatively, the patient was blind in the right eye. Ophthalmoscopy showed diffuse retinal infarction, sluggish arterial blood flow and many other emboli (Fig 6, B). Vision did not improve.

Fig 6. – **A,** after a carotid artery compression test, several highly refractile emboli were seen in the ipsilateral fundus. **B,** arrowheads mark two large fresh cholesterol emboli which were among many additional emboli noted throughout the fundus 2 hours after endarterectomy of the external carotid artery. This shower of emboli caused diffuse infarction of the superficial retina as occurs with occlusion of the central retinal artery. (Courtesy of Burnbaum, M. D., et al.: Arch. Neurol. 34:532–535, September, 1977; copyright 1977, American Medical Association.)

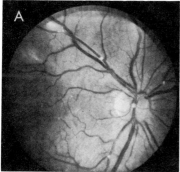 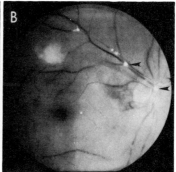

(5)   Arch. Neurol. 34:532–535, September, 1977.

An embolic origin for amaurosis through external carotid collaterals in this case is supported by the angiographic and surgical demonstration of an occluded internal carotid artery and pathologic demonstration of a source for the platelet-fibrin embolus observed during an amaurotic episode. Appearance of additional cholesterol emboli after carotid compression shows that the collaterals are large enough to allow passage of emboli. Widespread embolization to external carotid branches in the scalp explains the severe unilateral headache after carotid compression.

External carotid endarterectomy may be indicated to prevent retinal infarction when amaurosis fugax recurs in the presence of ipsilateral internal carotid occlusion and external or common carotid ulceration or stenosis. The risk of surgically induced embolization to the eye and possibly to the cerebral circulation should not be overlooked.

▶ [This is a fascinating case report showing that embolization can occur in arteries that are normally branches of the internal carotid artery after occlusion of the latter artery if there are abundant collaterals from the external carotid artery. — Ed.] ◀

Failure of Downward Gaze: Site and Nature of the Lesion. Isolated failure of downward gaze is a rare clinical finding. Only three reports that include autopsy examination have appeared. G. Michael Halmagyi, William A. Evans and John M. Hallinan[6] (Univ. of Sydney) report data on 4 patients with paralysis of downward gaze but intact upward gaze, 1 of whom had detailed clinicopathologic studies.

Woman, 65, with a history of gastric ulcer and two myocardial infarcts, was seen a month after the second infarct because of sudden dysarthria and loss of consciousness that lasted 20 minutes. A mild gait ataxia and a left carotid bruit were noted. Beats of spontaneous convergence nystagmus were seen, with skew deviation in left gaze with the left eye down. Over 10 degrees of upward gaze were present but there was no downward gaze on volition or on bilateral caloric testing. A brain scan was normal. Heparin therapy was given but the patient suddenly became dysarthric a week later, had left 6th and 7th nerve pareses and lost consciousness and died in apnea after 6 hours.

Autopsy showed a false aneurysm of the left cardiac ventricle and mural thrombus in the aneurysm. Bilateral areas of infarction were found in the rostral midbrain and the left ventral thalamus (Fig 7). The infarct was confined to the red nucleus on the right.

(6)   Arch. Neurol. 35:22–26, January, 1978.

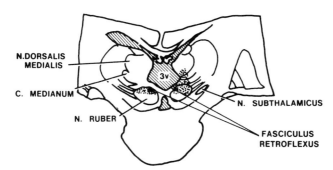

Fig 7.—Composite drawing of coronal section showing extent of lesions (*stippled areas*); 3v indicates 3d ventricle. (Courtesy of Halmagyi, G. M., et al.: Arch. Neurol. 35:22–26, January, 1978; copyright 1978, American Medical Association.)

The fasciculus retroflexus was involved on both sides. The 3d nerve nuclei and exit fibers were spared. Death was due to bleeding into a large unrecognized infarct of the left cerebellar hemisphere.

Isolated failure of downward gaze is much less common than failure of upward gaze. Selective downward gaze paralysis may be caused by bilateral lesions of the fasciculus retroflexus. Consciousness is usually transiently disturbed and the median thalami may also be involved by the infarction. The usual cause is embolization of the posterior thalamosubthalamic or rubral artery.

► [One wonders why these patients with bilateral red nucleus lesions had no tremors or other motor manifestations. — Ed.] ◄

Neurology of Aging

Neurologic Manifestations of Aging. Many neurologic functions are said to decline with aging, but it has been difficult to determine whether aging alone or associated diseases are responsible. Emre Kokmen, Robert W. Bossemeyer, Jr., Jane Barney and William J. Williams[7] (Univ. of Michigan) compared neurologic function and joint motion perception quantitatively in 51 socially active persons aged 61–85 years and living in the community with those of 11 subjects aged 21–30. The 31 women and 20 men in the older group had mean ages of 72.3 and 70.2 years, respectively. Most were retired.

Memory deficits in the older group were reportedly limited to not remembering names of persons and occasionally to misplacing objects; no subject had had significant disability from this deficit. Numbness and tingling of the digits were intermittent. Fainting spells were extremely unusual. Two subjects reported weakness and coordination problems, which were fairly transient. No trend toward an increasing number of signs and symptoms with advancing age was evident. No gaze palsies or individual muscle palsies were seen. No true dysmetria was observed. Abnormal face-hand test results were not clinically significant. No side differences in vibration perception were found. No subject exhibited a pattern of central or peripheral nervous system dysfunction. Several of the younger controls had similar signs and symptoms. Vibration sensation was better than in older subjects, but the difference was not impressive.

Many older subjects in this study had neurologic complaints, but none showed a pattern indicating a neurologic disease. The findings in these highly articulate, relatively well-to-do, socially active aged subjects indicate that many aspects of neurologic function are little affected by aging.

---

(7)   J. Gerontol. 32:411–419, July, 1977.

The study has not defined the progress of neurologic symptoms and signs in a life span.

► [The results obtained from this study of this relatively well-to-do, highly articulate and socially active group of aged subjects indicate that many aspects of neurologic function are affected little by the aging process. Caution must be used before attributing neurologic abnormalities to the aging process alone. – Ed.] ◄

Central Neurotransmitter Substances and Aging: Review is presented by T. Samorajski[8] (Texas Med. Center, Houston). In conjunction with hormones, neurotransmitters regulate physiologic activity throughout the body. Integration between brain neurotransmitters and hormones presumably occurs in the hypothalamus. The hypothalamus may be a critical site of selective cell death during aging. A decrease in neuroendocrine transducer cells, neurotransmitter cells or both may alter the hypothalamic threshold of responsiveness to circulating hormones. Another possibility is that different hypothalamic areas age in different ways and at different rates. The resultant disregulation of hypothalamic function may accelerate aging throughout the body and cause early onset of age-related pathologic conditions. Neurotransmitter function may be altered by changes in the amount of rate-limiting enzyme, replacement by a "false" transmitter or accumulation of metabolites. A decrease in number of synaptic processes might alter the sensitivity of the postsynaptic cells to the transmitter.

Changes in neurotransmitter substances have been described in Parkinson's disease and in patients dying of Huntington's chorea. Changes in brain monoamine metabolism also occur in senile dementia. Depressed mood is a common feature of old age, and depressive illness appears to be associated with changes in circulating hormones and depletion of norepinephrine and probably serotonin in the hypothalamus. Many elderly persons have learning and memory dysfunction. Age-dependent impairments of this type may be associated with a loss of synaptic contacts and their associated neurotransmitter substances. They may also be related to feedback deficiencies in circulating hormones and a decline in the number of neuron receptor sites responsive to hormones. Control of food intake may be another example of neurotransmitter influences on behavior. Reduced sexual

(8)   J. Am. Geriatr. Soc. 25:337–348, August, 1977.

function in the elderly may be related to fluctuations in brain levels of dopamine and serotonin.

► [This article raises many questions. It is apparent that further information is needed to determine the importance of neurotransmitters in aging and the degree of control that might be developed and imposed by their manipulation. — Ed.] ◄

Cytophotometric Mapping of Neuronal Changes in Senile Dementia. Mental deterioration in old age is one of the most common yet least well understood of neurologic conditions. D. M. A. Mann, P. O. Yates and C. M. Barton[9] (Univ. of Manchester) investigated senile dementia by using a technique that allows both major and minor disease in nerve cell groups to be detected. The method involves measurement of a number of nuclear and cytoplasmic features, including nerve cell cytoplasmic RNA content, an indicator of the capacity of such cells to form the proteins appropriate for neurophysiologic function. Nerve tissue was taken at autopsy from 10 patients with senile dementia and 15 controls of similar age without overt neurologic illness at death. Sections of tissue blocks were stained for cell RNA.

The difference in overall mean cell RNA content between the demented and control groups exceeded the 5% level of significance in all groups of neurons studied and the 0.1% level in most instances. Losses of cell RNA were found for all neuron types measured and ranged from 7% to 51%. The types studied included Betz's cells, Purkinje's cells, dentate and thalamic cells and cells of the olives, locus ceruleus and substantia nigra. Several groups of hippocampal cells were also evaluated.

The greatest losses of RNA occur in pyramidal cells of areas $h_2 - h_5$ of Ammon's horn in the hippocampus. The relation of hippocampal lesions to dementia is unclear. The finding of widespread reductions in cytoplasmic RNA in senile dementia indicates a general decline in metabolic levels, which may have followed or produced a reduction in dendritic arborization in affected neurons.

► [Although certain aspects of the symptomatology of senile dementia may be accounted for by lesions in particular anatomical sites, the principal factors in the neurologic disturbance are related to more broadly based changes in nerve cell metabolism affecting much, if not all, of the central nervous system. — Ed.] ◄

---

(9) J. Neurol. Neurosurg. Psychiatry 40:299–302, March, 1977.

Neurology of Behavior

Memory and Cognitive Function in Man: Does the Cholinergic System Have a Specific Role? Pharmacologic studies have increasingly supported anecdotal and clinical impressions that cholinergic neurons in the brain are involved in memory and learning, but the specificity of cholinergic neuronal function in memory-cognitive processes remains uncertain. David A. Drachman[1] (Northwestern Univ.) compared the effectiveness of physostigmine and *d*-amphetamine in reversing memory and cognitive impairment induced by scopolamine in human beings. Physostigmine acts by allowing acetylcholine to persist at synaptic sites, antagonizing the action of scopolamine within the cholinergic system, whereas *d*-amphetamine potentiates the release and interferes with the reuptake of dopamine and norepinephrine.

Subjects aged 19–26 years participated in the study. A dose of 1 mg scopolamine was given subcutaneously. Physostigmine was given subcutaneously in doses of 1 or 2 mg, and *d*-amphetamine was given orally in a dose of 10 mg. Tests of a single trial span, supraspan digit storage, free recall word storage and retrieval by category were given, as well as the Wechsler Adult Intelligence Scale.

Scopolamine profoundly impaired storage of both supraspan digits and words in the free recall paradigm and moderately impaired retrieval by category. It significantly impaired performance IQ and full-scale IQ. Immediate memory and verbal IQ were not impaired. Physostigmine produced no significant changes. Amphetamine produced a significant but small improvement in performance and full-scale IQ scores. Physostigmine largely reversed many of the features of scopolamine dementia, especially word storage. Amphetamine improved alertness in scopolamine-treated subjects, but did not significantly improve any aspect

---

(1) Neurology (Minneap.) 27:783–790, August, 1977.

of cognitive functioning, and led to further deterioration in word storage.

These findings support the view that the cholinergic system has a specific relationship to memory and other cognitive functions. Probably both the cholinergic nature of the hippocampal complexes and the plasticity of cholinergic synapses that store information are involved. Undoubtedly, neurons belonging to other transmitter systems play additional roles in other aspects of cognitive functions.

▶ [This study provides supportive evidence that the cholinergic system has a specific relationship to memory and other cognitive functions. – Ed.]

Presenile Dementia Presenting as Aphasia. Language disturbances are not uncommon in the presenile degenerative dementias, but usually they do not occur until relatively late in the course, and the type of disorder found most often differs from those usually observed in aphasics. Adam F. Wechsler[2] (Univ. of California, Los Angeles) describes a man with evidence of presenile dementia in whom progressive deterioration of behavior and intellectual function followed the onset of aphasia.

Man, 67, who was right-handed, had noticed trouble with speech for about 2 years, starting with the use of incorrect words in conversation, repetitiousness and a tendency to reverse word order. The disorder had progressed and he began to have trouble understanding what was said to him. His handwriting also deteriorated and he became more forgetful. A cerebral blood flow study, brain scan and EEG were normal. Personality changes developed a year after onset of symptoms. Behavior became inappropriate and stereotyped, and the patient became irritable and suspicious. His health had always been excellent. Glabellar and snout reflexes were present.

The patient was good-natured but seemed childlike at times and reported having a slight memory problem. He made errors in calculation on verbal instruction but not with problems on paper. Story recall was poor. There was occasional hesitation on attempts to initiate speech, and occasional perseveration and frequent paraphasia were evident. Echolalia and verbal stereotypy were also present. Some objects were incorrectly named. A computerized axial tomographic (CAT) examination (Fig 8) showed diffuse enlargement of cortical sulci and marked dilatation of the left sylvian fissure, especially posteriorly. The lateral ventricles were mildly to moderately enlarged. No mass was seen on contrast infusion.

(2)   J. Neurol. Neurosurg. Psychiatry 40:303–305, March, 1977.

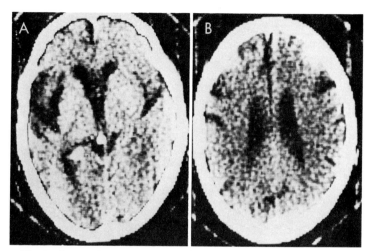

Fig 8.—Scan made with EMI instrument, showing striking dilatation of left sylvian fissure (A) in presence of diffuse sulcal enlargement (B). Lateral ventricles are moderately enlarged. (Courtesy of Wechsler, A. F.: J. Neurol. Neurosurg. Psychiatry 40:303–305, March, 1977.)

The findings in this case are most consistent with Alzheimer's disease or Pick's disease. Aphasia has not previously been reported as the initial symptom of presenile dementia. Early language involvement with relative sparing of constructional ability is more suggestive of Pick's disease than of Alzheimer's disease, as is the radiographic picture, but a definite diagnosis cannot yet be made of this case. Aphasia may be both the first and the most prominent symptom of degenerative dementia.

▶ [This case is an interesting one. Most neurologists with wide clinical experience, however, are aware of the frequency with which an aphasia-like picture may be the presenting symptom in patients with organic dementias. — Ed.] ◀

Developmental Dyslexia: Evidence for a Subgroup with Reversal of Cerebral Asymmetry. An estimated 1–3% of school-age children have developmental dyslexia, the cause of which is unknown. Daniel B. Hier, Marjorie LeMay, Peter B. Rosenberger and Vincent P. Perlo[3] (Harvard Med. School) used brain computerized tomography to assess the pattern of cerebral asymmetry in 24 dyslexic

(3) Arch. Neurol. 35:90–92, February, 1978.

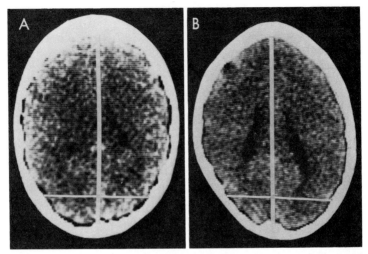

Fig 9.—Computerized brain tomograms of 2 dyslexic patients. Both transaxial sections are at the level of the bodies of the lateral ventricles. The heavy white stripe lies vertically along the interhemispheric fissure; the thin white stripe lies horizontally across the posterior parieto-occipital region. **A,** brain shows the common pattern of cerebral asymmetry with the wider left parieto-occipital region. **B,** brain shows a marked reversal of usual cerebral asymmetry with a wider right parieto-occipital region. (Courtesy of Hier, D. B., et al.: Arch. Neurol. 35:90–92, February, 1978; copyright 1978, American Medical Association.)

patients aged 14–47; the mean age was 25. Two patients were women; 6 were left-handed. All subjects either scored below the 5th-grade level on the Gray Oral Reading Test or had a history of reading at least 2 years below grade level while in school. All had normal neurologic findings. Cerebral asymmetry was assessed from computerized tomography scans, with four or six transaxial sections made through the hemispheres. The criterion of asymmetry was a 1-mm difference (Fig 9).

None of the tomograms showed evidence of brain injury. Ten patients had brains wider in the right than the left parieto-occipital region, 8 had brains wider on the left and 6 had approximately symmetric brains. Patients with brains wider on the right had a mean verbal IQ less than the others. Mean performance IQ scores were comparable. Four of the 10 patients with brains having a wider right parieto-occipital region reported delayed acquisition of speech, whereas only 1 other of 14 patients reported delayed speech; the difference was not significant.

An unexpectedly large number of dyslexic patients in this study exhibited reversal of the pattern of cerebral asymmetry found in most right-handed subjects. Only 9% of normal right-handed subjects and 27% of normal left-handed subjects have reversed cerebral asymmetry. The patients with reversed cerebral asymmetry had lower verbal ability than the other dyslexic patients. The reversal may have contributed to the reading disability and may reflect a mismatch between hemispheric specialization for language and structural asymmetry of the hemispheres. A reversal of cerebral asymmetry alone does not produce dyslexia or verbal disability. Reversed cerebral asymmetry may prove to be an important risk factor for dyslexia, much as male sex is a risk factor.

► [The authors postulate that reversal of cerebral asymmetry may result in language lateralization to a cerebral hemisphere that is structurally less suited to support language function. This may serve as a risk factor for the development of reading disability. — Ed.] ◄

Distribution of Cerebral Blood Flow in the Dominant Hemisphere during Motor Ideation and Motor Performance. David H. Ingvar and Lars Philipson[4] (Univ. of Lund) used radioxenon to measure regional cerebral blood flow (rCBF) with a multidetector device to analyze the events accompanying motor ideation in comparison with the rolandic flow changes induced by actual movements. A new technique of displaying two-dimensional color diagrams of the mean flow distribution in a group of patients is termed "cerebral ideography." Studies were done in 4 neurologically normal male psychiatric patients, 2 with chronic schizophrenia and 2 with suspected presenile dementia, and 2 patients with treatment-resistant focal cortical epilepsy. All 6 subjects had a normal mental state at the time of examination. Mean flow distribution was determined from the detector data with use of a smoothing procedure, color coding and color plotting performed by a Univac 1108 computer. Hand movements were first conceived and then carried out.

Values of rCBF were normal at rest. There was a moderate increase in mean gray matter blood flow during ideation

(4) Ann. Neurol. 2:230–237, September, 1977.

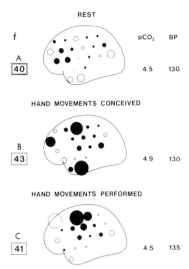

Fig 10. — The rCBF measurements in a woman, aged 25, with focal cortical epilepsy. Study was made in an interictal phase; the patient was fully lucid and cooperated excellently. Mean hemisphere rCBF at rest ($\bar{f}_{\text{init}}$, 40 ml/100 gm/minute) was subnormal but there was no focal hyperemia in the temporal region, where moderate paraoxysmal EEG changes had been recorded. **A** shows flow distribution at rest in relationship to the hemisphere mean flow of 40 ml/100 gm/minute. **B** and **C** are based on comparison of each regional flow value with flow at rest in the same position. **B** shows the frontal and temporal flow increase during motor ideation; increase in mean flow was moderate (43 ml/100 gm/minute). **C** shows the localized rolandic flow increase during hand movements; mean flow was 41 ml/100 gm/minute. (Courtesy of Ingvar, D. H., and Philipson, L.: Ann. Neurol. 2:230–237, September, 1977.)

and motor activity. A general flow increase of about 7% occurred with ideation, with no change in Pa_{CO_2} or blood pressure. The increase was most marked in the premotor and frontal regions, including the supraorbital parts. Postcentral-parietal and temporal flows were also increased. On hand movements the typical rolandic increase in rCBF emerged; the peak was localized at the vertex, with flow augmentations of over 50%. Motor ideation produced the most marked relative increase in flow in the temporal region where it amounted to 60–70% at several points. Similar results were obtained in the neurologically normal subjects and those with focal cortical epilepsy (Fig 10).

These findings support the view that ideation, or the formation of abstract concepts, is now accessible to direct quantitative studies. Measurements of the rCBF distribution at rest and during various forms of mental activation, including motor ideation, might be useful in studies of the cerebral pathophysiology of mental disorders.

► [The pattern of increase in cerebral blood flow in the left cerebral hemisphere during ideation (attempts to conceive movements of the right hand) and actual movements of the hand showed an interesting difference. During ideation the cerebral blood flow was increased most markedly in the temporal and frontal areas, whereas during actual movements the increase was most marked in the rolandic area. The results suggest that centers for motor ideation have a different location than those that control the actual hand movements. — Ed.] ◄

Recurrent Hypersomnia Secondary to Sleep Apnea. Henry M. Spira and Peritz Scheinberg[5] (Univ. of Miami) describe an unusual patient with severe hypersomnia who presented with episodes of falling thought to be epileptic. The symptoms were believed to be due to sleep deprivation secondary to cerebral hypoxia that occurred as the patient fell asleep and that was caused by upper airway obstruction.

Woman, 66, had had recurrent episodes of falling and had sustained injuries on several occasions. She had had no incontinence or postictal confusion; the period of unconsciousness did not last over 1 or 2 minutes. Most episodes occurred shortly after awakening. She had been hypersomnic for 5 years and this had progressed. Decreased memory and irritability were also reported. The patient had taken 20 mg methylphenidate 4 times daily for several years. Operations for diphtheria and "lockjaw" had left a facial deformity for which several attempts at correction had been made, resulting in left facial paresis and partial upper airway obstruction. A sleep EEG showed awakening after stage 2, recurring every minute or so; at no time was stage 2 sleep fully developed, and rapid eye movement sleep did not occur. The arterial pH fell to 7.30 during sleep and the Pa_{O_2} to 57 mm Hg, with a rise in the Pa_{CO_2} to 60 mm Hg. Improvement followed use of a cervical collar in sleep and pseudoephedrine administration. A reducing diet was prescribed. Falling spells have not recurred and the patient is much less sleepy in the daytime. A sleeping cap arrangement was substituted for the cervical collar.

Falling was presumably due to the patient entering sleep while upright. This case emphasizes the need to seek a respiratory cause of simple narcolepsy when other features of the narcoleptic syndrome are absent. The syndrome of sleep apnea is not benign. Some instances of hypersomnia may

(5) Arch. Neurol. 34:513–514, August, 1977.

have a simple mechanical cause and be curable, although the causes of most sleep disorders are obscure.

▶ [This case emphasizes the point that some instances of hypersomnia may have a simple, mechanical cause and be curable. – Ed.] ◀

Prosopagnosia: Clinical, Psychologic and Anatomical Study of Three Patients. Prosopagnosia is a rare condition in which recognition of faces is impaired. It is not clear whether bilateral lesions are necessary to produce this state. In several case reports, surgery on the right temporal and occipital lobes has been responsible, and a purely unilateral lesion is clinically suspected. A. M. Whiteley and Elizabeth K. Warrington[6] (London) studied data on 3 patients with prosopagnosia, 2 of whom had right occipital lesions. Analysis of visual and perceptual functions showed a defect in perceptual classification that appeared to be stimulus specific.

Woman, 49, right-handed, developed increasing occipital headache over 4 weeks, with blurred vision on the left, and a dense left homonymous hemianopia was discovered. Neurologic examination was otherwise normal. An EMI scan showed a tumor with extensive edema in the medial right parieto-occipital region and a shift

Fig 11.—Computerized axial tomography, **A,** preoperative (with enhancement) parieto-occipital tumor with surrounding edema. **B,** postoperative (with enhancement) area of right occipital lobectomy with residual tumor anterior to right glomus. (Courtesy of Whiteley, A. M., and Warrington, E. K.: J. Neurol. Neurosurg. Psychiatry 40:395–403, April, 1977.)

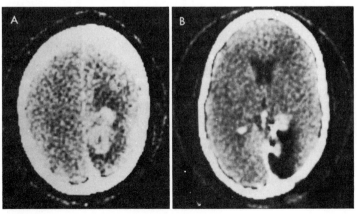

(6)   J. Neurol. Neurosurg. Psychiatry 40:395–403, April, 1977.

of midline structures to the left (Fig 11). Angiography showed a highly vascular tumor in the right occipital lobe, but no tumor in the left hemisphere. Craniotomy revealed a grade III astrocytoma on the medial surface of the occipital lobe, and an occipital lobectomy was done; further exploration was necessary to remove tumor deep in the parietal lobe. Postoperatively the patient reported that people looked strange, with ugly, distorted faces, and she could not recognize anyone until he or she spoke. A scan showed possible residual tumor but no midline displacement; the left hemisphere appeared normal. The tumor site was irradiated and the symptoms had largely resolved 2 months later.

Performance on a facial matching task was clearly impaired in all 3 patients but no consistent pattern of impairment was noted on other visual and perceptual tests. Ability to recognize famous faces was variable.

The critical cortical lesion in these patients is likely to be in the right occipitotemporal region; 2 patients seemed to have a purely unilateral lesion. One patient performed the memory for faces test quite well. Prosopagnosia can occur as a face-specific perceptual deficit; whether or not it also occurs as a face-specific memory deficit remains an open question.

▶ [Many have questioned whether prosopagnosia is actually a clinical entity. These well-studied cases suggest that it is and that it results from unilateral rather than bilateral cerebral disease. They indicate the importance of the right posterior portion of the brain in relation to the syndrome. — Ed.] ◀

Outline for Analysis of Dementia: Memory Disorder of Huntington's Disease. Eric D. Caine, Michael H. Ebert and Herbert Weingartner[7] (Natl. Inst. of Health) report on an analysis of memory dysfunction in patients with Huntington's disease. Subjects without advanced dementia or debilitating psychiatric disorder were used in the study. Generally they were in the early stages of the disease, most of them diagnosed in the past 5 years. Ten Huntington subjects were initially matched for age, sex and education with patients having Parkinson's disease and with normal subjects. An auditory presentation of categorized words and a serial learning task were administered, as well as a digit repetition test, two sorting tasks and a selective reminding task of categorized words. Seven Huntington's disease pa-

---

(7) Neurology (Minneap.) 27:1087–1092, November, 1977.

tients were then compared with 7 normal subjects on the Brown-Peterson paradigm.

The pattern of memory disorder was similar in the most and least affected Huntington's disease patients. Digit span with repetition forward was minimally reduced at most; repetition backward was significantly impaired. Immediate and delayed free recall were slightly impaired, but not at a significant level. Category cueing and reexposure of the stimulus word in a recognition task did not enhance recall, in marked contrast with both control groups. Huntington's disease patients could not master the serial recall task, despite repeated trials and regardless of list content. These patients were increasingly impaired with successively longer delay periods in the Brown-Peterson paradigm and could not complete the selective reminding tasks.

Patients with Huntington's disease exhibit mildly impaired registration, significant difficulty in encoding new information and marked impairment in consistently retrieving stored information. This approach of studying the breakdown of cognitive processes and strategies is recommended for systematically investigating other diseases with problems of remembering and forgetting.

► [This study describes methods for assessing impairment of memory and cognitive functions in patients with Huntington's chorea. The memory defect described, however, is probably not specific for Huntington's chorea, but is present in most, if not all, patients with organic dementias. More important would be a study of psychologic changes that could be found before other evidences of Huntington's chorea are evident, so that it would be possible to predict which children of a patient with Huntington's chorea will develop the disease and carry it on to their children. — Ed.]

Further Observations on Neurology of Music: Musical Notation and Pitch Discrimination. R. A. Henson[8] (London) observes that music is art in sound and is always an art, though sometimes debased. Music is a nonverbal language, and reading musical notation demands exclusive use of the language. The position of the musician is comparable with that of the verbal bilingual exponent who thinks and speaks both languages independently. Trained musicians think in musical terms. All musical experience depends on the ability to identify or discriminate the pitch of tones, a facility that is also engaged in hearing speech and

(8)   Br. Med. J. 1:1121–1125, Apr. 30, 1977.

natural sounds. It is impossible to determine with certainty whether there is an in-built tuning system. The normal range of heard frequencies is age dependent and contingent on what is meant by hearing a frequency. A sense of relative pitch is necessary to hear or sing a simple tune. Early training is necessary for the development of absolute pitch.

Understanding of the mechanisms of central auditory processing is quite deficient. Studies on the afferent auditory paths from the cochlea to the temporal lobe show that whereas the frequency organization of the cochlea is maintained, synchrony of neural discharges diminishes progressively. The template-matching hypothesis probably offers the firmest basis for understanding the process of pitch discrimination. A match between the sensory input and the stored "standard" derived from past experience is likely, however, to affect more than one memory code. Factors such as semantic memory, musical memory, prediction and set and bias can be expected to play important roles in the analysis of pitch discrimination and in other types of musical experience. The subject of musical memory is relatively unexplored, but it would be incorrect to ignore the remarkable way in which music can be analyzed, learned and stored.

► [There has been a recent announcement of the publication of a book on the neurology of music by this authority and another neurologist, Dr. Macdonald Critchley, who is also a student of this subject. – Ed.] ◄

Pediatric Neurology

Biochemical Basis of Minimal Brain Dysfunction.
Sally E. Shaywitz, Donald J. Cohen and Bennett A. Shaywitz[9] (Yale Univ.) assert that minimal brain dysfunction (MBD) is a common problem in pediatric practice, affecting an estimated 5–10% of the school-aged population. It is an ill-defined, poorly understood disorder and is often unrecognized by physicians responsible for the primary care of children. It is unclear whether the various cardinal symptoms coexist as unrelated symptoms or arise from a common pathophysiologic process and conform to a medical model. Support for the latter possibility is accumulating from several lines of investigation.

Findings of differences in blood or platelet serotonin concentrations in children with MBD have not been corroborated, and there are formidable theoretical obstacles to the assumption that demonstration of a serotonin abnormality may be extrapolated to include a defect in indoleamine metabolism in the central nervous system. Brain dopaminergic mechanisms may, however, play a fundamental role in the pathogenesis of MBD. Documentation of a genetic component may support a biochemical basis for MBD in children and there does appear to be a heritable component to some of the symptoms of MBD. An animal model conforming to minimal criteria for MBD was not developed until recently, when a system strikingly similar to the clinical disorder has been produced by selective depletion of brain dopamine with intracisternal administration of 6-hydroxydopamine. Central to such studies is the belief that particular behavior patterns may relate to damage to specified neural pathways.

Knowledge of the fundamental mechanisms underlying MBD is still far from complete, but there is clinical and laboratory evidence suggesting that brain monoaminergic

(9)   J. Pediatr. 92:179–187, February, 1978.

mechanisms may significantly influence the evolution of many clinical manifestations of MBD.

▶ [So-called minimal brain damage remains an ill-defined, poorly understood concept. These investigators seem to consider it an entity with a single pathophysiologic basis. It is still to be demonstrated, however, whether or not the varying aspects of the disorder—motor, sensory, behavioral and psychologic—stem from a single etiology. These various aspects of the disorder vary from patient to patient and consequently may have different causes.—Ed.] ◀

Megavitamins for Minimal Brain Dysfunction: Potentially Dangerous Therapy. Quasimedical treatments of chronic disease may be the immediate cause of severe illness. Children with chronic neuropsychiatric disorders are particularly subject to peculiar treatments. Bennett A. Shaywitz, Norman J. Siegel and Howard A. Pearson[1] (Yale Univ.) describe a boy with minimal brain dysfunction who received megavitamin therapy, with potentially disastrous consequences.

Boy, aged 4 years, had been febrile and irritable for about 4 months, and more so in the past week. He had been seen a year earlier for hyperactive behavior; abnormal liver function had been observed. The boy had then been seen 10 months earlier by a physician known to prescribe megavitamin therapy for hyperactivity. At the present examination the boy was very irritable and febrile, with fissures at the corners of the mouth, a grade 2/6 systolic murmur and a palpable liver edge at 3 cm. He reported pain on palpation of his body and refused to walk. The sedimentation rate was 44 mm/hour. Computerized tomography of the brain showed mild enlargement of the lateral ventricles. A polyphosphate bone scan showed increased uptake in the shafts of all long bones, especially the tibia. An echocardiogram was normal. The vitamin A level was 1,430 mg/dl, more than 10 times normal. It was learned that the child had eaten vitamin tablets continuously at nursery school. The symptoms abated over 4 weeks in the hospital, and the vitamin A level fell gradually to 110 mg/dl. A liver biopsy showed mild fatty infiltration with vacuolated cells. The child is now in a foster home and has not had recurrent symptoms.

The manifestations of hypervitaminosis A include bone pain and tenderness, anorexia, irritability and fissuring of the lips. Hepatic inflammation and dysfunction are less frequent findings. Megavitamin therapy is not only ineffective for such conditions as learning disabilities and childhood

(1) J.A.M.A. 238:1749–1750, Oct. 17, 1977.

psychoses, but potentially dangerous. If even a small proportion of children with minimal brain dysfunction receive megavitamin therapy, the potential for complications is substantial.

▶ [Although methods of treatment such as megavitamin therapy are not only ineffective but also potentially dangerous, physicians are often unsuccessful in preventing their patients from being recipients of such practices. A recent editorial (J.A.M.A. 238:761, 1977) discusses this subject and the indiscriminate use of megavitamins for the treatment of many organic and nonorganic conditions. In the health food stores there are preparations that contain 8,000%, 16,000%, and even 52,000% of the recommended daily dosage of the vitamin B complex and vitamin C as well as excessive amounts of vitamins A and D and folic acid. Such preparations are dangerous and their sale should be prohibited. — Ed.] ◀

Therapeutic Use of Glucocorticoid Hormones in the Perinatal Period: Potential Neurologic Hazards are discussed by Morton E. Weichsel, Jr.[2] (Univ. of California, Torrance). The therapeutic use of synthetic glucocorticoids in infancy and childhood has become widely accepted, but little is known of the potential hazards to human nervous system development. In addition to preventing respiratory distress syndrome by transplacental use, high-potency glucocorticoids are often used in infants to treat a number of neurologic conditions, including trauma, asphyxia and meningitis. Glucocorticoids are used for longer periods in neonatal hypoglycemia and infantile myoclonic seizures. The long-term use of glucocorticoids in childhood produces deficits in somatic growth, but developmental sequelae from perinatal glucocorticoid therapy have not been documented.

Studies in animals suggest a need for serious concern. Retardation of evoked responses in the rat sensory cortex has been noted with cortisol. Changes in biogenic amine levels in the hypothalamus have been described after the administration of hydrocortisone to rats at birth. The interaction of steroid hormones with target cells in brain tissue has been considered to influence neuroendocrine physiology and behavior. Marked behavioral changes outlasting the period of steroid administration have been seen in mice given corticosterone in infancy. Granule cells in the dentate gyrus of the hippocampus are subject to pathologic influences from glucocorticoids, and prevention of dentate gran-

(2) Ann. Neurol. 2:364–366, November, 1977.

ule cell multiplication in the hippocampus of irradiated infant rats has been followed by behavioral changes resembling those due to surgical destruction of the hippocampus in adult rats.

► [Glucocorticoids have become widely used in the perinatal period — antepartum to prevent the respiratory distress syndrome and postnatally for the treatment of widely varying conditions. Important developmental changes take place in the brain during this period. The glucocorticoids may alter these and exert irreversible effects on brain cell division and differentiation. These substances should be used with extreme caution during this period. — Ed.] ◄

Acute Confusional State in Children with Migraine. In 1970, Gascon and Barlow described 4 children who displayed acute confusional states during migraine attacks. E. Stanley Emery III[3] (Univ. of Vermont) reports similar episodes in 4 more children.

Girl, aged 8 years, fell and rolled down a hill and was found to be confused, fearful, agitated and combative. At age 5 years she had been found confused and combative for 60–90 minutes and had then slept for several hours. Her father had migraine. The girl was agitated and screaming at admission. Slight swelling was present over the right occiput. Skull films and a brain scan were normal. An EEG showed high-voltage polymorphic delta activity, of higher amplitude on the left side. Improvement was evident after the patient was mentally clear, and a third record obtained 5 months later was normal. The agitated behavior lasted about 9 hours until the girl was allowed to sleep. She was alert when she awoke 4 or 5 hours later, and the neurologic findings were normal. She had little recall of the past events. Intermittent severe headaches have continued over 3 years of follow-up.

A diagnosis of migraine was firm in 3 cases. The belief that confusion is a symptom of an acute migraine attack seemed to be justified in the 2 teenaged patients and in 3 of Gascon and Barlow's 4 patients. It seems to be unlikely that these episodes could represent merely a posttraumatic state; the head trauma was minimal, and there was an interval before any sensorial abnormality was observed. One of the present patients had cerebral vasoconstrictive symptoms preceding confusion and another has had multiple episodes of vasoconstrictive symptoms in a carotid and basilar distribution.

Recognition of this confusional disorder provides reassur-

(3) Pediatrics 60:110–114, July, 1977.

ance for children who have recurrent episodes. All the children have had self-limited courses and benign outcomes. A diagnosis of the disorder can avoid possibly hazardous diagnostic procedures such as angiography.

▶ [It has been recognized in recent years that acute confusional states may occur during an attack of migraine in children, but this has not been widely recognized. Although the children appear seriously ill, all of them had self-limited courses and benign outcomes. Of course, various infectious, metabolic or other etiologies must be suspected when this confusional state is seen initially, but if the child is observed over a period of time, it may be possible to avoid potentially hazardous diagnostic procedures. — Ed.] ◀

Chronic Progressive Poliomyelitis Secondary to Vaccination of an Immunodeficient Child. Larry E. Davis, David Bodian, Donald Price, Ian J. Butler and James H. Vickers[4] studied an immunodeficient child who developed a slowly progressive central nervous system disease after she received trivalent live poliovirus vaccine and who had lesions typical of poliomyelitis at autopsy. Poliovirus type II was isolated from the throat, stool and brain.

Girl, a short-limbed dwarf, became intermittently febrile at age 8 months, 3 months after the last of three doses of trivalent live poliovirus vaccine. Development regressed and the infant became irritable and withdrawn. Limb tremors and vermiform movements of the tongue appeared. Nystagmus was present at age 10 months, and persistent myoclonic activity was seen in all extremities, where muscle tone was increased. Ankle clonus was occasionally elicited. Serum IgG, IgA and IgD were absent and IgM was markedly reduced. No antibody titers to poliovirus, tetanus toxin or diphtheria toxin were found despite immunizations. A persistent blood lymphopenia was present. Skin tests to several antigens were negative. Phytohemagglutinin stimulation of the lymphocytes was low-normal. The patient's condition deteriorated despite γ-globulin treatment, and she died of acute *Pneumocystis carinii* pneumonia at age 11 months.

Autopsy showed defective endochondral ossification in all bones examined, an extremely small thymus and bilateral *P. carinii* pneumonia. Focal neuron loss was seen in the anterior horns, with collections of mononuclear cells and reduced numbers of axons. Muscle showed denervation atrophy. A focal loss of Purkinje's cells was seen in the cerebellar cortex. Scattered foci of reactive inflammation were present in the dentate nucleus and the other roof nuclei. Extensive necrosis and reactive astrocytosis were seen in the

(4) N. Engl. J. Med. 297:241–245, Aug. 4, 1977.

thalamus. Milder involvement of the globus pallidus was observed. Accumulations of inflammatory cells were seen near degenerating neurons in the premotor cortex. Betz's cells were not identified.

In this patient, poliovirus type II was isolated from throat and stool during life and from several brain sites at autopsy. The brain isolate was considered as vaccine-like from temperature sensitivity and antigenic marker studies, but in monkeys it produced moderately severe lesions in the spinal cord and brain stem.

Apparently, attenuated poliovirus can produce a chronic progressive neurologic disease under unusual circumstances, such as immunodeficiency. Immunodeficiency should be diagnosed early to avoid administration of live virus vaccines. Dissociation of in vitro and neurovirulence markers may occur because replication of poliovirus in the nervous system permits selection of the most neurovirulent populations.

► [This case demonstrates that under unusual circumstances such as immunodeficiency, attenuated poliomyelitis virus can produce a chronic progressive neurologic disease. This case also emphasizes the need to diagnose immunodeficiency as early as possible so that live virus vaccines will not be administered. — Ed.] ◄

Electroencephalogram in Childhood Basilar Artery Migraine.

Martin L. Lapkin, Joseph H. French, Gerald S. Golden and A. James Rowan[5] (Albert Einstein College of Medicine) describe 2 pediatric patients with basilar artery migraine in whom significant transient EEG abnormalities were documented in temporal proximity to the headache episodes.

Girl, 10, was admitted because of headache and lethargy 10 days after an episode of rotational vertigo, during which she fell, struck her head and had transient loss of consciousness. Two days before admission bilateral transient blindness lasting 10 – 15 minutes occurred, followed by a pounding occipital headache and nausea. The headache recurred intermittently over the next 2 days, with associated neck pain and tinnitus. Renal function had been impaired since ureterostomies were done for obstructive uropathy at age 7. Nuchal rigidity and a Kernig sign were present. The urinary diversions were functional. The child was sleepy and irritable but oriented.

The next day, diplopia and tinnitus were reported, and minimal 6th nerve paresis, right central 7th nerve palsy and nystagmus

(5) Neurology (Minneap.) 27:580 – 583, June, 1977.

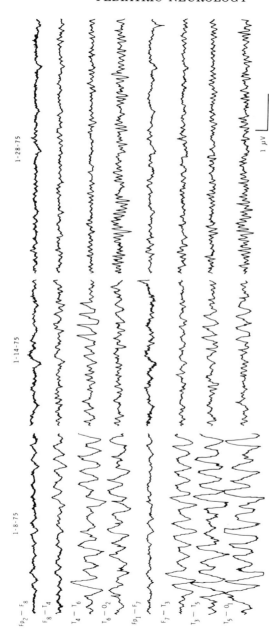

Fig 12. – Serial EEGs from 1 patient. Initial tracing (*left*) during height of the attack shows asymmetric 2- to 3-Hz high-voltage slowing posteriorly, with left-sided preponderance. Repeat EEG 4 days later (*center*) shows some return of normal background activity, which is interrupted by bilateral posterior rhythmic 3½-Hz slowing. Two weeks later (*right*), tracing is normal. (Courtesy of Lapkin, M. L., et al.: Neurology (Minneap.) 27:580–583, June, 1977.)

were noted. The right plantar response was extensor. Carotid and vertebral angiograms were normal. An EEG was poorly organized and diffusely slow (Fig 12), with rhythmic delta activity posteriorly and a paradoxic response to arousal. Bilateral bursts of diffuse delta activity were also noted. Gradual improvement occurred after 24 hours, with complete resolution of the neurologic abnormalities. An EEG done 4 days later showed improvement, but occasional paroxysmal slowing was seen occipitally. An EEG obtained 2 weeks later was entirely normal.

The presumed pathophysiology of basilar artery migraine, with sequential vasoconstriction and vasodilation, explains the type and potential transience of the EEG findings. An EEG showing occipital delta activity with or without generalized delta bursts is compatible with the diagnosis, and serial recordings showing resolution of the initial abnormalities can support the diagnosis. If clinical improvement is noted, the abnormal EEG itself need not dictate the performance of neuroradiologic contrast procedures.

▶ [There is controversy about whether this syndrome first described by Bickerstaff actually exists, but, as described, it is quite clear-cut, and many clinicians feel that it is an entity that occurs in childhood. This study gives further credence to its existence by describing a specific EEG picture during attacks. — Ed.] ◀

Effects of Decaffeinated Coffee versus Whole Coffee on Hyperactive Children. Schnackenberg (1973) reported relief from symptoms, without side effects, in hyperactive children given whole coffee. Huestis et al. (1975) failed to obtain a good therapeutic effect with pure caffeine in capsule form. D. H. P. Harvey (Monash Univ.) and R. W. Marsh[6] (Univ. of Wellington) performed a double-blind, crossover comparison of the effects of whole coffee and decaffeinated coffee on 12 children with symptoms of hyperkinetic impulse disorder. The 8 boys and 4 girls, with a mean age of 7.3 years, had been referred with chronic behavior problems at home or at school. Activity levels were well above average, but intelligence was normal. No medication had been prescribed. After baseline evaluation, coffee was dispensed twice daily. Either normal or decaffeinated coffee was given for 3 weeks before the crossover. The normal coffee regimen contained 175 – 200 mg caffeine daily. Decaffeinated coffee contains an average of 0.08 – 0.19% caffeine.

(6)   Dev. Med. Child Neurol. 20:81 – 86, February, 1978.

Whole coffee produced significant improvement, compared with both the baseline period and the decaffeinated coffee period. No sequential effect was observed in parent or teacher ratings. Eight children responded positively to caffeine, and 2 responses were marginal but in the desired direction. Two children responded equally well to placebo and caffeine. Only 2 children failed to improve their Digit Span scores while they were on caffeine. Most children showed marked improvement in the Porteus Maze Test while they were on whole coffee and lesser but significant improvement when they were on decaffeinated coffee. Differences in performance on the Twenty Second Clock Test were highly significant.

The findings suggest that whole coffee may be a useful first step in the treatment of hyperactive children. Treatment should be individualized, and it remains to be seen whether long-term use of whole coffee will maintain improvement.

▶ [Amphetamine and methylphenidate, the stimulant drugs used in the treatment of hyperactive children, are prescription drugs that are closely regulated and expensive. This study shows that a readily available and commonly used stimulant, caffeine, given as the beverage coffee, also brought about significant improvement in such children. There was lessening of motor activity and improvement in behavior and in the ability to perform psychologic tests. — Ed.] ◀

Hereditary Nonprogressive Athetotic Hemiplegia: New Syndrome. Floyd Haar and Paul Dyken[7] (Med. College of Georgia) report a previously undescribed syndrome of congenital familial unilateral neurologic deficit that occurs always on the same side. A male infant, the proband, had macrocephaly with mild left-sided weakness soon after birth and a ventriculogram showed aqueductal stenosis and obstructive hydrocephalus, more marked on the right. Five shunt revisions were necessary in 3 years. A static hypertonia of the arm persisted and definite hypoplasia of the left side of the body was noted at age 4, as was left esohypertropia. The Stanford-Binet IQ score was 47. The mother, aged 28, had a similar history but not stigmas of hydrocephalus. Athetoid movements of the left hand had developed at age 8. Right cerebral atrophy was noted on a computed axial tomographic (CAT) scan. The proband's maternal uncle, aged 22,

---

(7) Neurology (Minneap.) 27:849–854, September, 1977.

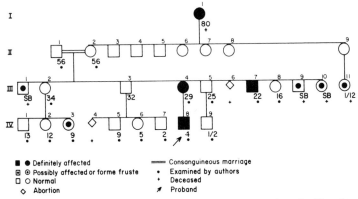

Fig 13.—Family pedigree. (Courtesy of Haar, F., and Dyken, P.: Neurology (Minneap.) 27:849–854, September, 1977.)

had had left-sided weakness shortly after birth and abnormal posturing of the left hand at age 10. The EMI showed an enlarged right lateral ventricle with a left-to-right shift.

The pedigree is shown in Figure 13. The proband's maternal great-grandmother was also affected. The syndrome is characterized by congenital left-sided weakness and hypertonicity, with the later development of athetosis and more evident hypoplasia. The life span is normal. Dysarthria and hydrocephalus are present in some cases. Right cerebral hypoplasia or atrophy was noted in the 3 patients studied. The syndrome is inherited as an autosomal dominant trait, probably with incomplete penetrance. This family may not be unique, but the concept of a genetic mechanism that could produce a benign congenital hemiplegia and later athetosis is a new one. The problem of identifying the genetic mechanism responsible for unilateral cerebral atrophy that is on the same side in each affected offspring remains.

► [Hereditary factors are not common causes for stereotyped unilateral neurologic motor defects. As a consequence, this family is a unique and interesting one. The authors, however, state that this complex is inherited in an autosomal dominant pattern, but autosomal dominant traits usually do not skip a generation, and in this family there was one unaffected generation. — Ed.] ◄

Significance of Positive Spike Bursts in Reye's Syndrome. The appearance of 14-cps and 6-cps positive spike bursts during coma has rarely been reported. Thoru Yamada, Samuel Young and Jun Kimura[8] (Univ. of Iowa) recorded EEGs daily on 3 consecutive patients with Reye's syndrome. The patients were initially studied during the acute phase of the disorder when they were in moderately deep or deep coma and they were followed until they regained consciousness.

Girl, aged 14 years, developed headache and sore throat 2 weeks after rubeola vaccination and became irritable and confused. The right pupil was dilated and underreactive and bilateral Babinski signs were present. The liver was enlarged. The girl became stuporous and was ventilated under therapeutic hypothermia. An EEG taken during moderately deep coma showed bursts of 50- to 100-μv, 2–2.5-cps delta waves. Improvement was observed the

Fig 14.—Second EEG (grade III) with 13-cps positive spike bursts (*underlining*). Note occurrence of bursts during suppressed delta activity induced by pinching right shoulder. (Courtesy of Yamada, T., et al.: Arch. Neurol. 34:376–380, June, 1977; copyright 1977, American Medical Association.)

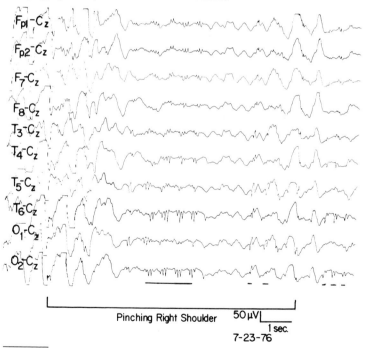

Pinching Right Shoulder 50 μV
1 sec.
7-23-76

(8) Arch. Neurol. 34:376–380, June, 1977.

next day, when stimulation suppressed delta activity, often in association with prominent 13-cps positive spike bursts (Fig 14). Subsequent recordings showed improvement, without positive spikes. The patient regained consciousness 5 days after the first recording. An EEG taken when she was fully recovered showed a few 14-cps positive spikes during light sleep. These were infrequent compared with those seen during coma.

The frequency of positive spikes in these cases was generally slower than the usual 14 cps and changed with EEG improvement or deterioration. At an appropriate stage of illness the positive bursts were much more frequent and prominent than the usual positive spike bursts seen in light sleep. The bursts were often precipitated by various stimuli. The incidence of positive spikes in patients with Reye's syndrome is high compared with that in other comatose patients. Whether the findings represent a specific biochemical or metabolic abnormality at a given stage of hepatic coma is unclear.

▶ [It appears that the presence of positive spikes in the EEG has diagnostic significance in Reye's syndrome. Undetermined metabolic or biochemical disturbances may be responsible for their presence. – Ed.] ◀

Juvenile Huntington's Chorea: Clinical, Ultrastructural and Biochemical Studies. A juvenile form of Huntington's chorea, with onset before age 20 years, has long been recognized. Hans H. Goebel, Rainald Heipertz, Wolfgang Scholz, Khalid Iqbal and Isabel Tellez-Nagel[9] report biochemical and ultrastructural studies of brain biopsy and autopsy tissues of a male patient aged 20 years.

Boy, 17, had had somewhat retarded speech development and had repeatedly failed at school. At age 11 his movements had become slow and his gait awkward. On admission he exhibited continuous choreoathetotic movements of the head and limbs and involvement of the neck and facial muscles. His speech was dysarthric. Intellectual functions were considerably reduced. An EEG was normal. Pneumoencephalography showed symmetric ventricular dilatation and widened cerebral sulci. His condition rapidly deteriorated 2 years later, and at age 20 years he could not walk or speak except in grunting sounds. He died in decerebrate rigidity 6 months later. His father had died at age 38 with a cerebral and motor condition diagnosed as Huntington's disease.

At autopsy the striate bodies appeared markedly atrophic (Fig 15). The caudate nuclei showed a complete loss of small neurons

(9) Neurology (Minneap.) 28:23–31, January, 1978.

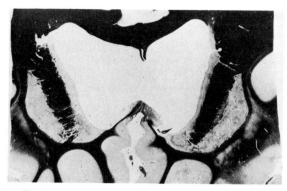

Fig 15.—Shrinkage of both corpora striata. Heidenhain-Woelcke myelin stain; reduced from ×6. (Courtesy of Goebel, H. H., et al.: Neurology (Minneap.) 28:23–31, January, 1978.)

and reduced numbers of large nerve cells, with marked astrocyte proliferation. Both putamens were similarly, but less markedly affected. Loss of cortical neurons was most marked in gyri around the sylvian fissures, also with fibrillary gliosis. Neurons were also reduced in number in the dentate nuclei and inferior olives. Ultrastructural study showed lipofuscin in neuron perikarya in the cortex and polygonal residual bodies in oligodendrocytes or microglia. Mitochondrial abnormalities were also observed. Degenerating neurites were frequent. Astrocytic perikarya and processes were often swollen. Abnormally high levels of three proteins were found in the neuron microsomal fraction on SDS polyacrylamide gel electrophoresis, as in adult cases of Huntington's chorea. Fatty acids were abnormal in white matter sphingomeylin.

The findings strengthen the concept of a uniform pathologic process in adult and juvenile Huntington's diseases despite some clinical and histologic differences.

► [These pathologic and biochemical studies tend to show that the juvenile and adult forms of Huntington's chorea are the same, despite some clinical and histologic differences. The clinical observation that juvenile Huntington's chorea is always inherited from the father is still unexplained.—Ed.] ◄

Epilepsy

Diagnostic and Therapeutic Reevaluation of Patients with Intractable Epilepsy. Roger J. Porter, J. Kiffin Penry and Joseph R. Lacy[1] (Natl. Inst. of Health) used intensive monitoring techniques in an attempt to improve seizure diagnosis and control in 11 male and 12 female patients aged 8 – 30, with intractable epilepsy. Most had a long history of uncontrolled epilepsy. Only 3 patients reported fewer than one seizure a day and most had 3 – 10 attacks daily. None had a definite cause of epilepsy. Three patients were retarded. Six-hour telemetered EEGs and video recordings were obtained from all patients. Plasma antiepileptic drug levels were frequently determined. Patients were monitored in the hospital for an average of 8 weeks and after discharge were followed for an average of 8 months. Carbamazepine was generally used to treat complex partial seizures and ethosuximide or sodium valproate, or both, for absence seizures.

At follow-up, 70% of patients continued to have improved seizure control compared with baseline studies. Toxicity was reduced in 83% of cases. About half the patients had made gains in social adjustment. One patient failed to maintain the good seizure control obtained in the hospital. Another was unable to sustain rehabilitation despite markedly improved seizure control.

Establishment of a seizure diagnosis by video and telemetered EEG recordings, alleviation of medication toxicity, tailoring of a specific regimen for the individual patient and frequent plasma drug level determinations have resulted in significant improvement in epileptic patients previously considered refractory to therapy. Good seizure control is a necessary but not sufficient criterion for reentry into society by epileptic patients. Attention also must be paid to the social adjustment of these patients, including assistance in

---

(1) Neurology (Minneap.) 27:1006 – 1011, November, 1977.

their continuing in school, vocational rehabilitation and recreational enjoyment.

▶ [The use of the techniques described in this article can result in significant improvement in patients previously thought to be intractable to therapy. — Ed.] ◀

Mesial Temporal Hemorrhage, Consequence of Status Epilepticus. Ischemic lesions and glial reactions in vulnerable regions of the brain are commonly held to be the result, not the cause, of status epilepticus, but in a number of cases this relation cannot be ascertained, especially when old gliotic hippocampal lesions are present. P. Noël, A. Cornil, P. Chailly and J. Flament-Durand[2] (Free Univ. of Brussels) report a case in which lesions were definitely acute and secondary to status epilepticus.

Woman, 52, was admitted in coma with seizures a month after pyrexia and exertional dyspnea developed. Headache and vomiting had occurred the day before admission, followed in a few hours by obtundation and recurrent generalized seizures. The rectal temperature was 38.2 C. The patient reacted to painful stimuli with semipurposeful movements. Coarse rales were heard throughout both lungs, and acrocyanosis was prominent. Phenobarbitone, phenytoin, dexamethasone and ampicillin were given, and the patient was ventilated. Subsequent seizures did not respond to intravenous diazepam or clonazepam. Decerebrate posturing developed, and seizures became permanent on the 4th day, interrupted only by short periods of total hypotonia. A brain scan and angiogram were negative. The EEG showed diffuse polymorphic slow waves on day 5, and the patient died the following day after the temperature had risen to 41 C.

Autopsy showed bronchopneumonia with filamentous fungi in the lesions, as well as large areas of hepatic necrosis. Hemorrhagic lesions were found in the anterior white commissure, amygdala and horn of Ammon (Fig 16). Recent hemorrhagic necrosis was observed without any glial reaction. A small solitary mycotic abscess was present in one horn of Ammon. Scattered ischemic lesions were seen in the Purkinje cells and temporal neurons. The hypothalamus, brain stem and basal ganglia were intact.

This patient had a severe encephalopathy with status epilepticus of 6 days' duration, associated with an acute, probably viral hepatitis, hyperammonemia and hyperventilation.

---

(2)   J. Neurol. Neurosurg. Psychiatry 40:932–935, September, 1977.

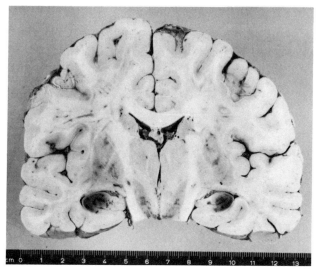

Fig 16.—Coronal section of brain showing symmetric hemorrhagic lesions of cornu Ammonis. (Courtesy of Noël, P., et al.: J. Neurol. Neurosurg. Psychiatry 40:932–935, September, 1977.)

The usual signs of hepatic coma were absent. The cause of the status epilepticus remains unclear. The fungal abscess in a horn of Ammon could possibly have been a critical factor in initiating the seizures.

▶ [In the case reported here the unusual character of the lesions leaves no doubt about the sequence of events. The medial temporal hemorrhagic lesions are acute ones and are secondary to the status epilepticus.—Ed.]

Natural History of Lactic Acidosis after Grand Mal Seizures: Model for Study of Anion Gap Acidosis Not Associated with Hyperkalemia. An acute metabolic acidosis secondary to lactic acid accumulation has been documented after grand mal seizures. Carl E. Orringer, John C. Eustace, Christian D. Wunsch and Laurence B. Gardner[3] (Univ. of Miami) sought to define the time course of this acidosis by obtaining serial blood samples from 8 consecutive patients immediately after a grand mal seizure lasting 30–60 seconds. No patient had more than one seizure within 1 hour. The 7 men and 1 woman had a mean age of 39.6

(3) N. Engl. J. Med. 297:796–799, Oct. 13, 1977.

years. Two had histories of alcohol abuse, but none had a history of any factor associated with elevated blood lactate levels. Arterial blood measurements were made within 4 minutes of the seizure and were repeated after 15, 30 and 60 minutes.

Metabolic acidosis was present immediately after the seizure, with a mean arterial blood pH of 7.14 and an anion gap of 19 mEq/L or greater. The mean lactate level was 12.7 mEq/L and fell to 8.9 at 15 minutes and to 6.6 at 60 minutes. The pH was 7.31 at 30 minutes and 7.38 at 1 hour. The carbon dioxide content, initially 17.1 mM/L, increased and was normal by 1 hour. The serum sodium concentration fell from 140 to 137 mEq/L at 30 minutes. Venous blood pyruvate and serum glucose values were consistently elevated. No significant interval respiratory changes were seen. There were no changes in arterial blood Pa_{O_2} or in venous blood concentrations of potassium, chloride, urea nitrogen or β-hydroxybutyrate.

Lactic acidosis occurs after a single grand mal seizure and resolves spontaneously within 1 hour. Resolution of the acidosis is primarily a metabolic event. No elevation of the serum potassium concentration is seen. This acute, self-limited but profound lactic acidosis may serve as a model for clarifying many of the phenomena accompanying this acid-base disorder.

▶ [The acute, self-limited, but profound lactate acidosis occurring in the patient after a seizure may serve as a unique model that may help to clarify further many of the phenomena that occur in lactate acidosis. — Ed.] ◀

Quantitative Analysis of Interictal Behavior in Temporal Lobe Epilepsy. Among neurologic diseases with confirmed anatomical localization, temporal lobe epilepsy has been most often associated with functional psychiatric disorders. David M. Bear and Paul Fedio[4] (Natl. Inst. of Health) attempted to determine the effects of a unilateral temporal epileptic focus on specific psychosocial aspects of behavior. Eighteen traits putatively associated with interictal behavior were evaluated by questionnaires in 48 subjects, including 27 with unilateral spike foci in the temporal lobe and psychomotor seizures, 9 with neuromuscular disorders and 12 normal adults.

(4)   Arch. Neurol. 34:454–467, August, 1977.

The epileptic patients self-reported a distinctive profile of humorless sobriety, dependence and obsessionalism. Raters discriminated the epileptics on the basis of circumstantiality, philosophical interests and anger. Right temporal epileptics exhibited emotional tendencies, in contrast to the ideational traits of left temporal epileptics. The former exhibited "denial," and the latter, a "catastrophic" overemphasis of dissocial behavior. Virtually no correlation between seizure frequency and behavioral variables was significant in this study. Duration of illness did correlate with most behavioral parameters.

The behavioral profile may reflect progressive changes in limbic structure secondary to a temporal lobe focus. The contrasting biases in self-profile, dependent on laterality of the epileptic focus, parallel observations on the reaction to deficits after unilateral cerebral lesions. The denial of physical or emotional deficits in patients with right hemisphere lesions may reflect a confabulatory response of the left hemisphere in the absence of reports from right hemisphere structures. Cognitive deficits in left hemisphere functions or verbal emotional associations established within the hemisphere will be readily apparent to "conscious verbal," injury. In the case of emotional tendencies, the immediacy of verbally expressible affect may lead the left temporal epileptic to exaggerate the behavioral severity of his emotions and he may be "hyperconscious" of such feelings.

► [The results support the hypothesis that sensory-affective associations are established within the temporal lobes and that, in man, there exists a hemispheric asymmetry in the expression of affect. — Ed.] ◄

Clinical Features and Ictal Patterns in Epileptic Patients with EEG Temporal Lobe Foci were reviewed by Don W. King and Cosimo Ajmone Marsan[5] (Natl. Inst. of Health). The 270 epileptics studied each had from 2 to 17 EEGs recorded. Electrocorticograms were obtained in 195 patients who underwent temporal lobe resection or exploration. Thirty-three patients had electrodes implanted in the temporal lobe for depth recording. The 162 male and 108 female epileptics had a mean age at first hospitalization of 29 years. The mean age at seizure onset was 14 years. Forty-five patients had a family history of epilepsy. Possible con-

(5) Ann. Neurol. 2:138-147, August, 1977.

tributory factors were present in most cases, usually in the form of early childhood seizures, trauma and perinatal complications. Ictal records were available for interpretation in 83 cases. Temporal lobectomy was performed in 173 patients.

Stereotyped sensations were reported by 83% of the patients; usually the sensations constituted an aura. Nearly half the patients reported more than one type of aura. Complex and visceral sensations were the most common subjective phenomena reported. Primary visual auras were reported by a third of the patients who had posterior foci. Focal motor activity as a manifestation of a partial seizure was seen in 80% of 199 evaluable patients and adversive phenomena in 61%. Half the patients had tonic limb movements, and a third exhibited clonic phenomena. The motor phenomena were not consistently lateralized to the side opposite the focus. Automatic behavior was present in 95% of the cases; often the automatisms were multiple. Autonomic changes were noted in 83% of the patients with well-observed seizures; half showed pupillary dilatation. A brief period of postictal confusion was usual. Twenty patients had a history of interictal violent behavior.

No ictal phenomenon is unique to patients with temporal lobe foci. The data do not support the concept of an association between temporal lobe epilepsy and violence. The similarities of these patients to those with foci elsewhere is slightly emphasized over the traditional view of them as having a unique type of epilepsy.

▶ [The clinical manifestations of epilepsy secondary to discharging temporal lobe foci vary widely from patient to patient. This study presents no evidence of any association between temporal lobe epilepsy and violence. – Ed.] ◀

Prolonged Epileptic Twilight States: Continuous Recordings with Nasopharyngeal Electrodes and Videotape Analysis. Prolonged twilight or fugue states may be a manifestation of a fixed epileptic condition. Most epileptic fugues result from absence status, but rarely similar conditions result from epileptic paroxysms originating in the temporal lobe. Melvin A. Belafsky, Sandy Carwille, Patricia Miller, Gwen Waddell, Jean Boxley-Johnson and A. V. Delgado-Escueta[6] report 3 cases of epileptic twilight states.

(6) Neurology (Minneap.) 28:239–245, March, 1978.

Man, 44, began in adolescence to have states of confusion lasting 18–72 hours. Speech was absent during the episodes and behavior was nonpurposeful. The spells were followed by sleep, vague headaches and no memory of what had occurred. About 10 episodes had occurred in 20 years. Observations during the current, prolonged episode showed lip smacking and eye blinks at a rate of 2 or 3 per second and the patient could feel pinpricks. Blood pressure was 160/120 mm Hg. The EEG is shown in Figure 17. Appropriate responses began in the 2d hour of recording. Lip smacking and eye

Fig 17. – Spike wave stupor. Eleven hours after onset of twilight state, patient was ambulatory but confused and did not speak. Every 2–20 seconds, lip smacking, eye blinks and pupil dilation were observed. (Courtesy of Belafsky, M. A., et al.: Neurology (Minneap.) 28:239–245, March, 1978.)

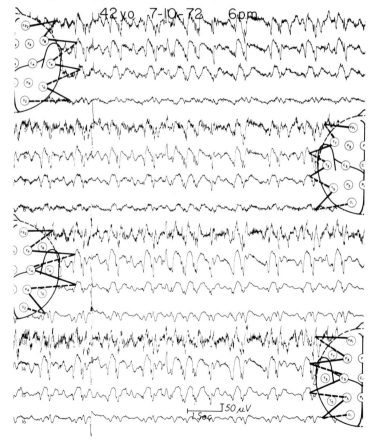

blinks were seen with diffuse rhythmic 3.5-Hz spikes and sharp waves. Stereotyped automatisms stopped after 20 hours of the twilight state, when bursts of slow waves began interrupting the continuous spike waves. Phenytoin and phenobarbital were given. The patient appeared to be alert and conversed fluently 47 hours after onset of the attack, but he was amnesic for all the recent events.

Two forms of epileptic twilight state can be distinguished clinically. Psychomotor status is manifested by recurrent cycles of a continuous twilight state with partial and amnesic responsiveness and quasipurposeful complex automatisms, often interrupted by staring, total unresponsiveness and stereotyped automatisms. In spike wave stupor only one continuous twilight state is manifested, with partial responsiveness of variable intensity. Both stereotyped and reactive automatisms are present. The EEG reflects these differences in psychomotor status and spike wave stupor. The presence of speech arrest and stereotyped automatisms strongly supports the existence of an epileptic fugue state.

► [Prolonged states of mental confusion, also termed prolonged twilight states, or "fugue states," may be a form of status epilepticus and represent either psychomotor status or spike wave stupor. — Ed.] ◄

Episodic Nocturnal Wanderings Responsive to Anticonvulsant Drug Therapy. It has often been assumed that somnambulism in older subjects is related to a disorder of non-rapid eye movement sleep, analogous to dyssomnias in children. Some adults scream and yell during their wanderings and they are referred for psychotherapy. Timothy A. Pedley and Christian Guilleminault[7] (Stanford Univ.) describe 6 patients aged 17 – 32 years who were seen because of repetitive abnormal, sometimes life-threatening behavior during sleep, for which they were entirely amnesic. One reported having sleep-walked in childhood. There was no family history of sleep disturbance or epilepsy, and no patient had used street drugs in the past 2 years. All patients had at least one all-night polygraphic monitoring study and a separate EEG investigation.

The abnormal behavior, which included abrupt arousal, violent ambulation, often with repetitive complex motor activity, and screaming, yelling or irrelevant phrases, first occurred at age 15 – 20 years. Episodes began after 2 – 4

(7) Ann. Neurol. 2:30 – 35, July, 1977.

hours of uneventful sleep, and they were often clustered. The patients seemed unusually strong when restrained. Often they were able to return to bed and would promptly fall asleep. Amnesia for the episodes was complete both immediately and subsequently. Neurologic examination was negative in all cases. Four patients injured themselves seriously during attacks. The patients behaved normally when awake. Recordings showed normal sleep cycles. Two patients had abortive attacks during stage 2 non-rapid eye movement sleep without any abnormalities on the tracings. Four patients had abnormal EEGs, 3 with focal epileptiform activity in the right anterior temporal region. No recurrences have been noted during follow-up for 6–48 months on treatment with phenytoin or carbamazepine.

It is likely that these patients have unusual complex partial seizures. The favorable response to anticonvulsants supports an ictal origin for the nocturnal wanderings. It is important to recognize this syndrome as an atypical form of epilepsy, because symptoms subside with anticonvulsant drug therapy.

► [This syndrome is distinct from the more typical types of non-rapid eye movement dyssomnia and appears to be an atypical form of epilepsy. – Ed.] ◄

Efficacy of Intravenous Phenytoin in Treatment of Status Epilepticus: Kinetics of Central Nervous System Penetration. B. Joe Wilder, R. Eugene Ramsay, L. James Willmore, George F. Feussner, Robert J. Perchalski and Jack B. Shumate, Jr.[8] (Univ. of Florida) attempted to verify the pharmacokinetics and clinical efficacy of intravenous phenytoin in the treatment of status epilepticus. Fourteen patients who had at least 20 minutes of continuous generalized motor activity or generalized seizures without recovery of consciousness, and who were going to have craniotomy or diagnostic pneumoencephalography, were studied. None had minor motor seizures. None had hepatic or renal disease or were on drugs that could interfere with phenytoin metabolism. A loading dose not exceeding 80 mg/minute was given, the mean being 13 mg/kg, followed by oral capsules for 5 days. Ten patients in status epilepticus received sufficient intravenous phenytoin to control seizure activity, but not more than 1,200 mg.

(8) Ann. Neurol. 1:511–518, June, 1977.

The mean plasma phenytoin level was 10.2 μg/ml 12 hours after infusion of the loading dose. Nine of 14 patients had therapeutic plasma levels. Studies of cortical samples from 3 patients given a mean of 9.2 mg/kg intravenously showed rapid drug penetration of the brain. Concentrations were comparable at the end of infusion and an hour later (16 and 23 μg/gm, respectively). In 6 patients given a mean of 10.9 mg/kg intravenously at pneumoencephalography, the cerebrospinal fluid phenytoin level gradually increased over 50 minutes to a plasma-cerebrospinal fluid ratio of 11. Of 10 patients given a mean of 12.2 mg phenytoin per kg intravenously, 9 were controlled within 30 minutes. No major side effects were noted.

Intravenous phenytoin rapidly enters the central nervous system and results in prompt, effective control of status epilepticus without suppressing higher cortical function or the cardiorespiratory centers. The rapid entry of phenytoin into brain parenchyma may help explain its effectiveness in controlling status epilepticus.

▶ [Intravenous phenytoin rapidly enters the central nervous system and results in prompt, effective treatment of status epilepticus without suppressing higher cortical functions or cardiorespiratory centers. – Ed.] ◀

Brain Lesions That Produce Delta Waves in the EEG. P. Gloor, G. Ball and N. Schaul[9] (Montreal) undertook a series of experiments in cats to determine what kind of localized brain pathology does and what kind does not produce localized or generalized polymorphic delta activity in the EEG. Localized destructive brain lesions were produced by thermocoagulation, with the use of an electrode 1 mm in diameter and an uninsulated tip 1 mm long. Cortical and white matter lesions (Fig 18) were produced, and vasogenic cerebral edema was created by cortical thermocoagulation. Radiofrequency lesions of the ectosylvian gyrus, thalamic lesions and lesions of the mesencephalic reticular formation and hypothalamus were produced in different groups of animals. Three animals had complete neuronal isolation of an area of cortex, encompassing the suprasylvian and ectosylvian gyri.

White matter lesions produced delta waves that were localized to the cortical area overlying the lesion. The waves

(9)   Neurology (Minneap.) 27:326 – 333, April, 1977.

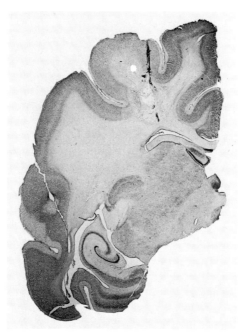

Fig 18. – White matter lesion below left middle suprasylvian gyrus. Electrode tract passes through superior border of this gyrus; cresyl violet stain. (Courtesy of Gloor, P., et al.: Neurology (Minneap.) 27:326–333, April, 1977.)

were polymorphic, about 500 μv at peak amplitude, and showed a predominant frequency of 1–2 cps. No delta activity appeared after the production of vasogenic cerebral edema, except in a few animals in which no wide craniectomy was done. Extremely variable delta activity was associated with thalamic lesions. Polymorphic delta waves were seen after bilateral lesions of the mesencephalic reticular formation, and a similar pattern resulted from bilateral lesions in the posterior hypothalamus. Unilateral hypothalamic lesions resulted in some ipsilateral delta activity. The slow waves seen in isolated cortex somewhat resembled the delta activity produced in cortex overlying a white matter lesion, but there were distinct differences.

White matter pathology is strongly correlated with the presence of polymorphic delta activity in the EEG. Midbrain and basal diencephalic lesions tend to produce delta activity. Total deafferentiation of the cortex does not result in the production of slow waves corresponding to the delta activity seen with the other types of brain lesion.

▶ [Many clinicians have the belief that the presence of delta waves in the EEG denotes the presence of a cerebral neoplasm. This extremely thorough and important article indicates that lesions of many types and in many different areas of the brain can produce delta waves. – Ed.] ◄

Slow Spike Wave Activity in EEG and Associated Clinical Features: Often Called "Lennox" or "Lennox-Gastaut" Syndrome. Patients with slow spike wave activity have been clinically distinguished from those with classic spike wave paroxysms. A high incidence of intellectual impairment and intractable seizures is associated with the abnormality. Omkar N. Markand[1] (Indiana Univ.) examined the clinical features of 83 patients, seen in 1972–75, with slow spike wave activity in the EEG. All had an interictal pattern of bisynchronous spike and slow wave activity with a frequency of less than 3 cps, awake or asleep, as well as paroxysms of slow spike wave activity lasting at least 2 seconds. Sixteen patients had both previous and follow-up EEG studies, whereas 16 had only an index study. The 45 male and 38 female patients had a mean age of $8\frac{1}{2}$ years at the time of the index EEG.

All patients but 1 had seizures; the mean age at onset in 81 patients was 3 years. Minor motor seizures occurred in (80%) 66 of 82 patients and tonic-clonic seizures in 63 (77%). Absences occurred in 44 patients and partial seizures in 8. Only 17 patients had had seizures of one particular type. Myoclonic seizures were the most frequent minor motor seizure. Different types of seizures tended to occur at different ages. Sixty-six patients were mentally retarded. Forty-nine patients had definite neurologic evidence of motor impairment; no obvious cause was apparent in 30 patients. Prenatal factors were considered etiologic in 13 patients, perinatal factors in 19 and postnatal factors in 21. The slow spike wave activity was commonly seen at 1.5–2.5 cps and 200–800 μv. Sleep had profound effects on the activity (Fig 19). Diazepam injection significantly reduced the slow spike wave activity in some studies. Ictal hypersynchronous EEG activity was typically seen during most absences. Ictal de-

(1)   Neurology (Minneap.) 27:746–757, August, 1977.

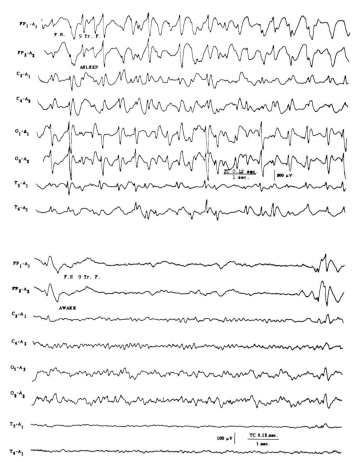

Fig 19. — Girl, aged 9, shows almost continuous slow spike wave activity during sleep but only occasional isolated spike wave paroxysms when awake. (Courtesy of Markand, O. N.: Neurology (Minneap.) 27:746–757, August, 1977.)

synchronization of EEG activity was the chief EEG change associated with clinical seizures. All but 11% of 60 follow-up studies in 37 patients showed continued slow spike waves.

There is a close relationship between the EEG patterns of hypsarrhythmia, slow spike waves and independent multi-focal spike discharges. The EEG abnormalities probably depend on cerebral maturation rather than on a particular kind of pathologic process. The Lennox-Gastaut syndrome is not a pathologic entity. The eponym seems most appropriate for patients with slow spike wave activity, mental retardation, intractable seizures and poor response to anticonvulsant medication. It identifies children who have a guarded prognosis with respect to intellectual performance and management of seizures.

▶ [Most authorities express the belief that it is appropriate to use the term "Lennox-Gastaut syndrome" for a patient who has slow spike wave activity in the EEG, exhibits mental retardation and has intractable seizures of various types. It must be remembered, however, that this is a syndrome and not a disease entity. Many disease processes, both static and progressive, can produce the syndrome. — Ed.] ◀

Epilepsia Partialis Continua: Review of 32 Cases. Epilepsia partialis continua (EPC) is now widely acknowledged to be a partial somatomotor status epilepticus. Whether cortical or subcortical mechanisms are responsible for the continuous epilepsy is unclear. Juergen E. Thomas, Thomas J. Reagan and Donald W. Klass[2] (Mayo Clinic and Mayo Med. School) reviewed the findings in 32 patients seen in 1950–73 with EPC, defined as regular or irregular, clonic muscular twitches of a limited part of the body, occurring for at least 1 hour and recurring at intervals of no more than 10 seconds. The 18 male and 14 female patients had a mean age of 37 years at onset of EPC.

Epilepsia partialis continua began suddenly in most patients. Both sides of the body were independently involved in 3. The territorial extent of the seizure activity varied markedly among patients, and seizure distribution and intensity varied even in the same patient. The speed and frequency of twitches were variable. Several patients still had EPC when last followed. Mean duration of EPC was 25 months. Seizures lessened or disappeared at rest or during sleep in 10 patients. Nine patients had twitching during coma. Only 3 patients were neurologically normal apart from the EPC. The rest had muscle weakness, sensory loss or reflex changes commensurate with the site and extent of the underlying brain disease. All but 7 of 245 EEGs were abnormal. Ten of 15 sleep recordings showed considerable reduction or abolition of muscle jerks during sleep. An active focal spike abnormality was recorded in all 5 patients

(2)   Arch. Neurol. 34:266–275, May, 1977.

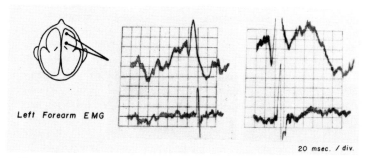

Left Forearm EMG

20 msec. / div.

Fig 20. – Two samples of oscilloscopic tracings from man, aged 25, with EPC of left arm. Upper trace in each sample is EEG activity recorded from pair of electrodes attached to scalp over right precentral region. Lower trace in each sample is electromyographic activity recorded from pair of leads attached to skin of left forearm. Note that onset of EEG spike precedes muscle jerk by 20 msec. (Courtesy of Thomas, J. E., et al.: Arch. Neurol. 34:266–275, May, 1977; copyright 1977, American Medical Association.)

who underwent electrocorticography. The findings in 1 patient are shown in Figure 20. An infarct or cerebral hemorrhage was the cause of 8 cases of EPC and presumed encephalitis was the cause of 5. For 9 cases the cause was indeterminate.

The results of treatment have been discouraging. Diazepam often stopped seizures temporarily in the acute stage. A few cases of EPC stopped for an apparent reason after years of unresponsiveness to drugs. Only 1 of 5 patients benefited from surgical exploration and excision. Mean follow-up was 37 months. Neither the presence of EPC, its distribution nor its clinical features carried reliable prognostic implications. Autopsy findings in 8 cases included consistent involvement of the motor cortex or closely adjacent areas.

The electrophysiologic and pathologic findings in these cases provide no evidence for a subcortical origin of EPC, but rather favor a primary role of the cerebral cortex.

► [In this extremely thorough clinical, electroencephalographic and pathologic study of 32 patients with epilepsia partialis continua, the data favor a cortical origin of the syndrome. – Ed.] ◄

Salivary Levels of Anticonvulsants: Practical Approach to Drug Monitoring. John J. McAuliffe, Allan L. Sherwin, Ilo E. Leppik, Shirley A. Fayle (McGill Univ.) and Charles E. Pippenger[3] (Columbia Univ.) attempted to devel-

(3) Neurology (Minneap.) 27:409–413, May, 1977.

op an accurate, practical method of calculating plasma phenobarbital levels from salivary measurements by correcting for variations in salivary pH. Techniques were developed to assay saliva either by the rapid, convenient immunoenzyme method or by gas-liquid chromatography. Simultaneous samples of saliva and venous blood were obtained at least 2 hours after the last dose of medication from 115 patients receiving anticonvulsant drugs. Salivary secretion was stimulated by having the patient chew paraffin.

Salivary phenobarbital levels were not equivalent to plasma free (dialysate) levels in many patients. Seventeen of the 42 patients studied produced saliva with a pH below 7.0, and their phenobarbital levels were 21.1% below their plasma dialysate levels. The levels of phenobarbital were equivalent to the plasma free fraction only when the salivary pH was close to 7.4, but there was a highly significant relationship between the log of the ratio of free plasma phenobarbital to salivary phenobarbital and salivary pH (Fig 21). Correlation between total plasma and salivary levels of phenytoin, carbamazepine and ethosuximide was close. More variability, not related to salivary pH, was seen for primidone.

Fig 21. — Correlation between measured total plasma phenobarbital levels and salivary concentration corrected for pH. (Courtesy of McAuliffe, J. J., et al.: Neurology (Minneap.) 27:409–413, May, 1977.)

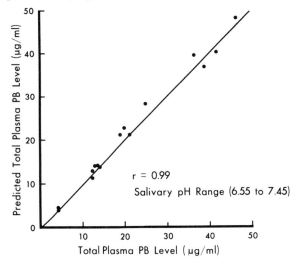

Salivary levels of phenytoin and carbamazepine agreed well with plasma free drug levels as determined by equilibrium dialysis. Excellent correlation was found between immunoassay and gas-liquid chromatographic values for phenytoin, phenobarbital and primidone in saliva.

Measurements of salivary drug levels provide an accurate index of both free and total plasma levels of phenytoin, carbamazepine, phenobarbital, primidone and ethosuximide. This approach may be particularly important in pediatric practice, especially when coupled with the rapid immuno-enzyme assay (Emit) technique.

► [Salivary concentrations of the usual anticonvulsant medications were found to be equivalent to the plasma free drug and to correlate closely with the total plasma levels. The availability of a rapid, painless technique for monitoring commonly used anticonvulsant drugs is of particular importance in pediatric practice. – Ed.] ◄

Distribution of Anticonvulsant Drugs in Gray and White Matter of Human Brain. The intensity and duration of action of anticonvulsant drugs in epilepsy depend on maintenance of an adequate drug concentration at hypothetical receptor sites. C. D. Harvey, A. L. Sherwin and E. Van Der Kleijn[4] studied the relative distributions of phenytoin, phenobarbital and carbamazepine between the gray matter of human cerebral cortex and subcortical white matter in 17 patients undergoing neurosurgery for focal epilepsy. Prolonged trails of various anticonvulsants had failed to produce adequate seizure control in all patients. All were at steady state, having received fixed doses for at least five half-lives before surgery. Temporal surgery was done in 14 cases and frontal surgery in 3. The excisions were done under local anesthesia.

Phenobarbital was distributed uniformly between the gray matter and the white matter. Plasma concentrations were significantly related to both gray matter and white matter contents. Plasma concentrations and gray matter phenytoin contents correlated well with a gray matter-plasma ratio of 1.44, 1.9-fold greater than that of phenobarbital. White matter contained an average drug concentration 1.4-fold higher than the gray matter of the cerebral cortex. Carbamazepine metabolite was not detected in samples from 2 subjects with temporal lobe epilepsy, but the metabolite was

(4)   Can. J. Neurol. Sci. 4:89 – 92, May, 1977.

not detected in the plasma of 1 of the patients at the time of operation.

The findings indicate substantial differences in the relative distributions of anticonvulsant drugs in the cerebral cortex, subcortical white matter and plasma. These differences must be taken into account in evaluation of pharmacologic or neurophysiologic studies that involve determinations of relative concentrations of these drugs in the brain.

► [These data show substantial differences in the relative distribution of anticonvulsant drugs among the cerebral cortex, the subcortical white matter and the plasma. These differences must be taken into account in evaluation of pharmacologic or neurophysiologic studies involving the determination of the relative concentrations of these drugs in the brain. — Ed.] ◄

Acetazolamide-Accelerated Anticonvulsant Osteomalacia. Long-term administration of anticonvulsants may cause osteopenic bone disease with florid osteomalacia or rickets, or simply with reduced bone density. Most patients reported to have severe osteomalacia took at least two anticonvulsant drugs concurrently. Lawrence E. Mallette[5] (Baylor College of Medicine) encountered 2 patients with severe osteomalacia who, in addition to standard anticonvulsant agents, were taking acetazolamide for control of atypical seizures. The patients, women aged 33 and 40 years who were using congeners of phenytoin and phenobarbital, had slightly low serum calcium and normal or low serum phosphate levels and normal parathyroid hormone levels. Discontinuance of acetazolamide produced an immediate threefold fall in urinary calcium excretion and a slight rise in tubular phosphate reabsorption, with no changes in serum calcium or phosphate levels. Both patients were misdiagnosed over many months of progressing morbidity.

The severe osteomalacia present in these patients is rather uncommon among patients who are taking anticonvulsants. The only common pharmacologic factor was the use of acetazolamide. Acetazolamide might have accelerated the development of osteomalacia through enhanced renal calcium excretion, increased renal phosphate excretion, a local excess of H^+ due to the induced systemic acidosis, or retardation of conversion of 25-hydroxyvitamin D_3 to 1,25-dihy-

(5)   Arch. Intern. Med. 137:1013–1017, August, 1977.

droxyvitamin D_3 by systemic acidosis. Regardless of the mechanism involved, the enhanced renal calcium excretion would make calcium balance more negative and thus accelerate the loss of bone mineral, unless intestinal calcium absorption were also increased by the drug. Clinicians should be especially alert to the possibility of osteomalacia developing in any patient who is taking acetazolamide and who might already have a reduced supply of 25-hydroxyvitamin D. Such patients include not only users of anticonvulsant drugs, but also patients with malabsorption or biliary disease and persons who avoid milk and receive little sunlight.

▶ [Patients receiving any medication or combination of medications over a long period of time should be reevaluated periodically because of the possibility of development of unexpected side effects or adverse reactions. — Ed.] ◀

Phenytoin, Phospholipids and Calcium. It has been suggested that the membrane-stabilizing effect of phenytoin results from a complex interaction with several membrane components. Several reports have attributed the pharmacologic properties of the drug to an interaction with Ca^{2+}. Mark A. Goldberg[6] (Univ. of California, Los Angeles) attempted to correlate properties of the phenytoin-phospholipid interaction with the pharmacologic properties of the drug. Studies were done using phenytoin (phenyl-4-^{3}H), phenobarbital (^{3}H-G) and $^{45}Ca^{2+}$ as $CaCl_2$.

Binding of phenytoin to phospholipid was found to be related to fatty acid composition. Dipalmitoyl and dioleoyl lecithins, the most abundant lecithins in the brain, showed the greatest binding activity. There was an exact correlation between binding activity and phosphorus content in lipids derived from fractionating total lipids of rabbit and human brain. Phenobarbital showed little interaction with phospholipids. Phospholipid binding of Ca^{2+} could be increased up to fivefold by adding 1×10^{-4}M phenytoin.

Enhancement of Ca^{2+} binding may explain the effectiveness of phenytoins in the treatment of hypocalcemic symptoms. Calcium and phospholipid binding may be important factors in the stabilizing action of phenytoin. A nonpolar, anionic molecule such as phenytoin would be expected to

(6) Neurology (Minneap.) 27:827–833, September, 1977.

orient itself with the two phenyl groups associated with the hydrophobic, fatty acid moiety of a phospholipid, whereas the polar hydantoin end reacts with the cationic amine group. Such a configuration could act to limit lateral diffusion of phospholipid molecules within the membrane, an activity that may be important in membrane stability. The proposed effect of phenytoin may only explain its actions in low-Ca^{2+} mediums.

▶ [The enhancement of calcium binding may explain the effectiveness of phenytoin in the treatment of hypocalcemic symptoms. Calcium and phospholipid binding may be important factors in the stabilizing action of phenytoin. — Ed.] ◀

Unnecessary Polypharmacy for Epilepsy. Epileptics are commonly treated with more than one anticonvulsant drug. In a prospective study of 31 patients given phenytoin alone for grand mal or focal epilepsy or both, only 3 required a second drug over a mean follow-up of nearly 15 months. S. D. Shorvon and E. H. Reynolds[7] (King's College Hosp., London) reviewed the records of all adult epileptics taking two anticonvulsants at a neurologic outpatient department in 1972–76. Of 276 patients, 82 were taking two drugs when most recently seen and 22 were taking more than two. The 50 evaluable epileptics included 27 female and 23 male patients with a mean age of 34.8 years. Twenty-six had grand mal seizures, 16 had focal minor seizures and 8 had mixed temporal lobe seizures. The most common drug combinations were phenytoin with phenobarbital and with primidone.

The interval between introduction of the first and second drugs was 2.4 years. Forty-four patients were given a second drug because of continuing seizures, but 6 were begun on two drugs. Sixteen of 44 patients had a 50% or greater reduction in seizure frequency on two drugs, but 28 others did not improve. Improved seizure control was clearly related to an optimum blood concentration of one or both drugs. All but 4 of the 28 improved patients had an optimum blood concentration of at least one anticonvulsant, compared with only 4 of 14 patients whose seizures were not improved.

The findings of this study cast some doubt on the assumption that institution of a second anticonvulsant drug will

(7)   Br. Med. J. 1:1635–1637, June 25, 1977.

improve seizure control. Patients should receive one drug initially, and this should be gradually increased in dosage until seizures are controlled or until the blood drug concentration is at the higher end of the optimum range. Only then can a second drug be considered. An alternative drug should also be considered. Much unnecessary polypharmacy can be avoided with this approach.

► [Much unnecessary polypharmacy in the treatment of epilepsy could be avoided by insuring an optimum blood concentration of one drug before considering the addition or substitution of a second one. – Ed.] ◄

Treatment of Epilepsy with Clonazepam and Its Effect on Other Anticonvulsants. A therapeutic range of serum clonazepam concentrations has not been established for use in epileptic patients. R. N. Nanda, R. H. Johnson, H. J. Keogh, D. G. Lambie and I. D. Melville[8] (Glasgow) measured serum clonazepam concentrations in 22 male and 8 female patients with a mean age of 27 years, on dosages of 3 – 12 mg clonazepam daily in a double-blind trial. Fifteen had generalized epilepsy with myoclonic jerks and tonic-clonic seizures, 4 had atypical absences and 11 had focal epilepsy with frontotemporal seizure source(s). Five patients were on no medication. Thirty-six others, 19 male and 17 female patients with a mean age of 27 years, were placed in an open trial of clonazepam. About half of these had focal epilepsy. All were being treated. In the double-blind trial, clonazepam was begun at 1 mg daily and increased every 3d day by 1 – 3 mg daily. The same maximum initial dosage was used in the open trial.

Clonazepam suppressed myoclonic jerks completely in 12 of 15 patients in the double-blind trial and abolished tonic-clonic seizures in 8 patients. Four patients received up to 12 mg daily without side effects. In 4 patients, other anticonvulsants could be reduced or stopped. Atypical absences were suppressed in all patients but 1. A minority of patients with focal attacks and tonic-clonic seizures responded to clonazepam. Clonazepam controlled myoclonic epilepsy and photosensitive epilepsy in most patients in the open trial, but it was less effective in patients with only tonic-clonic seizures. Most patients had drowsiness on initial treatment and some were ataxic. Clonazepam suppressed the EEG

(8)   J. Neurol. Neurosurg. Psychiatry 40:538 – 543, June, 1977.

photosensitive response in patients with photosensitive epilepsy. Patients in the open trial who were well controlled on 2 – 12 mg clonazepam daily had serum drug concentrations of 17 – 330 nM/L. Other anticonvulsants appeared to reduce serum clonazepam concentrations.

Clonazepam is highly effective in the treatment of generalized epilepsy with myoclonic jerks alone or with tonic-clonic seizures. It is also effective in the treatment of photosensitive epilepsy and it may help some patients with temporal lobe epilepsy. Other anticonvulsants taken in conjunction with clonazepam may reduce serum clonazepam concentrations.

► [It appears that clonazepam is particularly valuable in the treatment of epilepsy with associated myoclonus and in photosensitive epilepsy. – Ed.]

Carbamazepine: Double-Blind Comparison with Phenytoin. Allan Troupin, Linda Moretti Ojemann, Lawrence Halpern, Carl Dodrill, Robert Wilkus, Patrick Friel and Polly Feigl[9] (Univ. of Washington) compared carbamazepine and phenytoin as single anticonvulsant agents in a double-blind, crossover study of 47 patients with focal and major generalized seizures. All were aged 18 years and over (mean age, 29); a few were clinically retarded. Overall, they had moderately severe seizure disorders but could care for themselves adequately. All patients regularly had four or more seizures monthly. Mean duration of the seizure disorder was 15.9 years. The study lasted 10 months. A dosage change of 300 mg carbamazepine was taken as clinically equivalent to a 100-mg change in phenytoin dosage. The maximum dosages were 800 mg phenytoin and 2,400 mg carbamazepine daily.

Little difference was found between the two drugs in control of seizures, as measured by the average number of seizures monthly for the last 3 months of each treatment. About half of each group had a greater than 50% reduction in seizure frequency. Five patients were seizure free in the phenytoin trial and 4 in the carbamazepine trial. Some patients tended to emphasize dulled mentation and unsteadiness of gait on phenytoin and nausea on carbamazepine. No patient had marked side effects when using either drug, but more patients had higher-grade objective side effects when

(9)   Neurology (Minneap.) 27:511 – 519, June, 1977.

on phenytoin. No patient was withdrawn from the study because of hematologic problems. Psychometric studies showed better results in carbamazepine-treated patients. Minnesota Multiphasic Personality Inventory scores were slightly better with carbamazepine therapy, but the difference was significant only for the scale most indicative of overall psychopathology (F scale). Mean serum phenytoin and carbamazepine concentrations were 31.2 and 9.3 μg/ml, respectively.

Carbamazepine and phenytoin do not differ significantly in anticonvulsant efficacy. The side effects of carbamazepine are generally similar to those of phenytoin but tend not to become prominent in most patients before optimum serum drug concentrations are reached. A possibility of serious hematologic reactions to carbamazepine exists.

► [Carbamazepine offers an independent choice of improved seizure control with a possibility of fewer side effects. – Ed.] ◄

Carbamazepine as an Anticonvulsant in Children. There has been considerable interest in the anticonvulsant properties of carbamazepine because of its relatively low sedative actions and the rarity of serious somatic side effects. Richard J. Schain, Joseph W. Ward and Donald Guthrie[1] (Univ. of California, Los Angeles) used carbamazepine in 45 children with convulsive disorders and evidence of learning or behavior problems that were thought to be due at least partly to sedative anticonvulsants. Loss of alertness, poor school work, hyperactivity and impulsiveness were common signs. Mean age was 10.8 years. Mean age at onset of seizures was 4.3 years. Some patients were inadequately controlled at entry into the study. Treatment was begun with a dosage of 10 mg/kg in two doses and was increased to a maximum of 30 mg/kg daily as needed to control seizures. Sedative anticonvulsants were concurrently reduced over 2- to 4-week intervals. Phenytoin was continued in 26 cases during the initial crossover and was later withdrawn or reduced if seizure control was complete on carbamazepine.

Thirty-seven patients were continued on carbamazepine after the study because of reduced seizure frequency, improved mental function or both. Carbamazepine was stopped in 2 patients because of a rash and in 3 because of behav-

---

(1) Neurology (Minneap.) 27:476–480, May, 1977.

ioral deterioration. Three subjects withdrew from the study, 1 because of worsening seizures. The most common side effects were dizziness, diplopia and blurred vision; these were usually transient. There were no serious side effects. There was substantial improvement in psychometric measures dependent on cognitive styles facilitating problem solving but no significant change in Wechsler Intelligence Scale for Children scores. Attentiveness and alertness were improved at the end of the study.

These findings indicate the usefulness of carbamazepine in the management of seizure disorders in childhood. It is equivalent in efficacy to phenobarbital or phenytoin in preventing seizures, and adverse mental and somatic side effects are less frequent. Carbamazepine can be freely administered as a primary anticonvulsant to children with grand mal, focal motor or psychomotor seizure disorders.

► [This study indicates that therapeutic regimens of carbamazepine are less likely to interfere with mental functions in children than are equivalent doses of sedative anticonvulsants. — Ed.] ◄

Psychotropic Effects of Carbamazepine in Epilepsy: Double-Blind Comparison with Phenytoin. Most studies of carbamazepine in epilepsy have not used objective test measures. Carl B. Dodrill and Allan S. Troupin[2] (Univ. of Washington) performed a double-blind crossover comparison between carbamazepine and phenytoin in adult epileptic out patients, with use of a series of objective measures of performance and emotional status. Forty patients, 25 men and 15 women with an average age of 28.6, took part in the trial. Twenty-eight had complex partial seizures; 20 of these had generalized seizures at some time. The average duration of seizures was about 15 years. Patients were stabilized for 2 months on phenytoin alone before two 4-month double-blind study periods.

No differences in scores on the Wechsler Adult Intelligence Scale (WAIS) or Halstead's battery were found in the comparison of the two drugs. All significant differences on other measures favored carbamazepine. The tasks involved efficiency in concentration and mental manipulation and did not rely on simple perceptual or motor abilities. No biodata or seizure history variable was significantly related with

---

(2) Neurology (Minneap.) 27:1023–1028, November, 1977.

neuropsychologic improvement, although patients who improved the most tended to have had a longer illness. Patients who improved were below average in intelligence and had significantly more elevated scores on the Minnesota Multiphasic Personality Inventory (MMPI) than those not showing such improvement. In the MMPI, only the F scale showed a significant difference between the two treatments. The findings were suggestive but not truly demonstrative of a slight improvement in emotional status during carbamazepine administration.

Most tests failed in this study to identify differences in psychologic functions with carbamazepine administration. Those that were identified were selective as to functions and patients. The study does not provide evidence for a general "psychotropic" effect of carbamazepine. Reports of enhanced functioning with carbamazepine will continue to appear, but these will likely be only with respect to select patient populations and with respect to select functions.

► [Whereas objective evidence of a "psychotropic" effect of carbamazepine was not demonstrated, most patients reported improvement in alertness and mental functioning while taking the drug. This, along with its anticonvulsant action, warrants the use of carbamazepine in the treatment of epilepsy. – Ed.] ◄

Valproic Acid in Epilepsy: Clinical and Pharmacologic Effects. Valproic acid is a promising antiepilepsy drug with a chemical formula unlike that of other antiepilepsy drugs, which appears from animal studies to increase brain levels of γ-aminobutyric acid, inhibiting seizures. Richard H. Mattson, Joyce A. Cramer, Peter D. Williamson and Robert A. Novelly[3] (Yale Univ.) studied valproic acid in 23 adults participating in an open 3-month clinical study. The 20 men and 3 women were subject to uncontrolled seizures despite therapeutic serum concentrations of two or three antiepilepsy agents. They had no evidence of progressive medical or neurologic disorder. Partial complex and partial elementary seizures were the most common types. In 2 patients absence attacks were quantified during valproate therapy. The drug was given in syrup form or in capsules in daily doses of up to 2 gm as tolerated.

The mean monthly seizure frequency was reduced by more than 75% in 8 patients and by 50 – 74% in 5 others. Six

(3)   Ann. Neurol. 3:20 – 25, January, 1978.

patients had minimal or no reduction in seizures. Nine of 16 patients with partial seizures and elementary or complex symptoms had a 50% or greater reduction in seizure frequency. Seven patients had side effects, but only 2 had to withdraw during the 1st month of the trial. The EEGs showed a decrease in interictal abnormalities, primarily in patients with absence attacks. The use of gelatin capsules resulted in slower absorption than did use of the syrup. Phenytoin levels fell rapidly in many patients during valproate therapy.

The findings confirm the clinical efficacy of valproate. It decreases absence attacks and relieves partial seizures. Side effects are annoying but not serious. Valproic acid competes with phenytoin for access to binding sites on plasma proteins, but the dose of phenytoin may not have to be increased because the fall in plasma concentration from displacement by valproic acid is compensated by a proportional increase in the ratio of free drug.

► [Valproic acid is finally available for general use as an anticonvulsant, and many articles on its pharmacology and usefulness are to be expected. The study herein reported suggests that valproic acid competes with phenytoin for access to plasma binding sites and during valproate therapy the serum phenytoin concentration levels decline, but the percentage of free phenytoin increases. — Ed.] ◄

Sodium Valproate in Treatment of Intractable Seizure Disorders: Clinical and Electroencephalographic Study. Sodium valproate is a new antiepilepsy agent that has proved to be most effective in typical absence and tonic-clonic seizures, but it can benefit virtually all seizure types. An action through elevation of brain γ-aminobutyric acid content has been postulated but not proved. David J. Adams, Hans Luders and Charles Pippenger[4] (Columbia Univ.) studied the effects of valproate in 10 men, aged 21–50 years, with intractable epilepsy. Each had at least two seizures a week despite maximum tolerated dosages of conventional antiepilepsy drugs. Dosages of antiepilepsy drugs were stabilized 4 weeks before the start of valproate therapy. Valproate was given as a syrup, starting with a dose of 300 mg every 8 hours. At each visit until the 12-week visit, dosage was increased, unless control was obtained or intolerable side effects developed.

(4) Neurology (Minneap.) 28:152–157, February, 1978.

Patients with generalized seizures responded best to valproate; all 4 had at least a 50% reduction in seizure frequency. Patients with partial seizures had varied responses. Adverse effects were easily managed by dose reduction; no patient had to be withdrawn from the study. Reductions in EEG epileptiform activity were roughly correlated with decreases in seizure frequency. All 5 patients with a 50% or greater reduction in seizures had plasma drug concentrations of about 40 μg/ml or above. Three of 5 with less improvement had lower plasma drug concentrations. Five of 6 patients receiving phenytoin showed a marked reduction in phenytoin concentrations which was unaffected by the duration of valproate therapy.

Although the complete spectrum of usefulness of valproate remains to be fully defined, it is clearly a significant addition to the drugs available for treatment of epilepsy. Serum concentrations of all drugs must be monitored in patients receiving valproate.

► [This is another report on the use of sodium valproate in epilepsy and its interactions with other drugs. It appears that the serum concentration of all anticonvulsants must be monitored in patients receiving sodium valproate. — Ed.] ◄

Extrapyramidal Disease

Parkinson's Disease: Overview of Its Current Status is presented by Melvin D. Yahr[5] (Mount Sinai School of Medicine). Among the disorders of the nervous system in which parkinsonism symptoms occur, Parkinson's disease is separable as a distinctive clinical entity. There is now general agreement that loss of pigmented neurons, especially in the substantia nigra, occurs in the brains of those who have Parkinson's disease. Dopamine is selectively depleted in the neostriatum in this condition, and the depletion can be correlated with the degree of degeneration of the substantia nigra. Parkinson's disease can now be defined as a dopamine deficiency state resulting from disease or injury to the dopaminergic neuron system. To the classic triad of tremor, rigidity and akinesia may be added abnormalities of posture, equilibratory disturbance and autonomic dysfunction. Muscle rigidity is present in nearly all cases. Inability to initiate and maintain volitional motor activities is one of the most disabling features of the disease. The occurrence of dementia is not certain.

Though a variety of toxic, infective and other agents have induced parkinsonism, the cause of Parkinson's disease is unknown. Up to 15% of family members may have the disease. Considerable effort has been made to relate the disease to an epidemic of encephalitis lethargica occurring in 1918–26. Conceivably the loss of dopamine could result from a primary defect in its metabolism, rather than being secondary to degeneration of cells responsible for its production.

Levodopa, given alone or with a peripheral dopa decarboxylase inhibitor, is the treatment of choice for Parkinson's disease, but when treatment should be started and whether its beneficial effects are sustained on long-term administration are unclear. Progress of the disease occurs during levo-

---

(5) Mt. Sinai J. Med. N.Y. 44:183–191, Mar.–Apr., 1977.

dopa therapy. The major impact of this treatment is an improved quality of life. Judicious use of levodopa benefits a large proportion of patients with Parkinson's disease.

▶ [At present, levodopa, though far from being the ideal antiparkinsonism agent, is the best therapy available. Its judicious use effectively benefits a large proportion of those suffering from Parkinson's disease. — Ed.]

Hypothalamus in Parkinson's Disease. J. William Langston and Lysia S. Forno[6] examined the hypothalamus

Fig 22.—A, Lewy body (*arrow*) in nerve cell perikaryon in the lateral hypothalamus. Note central core and peripheral halo. Hematoxylin-eosin; reduced from ×720. B, elongated Lewy body in lateral hypothalamus. Note central core and peripheral pale zone. Hematoxylin-eosin; reduced from ×720. (Courtesy of Langston, J. W., and Forno, L. S.: Ann. Neurol. 3:129–133, February, 1978.)

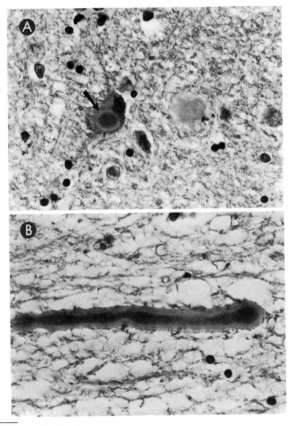

(6) Ann. Neurol. 3:129–133, February, 1978.

systematically in 30 patients with pathologically documented idiopathic parkinsonism, who died in 1961–74. At least
two classic clinical findings had been present in all cases
and autopsy had shown degeneration of pigmented nuclei
with Lewy body inclusions. The average age at death was
70.4. Only 1 patient was female. Only 1 patient had received
L-dopa for a prolonged period. The duration of illness was
less than 12 years, except in 1 patient with 22 years of disease. One patient had the Shy-Drager syndrome. Lewy body
formation was used as a marker for nerve cell degeneration
(Fig 22).

Every hypothalamus showed some degree of Lewy body
degeneration. Over 60 Lewy bodies per hyperthalamus were
found in 20% of the patient material. The tuberomamillary
nucleus and the lateral and posterior hypothalamic nuclei
contained the highest concentrations of Lewy bodies, but no
nucleus was consistently free from Lewy bodies. The size of
the nucleus alone did not appear to determine total Lewy
body counts.

Hypothalamic nerve cell degeneration was consistently
observed in this series of cases of Parkinson's disease. Recent endocrine studies appear to indicate it to be a disease
that affects primarily catecholamine nerve cells. These
study findings may help in interpreting the autonomic and
endocrine abnormalities in patients with Parkinson's disease.

▶ [This is an important and original study that gives information about
the underlying cause for the autonomic and endocrine abnormalities in
Parkinson's disease. Because such abnormalities occur (or occurred) so
much more frequently in postencephalitic parkinsonism, one wonders
how many of these patients had postencephalitic parkinsonism. – Ed.] ◀

**Brain Dopamine Turnover and Relief of Parkinson-
ism.** Urpo K. Rinne, Reijo Marttila and Vesa Sonninen[7]
(Univ. of Turku) studied the possible relationship between
dopamine receptor activation and relief from parkinsonian
features in 40 patients with Parkinson's disease. Changes in
basal and probenecid-induced levels of homovanillic acid
(HVA) and 5-hydroxyindole acetic acid (5-HIAA) in the cerebrospinal fluid during treatment with piribedil and bromocriptine were examined. No patient had previously received
levodopa. Anticholinergic therapy was continued during the

(7)   Arch. Neurol. 34:626–629, October, 1977.

study. Piribedil was given orally in a dose of 20 mg twice daily and was increased by 20 mg every 3d day to a maximum of 120 mg daily. Bromocriptine was started in a dose of 2.5 mg for 3 days and 2.5 mg for the rest of the 1st week. Then the dose was raised by 2.5 mg every week to a maximum of 30 mg daily. Probenecid tests were done before treatment and after 4 weeks of piribedil and after 20 weeks of bromocriptine therapy, using 100 mg/kg orally in 8 doses over 24 hours.

Both dopamine receptor agonists led to significant improvement in the patients. The basal cerebrospinal fluid HVA level decreased during piribedil therapy, and probenecid-induced accumulation of HVA was reduced after 1 month of treatment. No significant changes in basal or induced 5-HIAA levels were noted. Improvement in total disability was significantly related to HVA accumulation in the cerebrospinal fluid after probenecid, the increase being less in patients with clear improvement. Bromocriptine therapy caused similar changes in dopamine turnover. Patients who responded had significantly lower HVA responses to probenecid and had less severe disease than those who did not respond to bromocriptine.

The relationship between dopamine receptor activation and improvement in parkinsonian disability seen in this study suggests that the therapeutic efficacy of dopamine receptor agonists depends on the functional capacity of brain dopaminergic mechanisms. It appears that the effect of these agents on brain dopaminergic mechanisms is more specific than that of levodopa. It is important to clarify whether this is involved in the long-term clinical responses to dopamine receptor agonists as opposed to levodopa.

▶ [The demonstrated relationship between dopamine receptor activation and improvement of parkinsonian disability suggests that therapeutic efficacy of dopamine receptor agonists depends on the functional activity of brain dopaminergic mechanisms. — Ed.] ◀

Factors Influencing Occurrence of "On-Off" Symptoms during Long-Term Treatment with L-Dopa. Ann-Kathrine Granérus[8] (Univ. of Göteborg) followed 134 patients with Parkinson's syndrome for up to 91 months after they had received L-dopa therapy in 1968–70. Eighty-five

(8)   Acta Med. Scand. 203:75–85, 1978.

patients received L-dopa alone or with a peripheral dopa decarboxylase inhibitor for 5 years or longer. Forty-seven patients have died since the start of the study, and autopsies were performed on 22.

The "on-off" phenomenon appeared in 48 patients, the number of patients with on-off symptoms increasing with the duration of L-dopa treatment. Usually the phenomenon appeared after more than a year of treatment. Most patients continued on L-dopa despite the on-off symptoms. Forty-two patients received L-dopa for 5 years or longer without developing on-off symptoms. Patients with on-off symptoms were younger than the others at the start of the disease and at the start of L-dopa therapy. Maintenance dosages of L-dopa were higher in this group. Maintenance dosages did not correlate with the degree of improvement in either group, and the dosage was not related to the time when on-off symptoms began to appear. Initial improvement was more marked in the on-off group. Dyskinesia appeared earlier and more frequently in this group. Fewer on-off patients had dementia at follow-up. At follow-up, 26 on-off patients and 16 others were on combined treatment with dopa and an inhibitor.

It could be assumed that a good initial effect of L-dopa therapy in presumptive on-off patients might be associated with early parkinsonism, the other neurons being able to function almost adequately. Development of on-off symptoms appears to represent more advanced disease, with progression of damage to neurons in the basal ganglia. The magnitude of the L-dopa dosage appears to have some bearing on the appearance of the symptoms.

▶ [Those patients with Parkinson's disease who developed "on-off" symptoms had received higher dosage levels of levodopa therapy throughout treatment than those maintaining an even effect. They also had had more marked early improvement, and dyskinesias had appeared earlier and were more frequent. – Ed.] ◀

Levodopa-Induced Dopamine Receptor Hypersensitivity. Levodopa-induced dyskinesias are among the most common side effects of long-term levodopa therapy. Apomorphine and *d*-amphetamine induce stereotyped behavior and help distinguish between presynaptic and postsynaptic dopaminergic mechanisms. Harold L. Klawans, Christopher Goetz, Paul A. Nausieda and William J. Weiner[9] (Rush-

(9) Ann. Neurol. 2:125–129, August, 1977.

Presbyterian-St. Luke's Med. Center) studied the effects of chronic levodopa exposure on the thresholds for d-amphetamine- and apomorphine-induced stereotyped behavior. Guinea pigs received 200 mg levodopa per kg orally for 2 weeks. Carbidopa was given simultaneously in a dose of 20 mg/kg to maximize the central dopaminergic effects of levodopa. Apomorphine and d-amphetamine were injected subcutaneously.

None of the 6 animals given 200 mg levodopa per kg acquired full-blown stereotyped behavior, whereas all 6 given 300 mg/kg and 2 of 6 given 250 mg/kg did. Significant stereotyped behavior was seen after 7 days of treatment with carbidopa, 200 mg/kg daily. The latency period was reduced by chronic levodopa administration. Levodopa-treated animals showed marked sensitivity to a low dose of d-amphetamine. The threshold dose for apomorphine-induced stereotyped behavior was lowered in animals given levodopa and carbidopa for 2 weeks. With neither drug did chronic levodopa administration alter the latency or character of the induced stereotyped behavior.

Several observations are compatible with a concept of chronic agonist-induced hypersensitivity. This animal model of chronic agonist-induced hypersensitivity may be of use in evaluating new therapeutic agents for levodopa-induced dyskinesias.

▶ [The results reported here suggest that receptor site hypersensitivity may play a role in levodopa-induced dyskinesias and that chronic levodopa agonism may itself be involved in the pathogenesis of this movement disorder. – Ed.] ◀

Comparison of Effects of Bromocriptine and Levodopa in Parkinson's Disease. Both bromocriptine, a dopamine agonist, and levodopa are thought to act in Parkinson's disease by an effect on dopamine receptors in the striatum. R. B. Godwin-Austen and N. J. Smith[1] (Derby, England) compared the effects of these agents in 24 patients with idiopathic Parkinson's disease in a double-blind study. Disability ranged from mild to severe. Age range was 50 – 73 years. Most patients were receiving anticholinergic drug therapy at the time of the study, and a few were taking amantadine. Bromocriptine was begun in a dosage of 2.5 mg

(1)   J. Neurol. Neurosurg. Psychiatry 40:479 – 482, May, 1977.

3 times daily and increased weekly as levodopa was gradually withdrawn. The blind phase of the trial involved 2.5 mg bromocriptine and 250 mg levodopa in two treatment phases with each drug. The drugs were switched twice at random intervals during a 3-month trial.

Four patients did not tolerate bromocriptine. The optimal dose of bromocriptine was 7.5 – 40 mg, and the dose of levodopa was 1 – 4.5 gm. Seven patients had greater benefit from bromocriptine and 11 from levodopa; the difference was not significant for total disability scores. Symptom subscores also did not differ significantly. Bromocriptine caused severe nausea and vomiting in only 1 patient. Two withdrew because of colicky abdominal pain. Four had occasional hallucinations, nightmares and confusion, and 2 of them had brief episodes of severely disturbed behavior. Three patients had blurred vision while receiving bromocriptine. Two had abnormal limb movements. One patient had "on-off" attacks on bromocriptine. One patient became dysarthric after the first dose.

Bromocriptine has therapeutic effects comparable to those of levodopa in most patients with idiopathic Parkinson's disease. Side effects are similar except for more intestinal complaints and the occurrence of severely disturbed behavior with bromocriptine. There are individual variations in response to each drug. If levodopa therapy is associated with intolerable or dose-limiting side effects, bromocriptine may produce greater benefit.

▶ [Side effects occur more frequently with the use of bromocriptine than when levodopa is administered. The side effects are similar, but both intestinal and behavioral side effects develop more often in patients taking bromocriptine, and the latter may be quite severe. Bromocriptine, however, may be used effectively in many patients who have intolerable or dose-limiting side effects when using levodopa. – Ed.] ◀

Interaction between Bromocriptine and Levodopa: Biochemical Basis for an Improved Treatment for Parkinsonism. Side effects of levodopa and the possibility of a further reduction of brain serotonin levels in parkinsonism have encouraged the study of other drugs, including bromocriptine, which has a dopamine-mimetic action in inhibiting prolactin secretion. Cheryl S. Hutt, Stuart R. Snider and Stanley Fahn[2] (Columbia Univ.) studied the effects

(2) Neurology (Minneap.) 27:505 – 510, June, 1977.

of bromocriptine on brain monoamine metabolism and its interaction with levodopa in male Sprague-Dawley rats. Some rats received 5 mg bromocriptine per kg in 5% ethanol intraperitoneally 4 hours before they were killed. Others also received 250 mg levodopa per kg, with or without 25 mg carbidopa per kg, 1 or 2 hours before they were killed. Control rats received an intraperitoneal injection of 5% ethanol or 1% methylcellulose or both.

All levodopa-treated rats showed signs of sympathetic stimulation. Motor activity was slightly less in rats given bromocriptine plus levodopa. Bromocriptine led to a relative increase in whole brain 5-hydroxytryptamine (5-HT) levels and a decrease in 5-hydroxyindoleacetic acid (5-HIAA) values. A slight increase in γ-aminobutyric acid was also found. Tryptophan was unaltered. Levodopa, with or without carbidopa, led to 5-HT depletion at 1 or 2 hours, with no significant increase in endogenous 5-HIAA. When bromocriptine was also given, 5-HT levels shifted toward normal and the brain level of 5-HIAA increased. Whole brain dopa and dopamine levels increased more when carbidopa was given with levodopa. Brain dopamine was slightly reduced at 1 hour with bromocriptine-levodopa treatment. Epinephrine was detectable in the blood of these rats, but there was no significant change in brain norepinephrine. Combination treatment led to a slight increase in brain homovanillic acid levels relative to levodopa at 1 hour.

Concurrent bromocriptine and levodopa therapy may produce beneficial biochemical changes in brain during treatment of parkinsonism. The reduction in 5-HT from levodopa tends to be normalized, and the duration of action of dopamine and 5-HT is probably prolonged. The motor deficit may be further reduced by this combination, and the side effects of levodopa that are due to 5-HT deficiency may be decreased.

► [Results suggest that bromocriptine may not only improve the motor disorder of Parkinson's disease but also reduce some side effects of levodopa therapy such as depression, which could be due to serotonin depletion. — Ed.] ◄

Treatment of Parkinson's Disease with Lergotrile Mesylate. Bromocriptine and lergotrile both stimulate dopamine receptors directly and effectively reduce serum prolactin levels. Abraham Lieberman, Eli Estey, Mark Kupersmith, Govindan Gopinathan and Menek Goldstein[3] (New York Univ.) evaluated high doses of lergotrile in 20 patients with advanced Parkinson's disease who had become increasingly disabled on levodopa-carbidopa therapy. All 13 men and 7 women had previously received these drugs and had initially responded. Seven had also received bromocriptine but had had abnormal involuntary movements. All had such movements at the start of the trial, and 17 showed an on-off effect. None was demented. Lergotrile was begun in a dose of 5 mg and increased by 5 or 10 mg weekly until an optimal effect was obtained, adverse effects occurred or a dose of 150 mg daily was reached.

The group as a whole had significant reductions in rigidity, tremor, bradykinesia, gait disturbance and abnormal involuntary movements. Improvement usually occurred within 1–2 months of the start of treatment with over 20 mg lergotrile mesylate daily. Levodopa-carbidopa therapy usually had to be reduced at this dosage. Eleven patients were considered to be responders; their mean daily dose of lergotrile was 59 mg. The on-off effect was greatly reduced in these cases. In only 2 cases did levodopa have to be completely replaced with lergotrile. Three other patients improved to a lesser degree, whereas 6 did not respond. The results were corroborated by a double-blind crossover trial in 10 patients. Involuntary movements were reduced in 10 cases and increased in 3 on lergotrile therapy. Mental changes appeared in 6 patients, 4 of whom had had similar changes on levodopa-carbidopa therapy. The changes resolved when the dose of lergotrile was reduced or the drug discontinued. Six patients had symptomatic orthostatic hypotension, but only 1 was withdrawn from therapy. Persistent elevations in liver enzymes in 3 patients resolved when drug therapy was stopped. The daily dose of lergotrile in nonresponders was 38 mg.

Ergot alkaloids promise to be an important new class of antiparkinsonian drugs. The significance of the elevated transaminase levels is not clear. At present, lergotrile should be discontinued when such elevations last for over 2 months.

▶ [The finding that some drugs that inhibit prolactin secretion have the

(3) J.A.M.A. 238:2380–2382, Nov. 28, 1977.

ability to stimulate dopamine receptors (dopamine agonists) was an important one in the development of antiparkinson drugs. Both bromocriptine, a peptide-containing ergot alkaloid derivative, and lergotrile, a synthetic nonpeptide ergot derivative, stimulate dopamine receptors directly and are effective in relieving parkinsonian symptoms. – Ed.] ◀

Huntington's Disease: Clinical and Chemical Effects of Choline Administration. Brain levels of choline acetyltransferase are reduced in the corpora striata of patients with Huntington's disease which suggests impaired acetylcholine synthesis. John H. Growdon, Edith L. Cohen and Richard J. Wurtman[4] (Massachusetts Inst. of Technology) administered oral doses of choline over extended periods to 10 patients with Huntington's disease to test the efficacy of raising brain acetylcholine levels. All patients had a family history of Huntington's disease consistent with autosomal dominant transmission. Choline was given in a dose of 1 – 2 gm 4 times daily and the dose was increased every 2 days, to a maximum of 2 – 5 gm 4 times daily. Five patients received physostigmine after an oral dose of propantheline was given to block the effects of peripheral cholinergic activation.

Maximal oral dose of choline increased the mean serum choline level from 13.6 to 39.7 nmol/ml and the mean cerebrospinal fluid level from 1.8 to 3.1 nmol/ml. The choline was well tolerated, although a fishy body odor developed. No patient showed suppression of signs of Huntington's disease. Four patients who reduced the dose of haloperidol or discontinued it showed abrupt increases in symptoms and signs within 2 weeks. The original level of disability returned when choline was stopped and the original dose of haloperidol reinstituted. Physostigmine did not relieve any features of Huntington's disease in the 5 patients evaluated.

Oral choline increases the amount of acetylcholine precursor delivered to the brain but, although some of the present patients showed transient improvement in speech, balance and gait, choline treatment failed to lead to consistent or lasting improvement in any subject.

▶ [The choline levels in the blood and cerebrospinal fluid increased markedly during the study, affirming that oral choline administration does increase the amount of acetylcholine precursor delivered to the brain. There was not, however, evidence of lasting improvement in any of the

(4)   Ann. Neurol. 1:418 – 422, May, 1977.

patients. Oral choline administration is without value in the treatment of Huntington's chorea. — Ed.] ◄

Valproate Sodium in Huntington's Chorea. The brains of patients with Huntington's chorea show substantial reductions of γ-aminobutyric acid (GABA) and glutamic acid decarboxylase, its synthesizing enzyme. Deficiency of GABA may explain the release of involuntary movements such as chorea. Iris Pearce, Kenneth W. G. Heathfield and John M. S. Pearce[5] report results of an open trial of valproate sodium in 14 patients. Valproate elevates brain GABA levels by inhibiting the transaminating enzyme in animals. Ten patients on other drugs were observed for 9 – 30 months, whereas 4 given no other drug were followed for 3 – 6 months. The latter patients received a high-dose regimen for a short time, whereas the others received a lower dosage for a longer time.

No otherwise untreated patient showed significant improvement in chorea, other neurologic signs, affect, memory or behavior. No adults on other medication improved, but transient amelioration was noted in 2 juvenile patients, 1 of whom subsequently relapsed. Chorea increased over a 2-year period in 3 otherwise treated patients. Dementia increased in 7 patients in this group and in 2 otherwise untreated patients.

There is little additive effect of valproate sodium in patients with Huntington's chorea treated with dopamine antagonists. The maximal dose of valproate in man may be insufficient to increase basal ganglia GABA levels enough to inhibit chorea, or the inhibitory action of GABA may be relatively unimportant at the level of the basal ganglia. Alternately, the lack of both glutemic acid decarboxylase and GABA in Huntington's chorea may imply a basic defect in synthesis, making blockade of a degradative enzyme ineffective.

► [The brains of patients with Huntington's chorea have been shown to have substantial reductions of γ-aminobutyric acid and its synthesizing enzyme, glutamic acid decarboxylase. Because γ-aminobutyric acid is essentially inhibitory, its deficiency may explain the release of involuntary movements. Because valproate sodium elevates brain γ-aminobutyric acid in experimental animals by inhibition of its transaminating enzyme, it was tried in 14 patients with Huntington's chorea. The drug was not effective.

(5) Arch. Neurol. 34:308 – 309, May, 1977.

T. L. Perry and S. Hansen (N. Engl. J. Med. 297:840, 1977) found that isoniazid acted as an inhibitor of γ-aminobutyric acid aminotransferase, the first enzyme in the degradation pathway of γ-aminobutyric acid. In an extremely preliminary study, not controlled, they found that 5 of 6 patients with Huntington's chorea given large doses of isoniazid showed amelioration of symptoms. Other negative therapeutic studies include one using lithium (Vestergaard, P., Baastrup, P. C., and Peterson, H.: Acta Psychiatr. Scand. 56:183, 1977) and one using choline (Aquilonius, S-M., and Eckernas, S-A.: Neurology (Minneap.) 27:882, 1977). — Ed.] ◄

Familial Paroxysmal Dystonic Choreoathetosis and Its Differentiation from Related Syndromes. James W. Lance[6] (Univ. of New South Wales) describes four generations of a family in which 7 of 8 affected members had prolonged dystonic seizures, whereas 1 had attacks of paroxysmal choreoathetosis. The attacks lasted up to 4 hours, were precipitated by alcohol, emotion or fatigue and responded poorly to phenytoin and barbiturates. They were controlled by clonazepam. Autopsy of an affected child who died a "crib death" at age 2 showed no major brain abnormality.

Man, 56, had his first episode of muscle spasm shortly after he began walking. Attacks recurred every few months in childhood and have continued throughout adult life, increasing to one every 2d day when he is working particularly hard. Clenching of the fingers of one hand is followed by elbow flexion and flexion of the foot, knee and hip. The episodes last from 5 to 50 minutes. The voice is slurred and the patient becomes completely mute, but can see, hear and move his eyes. His mind remains clear. He cannot cough or swallow, but can urinate normally during an attack. Recently the attacks have become milder, and writhing movements of the limbs have been noted. The attacks occur during relaxation after a state of tension, excitement or exhaustion, especially if alcohol is taken. Examination, skull radiography and an EEG were negative.

This family appears to have the same condition as that described by Mount and Reback in 1940, Forssman in 1961 and Richards and Barnett in 1968, which the last authors termed "paroxysmal dystonic choreoathetosis." Analysis of reports of 100 cases of paroxysmal kinesigenic choreoathetosis indicates that the attacks last less than 5 minutes, are precipitated by sudden movement or startle and usually respond well to phenytoin or barbiturates. Most workers have considered paroxysmal kinesigenic choreoathetosis a

---

(6) Ann. Neurol. 2:285–293, October, 1977.

form of reflex epilepsy involving the thalamus and basal ganglia. Presumably any disturbance of cortical control of the neostriatum and its thalamic connections can induce paroxysmal choreoathetosis either transiently as an epileptiform phenomenon or prolonged as in paroxysmal dystonic choreoathetosis. The present family has an intermediate form of the disorder.

► [This interesting syndrome is to be differentiated from paroxysmal kinesigenic choreoathetosis in which the attacks are briefer (less than 5 minutes), are precipitated by sudden movement and respond to phenobarbital or phenytoin. The longer attacks of paroxysmal dystonic choreoathetosis are precipitated by alcohol, emotion or fatigue and respond poorly to phenytoin but are controlled by clonazepam. — Ed.] ◄

Headache and Head Pain

Clinical Link between Migraine and Cluster Headaches. Most workers believe that both cluster and migraine headaches are vascular in origin, but are not in agreement as to whether cluster headaches are a variant of migraine. Jose L. Medina (Loyola Univ.) and Seymour Diamond[7] (Chicago Med. School) report data on 7 patients whose headaches presented features common to both cephalalgias and who are thought to represent a clinical link between the disorders. Five patients had cluster headaches. These were preceded by migrainous scotomas in 2 patients and contralateral weakness in 1 and were accompanied by ipsilateral photopsias in 1 and contralateral paresthesias in 1. Two patients had "clusters" of daily common migraine headaches separated by long free intervals.

Contralateral sensory and motor symptoms commonly precede or accompany migraine. Cluster headaches typically occur in groups for several weeks, followed by long free periods, but this pattern is not pathognomonic for them. The present cases point to a common root for both cluster and migraine headaches. Pathophysiologic and biochemical studies have not conclusively shown a difference between cluster and migraine headaches; clinical symptoms provide the basis for classifying these conditions. Manifestations considered almost pathognomonic for migraine have also occurred with cluster headaches, and the grouping of headaches characteristic of clusters occurs with migraine.

▶ [The clinical course in these 7 patients suggests that it may not always be possible to distinguish between migraine and cluster headaches. They may represent clinical variations of the same underlying process.—Ed.]

Cluster Headache Syndrome and Migraine: Ophthalmologic Support for a Two-Entity Theory. The question of whether cluster headache is a separate clinical entity or a migraine variant has been controversial. I. Hørven and O.

---

(7) Arch. Neurol. 34:470–472, August, 1977.

Sjaastad[8] (Rikshosp., Oslo) evaluated 18 patients with typical cluster headache, 6 with atypical cluster headache and 22 with migraine. The group with typical cluster headache included 15 men and 3 women with an average age of 53.5 years. The group with migraine included 13 female and 9 male patients with an average age of 36.6 years. Thirteen had classic and 9 had common migraine. Four had bilateral headache. Dynamic tonometry was carried out during and between attacks, and corneal temperature was registered with a special thermometer probe.

A significant increase in intraocular pressure occurred on the symptomatic side during attacks of cluster headache, and a similar trend was found in the group with atypical cluster headache. No change in intraocular pressure occurred in the migraine patients. No change in corneal indentation pulse amplitudes was observed during migraine attacks. Amplitudes of sizes similar to those seen in migraine were found in the interparoxysmal period in patients with ordinary cluster headache. Patients with atypical cluster headache had corneal indentation pulse amplitudes about twice as large as those in patients with ordinary cluster headache. Slight bradycardia was found in most patients with either type of cluster headache, whereas pulse rate was increased in classic migraine. A significant side difference in pulse-synchronous change in intraocular volume was found in both cluster headache groups but not in the migraine group. Corneal temperature rose during attacks of cluster headache.

The findings indicate major differences between migraine and cluster headache patients and support the concept that migraine and cluster headache are different pathologic states. These disorders should be classified and studied separately, not lumped together as "vascular headache."

► [The point is stressed that migraine and cluster headache probably represent different pathogenetic entities and should be classed as such and not grouped together within an ill-defined group of vascular headaches. — Ed.] ◄

Potentiation and Antagonism of Serotonin Effects on Intracranial and Extracranial Vessels: Possible Implications in Migraine. Serotonin (5-HT) is thought to play

(8)   Acta Ophthalmol. (Kbh.) 55:35–51, February, 1977.

an important role in the pathogenesis of migraine attacks. J. E. Hardebo, L. Edvinsson, Ch. Owman and N.-Aa. Svendgaard[9] (Univ. of Lund) undertook to characterize the interaction of drugs with 5-HT antagonistic properties with the vasomotor action of 5-HT on isolated cranial vessels from cat and man. Studies were done on vessels from 20 adult cats and on material from 12 patients taken at neurosurgery. Segments of pial arteries were taken from normal parts of resected temporal and frontal lobes, and superficial temporal artery branches were also sampled. The effects of 5-HT and 5-HT antagonists on resting vessels were examined.

A contraction resulted from 5-HT application to the organ bath. Methysergide, pizotifen and cyproheptadine did not induce vascular contractions, but ergotamine and dihydroergotamine produced contractile responses, which developed rather slowly, in both types of artery. Methysergide in increasing doses produced a shift of the dose-response curve of the 5-HT-induced contraction in the extracranial arteries. Pizotifen, cyproheptadine, ergotamine and dihydroergotamine reduced the 5-HT-induced contraction of intracranial and extracranial vascular segments. Norepinephrine, histamine and potassium chloride induced dose-dependent contractile effects in intracranial and extracranial vessels.

Serotonin antagonists impair serotonin-induced contractions of intracranial and extracranial vessels. In minute doses they potentiate the contraction produced by serotonin. There is reason to believe that the mechanism responsible for this interaction is selective for tryptaminergic agents. This dual action of serotonin antagonists may contribute to a beneficial effect in migraine by interference in both the vasoconstrictor and vasodilatory phases.

► [This dual action of the serotonin antagonists may contribute to a beneficial effect in migraine by an interference during both the vasoconstriction and vasodilation phases. — Ed.] ◄

(9) Neurology (Minneap.) 28:64–70, January, 1978.

Infections of the Nervous System

Progressive Rubella Virus Panencephalitis: Synthesis of Oligoclonal Virus-Specific IgG Antibodies and Homogeneous Free Light Chains in the Central Nervous System. A chronic rubella virus infection causing progressive encephalitis in children in the 2d decade of life was recently described. Bodvar Vandvik, Marvin L. Weil, Monica Grandien and Erling Norrby[1] report the occurrence of oligoclonal IgG and homogeneous free lambda light chains in the cerebrospinal fluid (CSF) of a patient with progressive rubella virus panencephalitis. Serums and lumbar CSF samples were obtained from the patient described by Weil et al. Samples from a patient with subacute sclerosing panencephalitis and a pool of normal serums were used as control material.

The patient's CSF had an abnormal γ-globulin pattern with a marked increase in the gamma fraction and several homogeneous gamma bands (Fig 23). Similar bands were found in the serum of the patient. A marked selective increase in CSF IgG was observed, with no detectable IgM and no increase in IgA. Two distinct bands of free lambda light chains migrated with the β_2-globulin fraction. The serum contained oligoclonal IgG without free light chains. The light chain characteristics of the serum IgG corresponded to those of the major bands of IgG in the CSF. Serum CSF ratios of rubella virus-specific antibodies were significantly reduced compared with ratios of other types of antibodies. Antibody activity to theta antigen was present in both CSF and serum.

Oligoclonal virus-specific IgG antibodies occurred predominantly in the CSF in this case of progressive rubella encephalitis. The findings are consistent with local antibody synthesis within the central nervous system. Different populations of oligoclonal IgG appear to be associated with anti-

---

(1) Acta Neurol. Scand. 57:53–64, January, 1978.

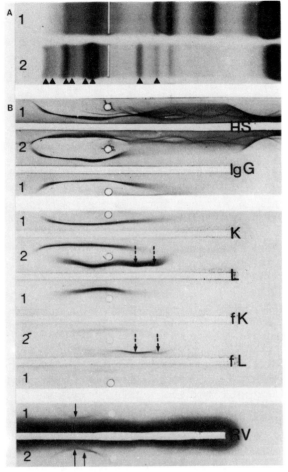

Fig 23.— **A,** agarose electrophoresis of serum (*1*) and concentrated CSF (*2*) from a patient with progressive rubella virus panencephalitis. Arrowheads indicate abnormal proteins of the β- and γ-globulin fractions. The serum and CSF samples were adjusted to IgG of approximately 5 mg/ml before being examined. Electrophoresis was carried out for 45 minutes. **B,** immunoelectrophoresis of the same samples carried out under conditions identical to the agarose electrophoresis. The troughs were filled with antiserums to human serum *(HS),* IgG, IgA, IgM, free and bound kappa *(K)* and lambda *(L)* light chains, free kappa *(fK)* and lambda *(fL)* light chains and with Brij-extracted rubella virus *(RV)* antigen. Broken arrows indicate positions of free lambda light chain bands. Unbroken arrows show gel-precipitating rubella antibody. (Courtesy of Vandvik, B., et al.: Acta Neurol. Scand. 57:53–64, January, 1978.)

body specifications to different antigenic components of the virus. Whether the serum oligoclonal antibodies are synthesized outside the central nervous system or represent antibodies resorbed from the CSF or central nervous system in unclear.

► [There have been recent reports of instances in children of a chronic progressive encephalitis due to rubella virus infection (Townsend, J. J., et al.: N. Engl. J. Med. 292:990, 1975; and Weil, M. L., et al.: ibid., p. 994). Study of these patients showed them to be extremely similar clinically to patients with subacute sclerosing panencephalitis, which is associated with measles virus infection. In this disorder, local synthesis of oligoclonal IgG virus-specific antibodies in the central nervous system is a prominent feature. In this study it is reported that there is oligoclonal IgG present in the cerebrospinal fluid and serum in patients with rubella virus panencephalitis and that this oligoclonal IgG represents rubella virus-specific antibodies. These same investigators have also reported similar findings in mumps meningitis and chronic meningoencephalitis (Vandvik, B., et al.: Eur. Neurol. 17:13, 1978; and Vandvik, B., and Nordal, H.: ibid., p. 23). — Ed.] ◄

Recommendations for National Policy on Poliomyelitis Vaccination are presented by Elena O. Nightingale[2] (Washington, D. C.). Public health officials are concerned that the troubled swine influenza vaccination program of 1976 may encourage the tendency of Americans to disregard preventive measures. Serious questions have arisen regarding the present policy that advocates the use of live attenuated oral poliovirus vaccine (OPV) to the virtual exclusion of killed, or inactivated, vaccine (IPV). The estimated risk of paralytic poliomyelitis is 1 case in a recipient for every 20 million doses of OPV distributed and 1 case in a contact for every 6 million doses of OPV distributed, or about 1 case in a recipient for every 11.5 million persons vaccinated with OPV. Both OPV and inactivated vaccine are remarkably safe vaccines.

The continued use of OPV as the principal vaccine is recommended at present, with provision of inactivated vaccine for persons relatively susceptible to infection, including immunodeficient children and their siblings, immune-suppressed persons and adults who are having an initial vaccination and then traveling to areas with a high rate of disease. This policy option should eventually reduce or eliminate cases among parents and other household contacts of

(2) N. Engl. J. Med. 297:249–253, Aug. 4, 1977.

persons given OPV. It also allows some choice for the public and for the provider. It is considered imprudent to select any other option until at least 90% of the population are adequately immunized. Informed-consent forms for poliomyelitis vaccination should be made as brief as possible. Education programs are needed to encourage vaccination for poliomyelitis.

▶ [Only about 60 – 70% of the people in the United States have been vaccinated against poliomyelitis. Until about 90% are vaccinated, this study advocates live virus vaccines be administered to infants with provision that certain categories of persons receive killed virus vaccine. Vaccination with an attenuated live virus for children aged 11 – 12 years is suggested in order to reduce vaccine-associated disease when they become parents of vaccinated infants. — Ed.] ◀

Adenine Arabinoside Therapy of Biopsy-Proved Herpes Simplex Encephalitis: National Institute of Allergy and Infectious Diseases Collaborative Antiviral Study. Encephalitis due to herpes simplex virus is considered the most common cause of sporadic fatal encephalitis in the United States. Richard J. Whitley, Seng-jaw Soong, Raphael Dolin, George J. Galasso, Lawrence T. Ch'ien, Charles A. Alford and the Collaborative Study Group[3] evaluated adenine arabinoside in the treatment of herpes simplex encephalitis in patients who had had a brain biopsy. Adenine arabinoside or placebo were given intravenously, the former in a dose of 15 mg/kg daily over 12 hours, in a concentration not exceeding 0.7 mg/ml. Biopsy-positive patients received either drug or placebo for 10 days, whereas biopsy-negative patients were treated for 5 days.

Twenty-nine of 50 patients in the study received the drug, and 21, placebo. Eighteen of 28 patients who had had a brain biopsy received the drug. Adenine arabinoside significantly reduced mortality from proved herpes simplex encephalitis from 70 to 28%, and the difference was greater when the data were adjusted for increased severity. The death rate in biopsy-negative cases was not significantly altered. The results are shown in Figure 24. Four survivors recovered completely, and another had only minor impairments. The prognosis depended on treatment and on the level of consciousness at the time of treatment. The treatments groups were comparable in most respects. All brain isolates were herpes

(3) N. Engl. J. Med. 297:289 – 294, Aug. 11, 1977.

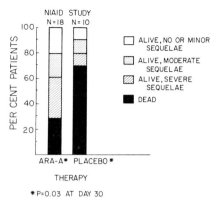

Fig 24. – Morbidity and mortality in biopsy-proved herpes simplex encephalitis. (Courtesy of Whitley, R. J., et al.: N. Engl. J. Med. 297:289–294, Aug. 11, 1977.)

simplex type 1. Adverse clinical drug reactions did not occur, and no serious adverse effects on the bone marrow, liver or kidneys were noted. No treated patients had absolute granulocytopenia, and only 4 were leukopenic. Two had thrombocytopenia alone. These changes did not lead to clinically significant sequelae.

Adenine arabinoside represents a major breakthrough in systemic antiviral therapy. It is hoped that more precise definition of its action on viral replication at the molecular level will lead to the development of even more specific and potent chemotherapeutic agents. The daily dose of adenine arabinoside should not be increased at present.

► [Whereas this drug is of value in the treatment of type I herpes simplex encephalitis, it must be given early in the course of infection, before the advent of coma, if it is to have a beneficial effect. Moreover, it should be coupled with brain biopsy for specific diagnosis to avoid unnecessary treatment of nonresponsive encephalitides that can mimic herpes simplex. – Ed.] ◄

Persistent and Fatal Central Nervous System Echovirus Infections in Patients with Agammaglobulinemia. Catherine M. Wilfert, Rebecca H. Buckley, T. Mohanakumar, John F. Griffith, Samuel L. Katz, John K. Whisnant, Peyton A. Eggleston, Marcie Moore, Edward Treadwell, Michael N. Oxman and Fred S. Rosen[4] observed persistent

(4) N. Engl. J. Med. 296:1485–1489, June 30, 1977.

echovirus infection of the central nervous system, defined as the continued presence of isolatable virus in cerebrospinal fluid (CSF), in 5 agammaglobulinemic patients. Three similar cases have previously been reported.

The immunologic defect was characterized by absence of B lymphocytes and of lymph node cortical follicles but normal T cell function. The echoviruses 30, 19, 9 and 33 were recovered from CSF for periods of 2 months to 3 years. The patients had few signs of acute central nervous system infection. Three had a dermatomyositis-like syndrome, with peripheral lymphocytes that reacted with anti-human leukemia-specific primate and rabbit serums in a cytotoxicity assay. Interferon levels in the CSF in 1 patient were in the range reported for patients with viral meningitis.

The persistent central nervous system echovirus infections seen in these patients with absent peripheral immunoglobulin-bearing lymphocytes strongly suggest that intact B cell function is essential for termination of enterovirus infection of the central nervous system. Infection with enteroviruses is potentially hazardous to these patients, and every effort should be made to prevent contact with and prohibit administration of attenuated poliovirus vaccines to these children. This precaution applies to those with severe humoral immunodeficiency as well as to those with deficits in cell-mediated immunity.

► [These data suggest that intact B cell function is essential for eradication of echovirus infection of the central nervous system. – Ed.] ◄

Saint Louis Encephalitis: The 1975 Epidemic in Mississippi was reviewed by Kenneth E. Powell and Durward L. Blakey[5] (Jackson, Miss). In 1975, 229 documented cases of St. Louis encephalitis, 36 of them fatal, occurred in Mississippi. Persons with documented cases were contacted 6 and 10 months after the epidemic. A total of 132 patients (58%) had encephalitis, 15% had aseptic meningitis, 21% had had a febrile illness with no reported central nervous system abnormality and 6% had other or unreported syndromes. Most patients with documented cases were febrile. A triad of lymphocytic pleocytosis and elevated cerebrospinal fluid protein and normal glucose concentrations was common in documented cases. Pleocytosis generally was not

(5) J.A.M.A. 237:2294–2298, May 23, 1977.

severe. Hemagglutination inhibition antibody appeared early in the course and peaked at about 3 weeks. The rates of inability to work or resume routine activities were 20% at 6 months and 9% at 10 months.

The attack rate, case-fatality ratio, proportion of patients with encephalitis and proportion with residual defects increased substantially with age. Attack rates did not differ by sex. Blacks had a significantly greater attack rate than whites (16.5 vs. 6.5 per 100,000). The epidemic spanned the period June through October (Fig 25).

Fig 25. – Epidemic of Saint Louis encephalitis in Mississippi, 1975. Cases given by date of onset of symptoms. (Courtesy of Powell, K. E., and Blakey, D. L.: J.A.M.A. 237:2294 – 2298, May 23, 1977; copyright 1977, American Medical Association.)

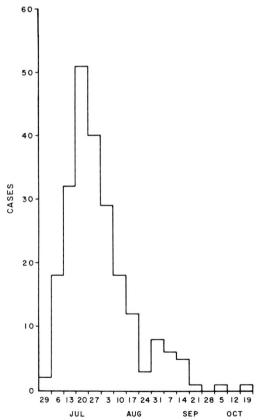

The most useful immediately available laboratory test is examination of the cerebrospinal fluid. The higher attack rate observed in blacks in comparison with whites is presumably related to blacks' increased exposure to infected mosquitoes. Although virus activity varies in poorly understood meteorological patterns and with other unknown factors, epidemics of St. Louis encephalitis can be reduced in magnitude or prevented by mosquito control. During a known epidemic, space spraying of an appropriate insecticide with ground or aerial equipment promptly reduces the density of adult mosquitoes and presumably the number of human infections, but sporadic cases continue.

▶ [It is of interest that the epidemic erupted almost simultaneously, with variable intensity, in widely separated areas. Mosquito control appears to stop the spread of the disease, but the results of such measures could not be quantified. — Ed.] ◀

Neonatal Meningitis: The Ventricle as a Bacterial Reservoir. Meningitis in the neonate is a formidable challenge despite apparently appropriate parenteral antibiotic therapy. Plexitis or ventriculitis is frequent in neonatal meningitis. Floyd H. Gilles, Juan L. Jammes and William Berenberg[6] (Harvard Med. School) evaluated the potential role of bacterial exudate in and around the choroid plexuses in the pathogenesis and evolution of neonatal meningitis. Data were reviewed on 25 infants under age 1 month at the onset who died before week 5 of meningitis in 1962–71. Those with a direct cutaneous-leptomeningeal communication were excluded. The prosencephalic choroid plexuses of the lateral and 3d ventricles were examined for purulent exudate, necrotic debris and bacteria. The neonates had gestational ages of 28–40 weeks; half were mature. Postnatal ages were 2–30 days.

The most common organisms isolated were *Escherichia coli*, β-hemolytic streptococci and *Klebsiella* species. Plexitis (Fig 26) was present in 21 of the 25 cases. The amount of cellular exudate, fibrin and plexus necrosis varied considerably from 1 case to another. In several cases the ventricular exudate was organized into layers. Bacteria were sometimes demonstrated within and outside the plexus, with or without an inflammatory infiltrate in the plexus. Four cases ex-

(6) Arch. Neurol. 34:560–562, September, 1977.

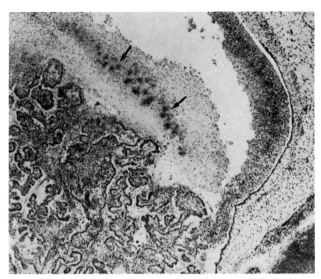

Fig 26.—Choroid plexus is in lower left corner. Plexus stroma is filled with cellular exudate. In many sites, plexus epithelium has been eroded. Lateral ventricle contains mass of protein-rich cellular exudate and necrotic debris organized into layers. Middle layer (*arrows*) is composed of colonies of bacteria. Hematoxylin-eosin; reduced from ×60. (Courtesy of Gilles, F. H., et al.: Arch. Neurol. 34:560–562, September, 1977; copyright 1977, American Medical Association.)

hibited no involvement of the supratentorial choroid plexus. The ventricles were enlarged in several cases and collapsed in several others. Collapse was often associated with a patchy, widespread necrosis of the brain.

A purulent exudate in the meninges has been associated with an exudate in or around the choroid plexuses of the lateral ventricles in neonatal meningitis. Possibly the glycogen-rich choroid plexus of the lateral ventricles not only facilitates local bacterial growth, but also acts as a bacterial reservoir relatively resistant to antimicrobial agents. More drastic approaches than parenteral antibiotic therapy may be indicated to reduce the morbidity and mortality of neonatal meningitis. Ventricular lavage or direct intraventricular instillation of antibiotics should be reconsidered in this setting.

▶[More drastic approaches than parenteral antimicrobial therapy may be indicated to reduce further morbidity and mortality of neonatal meningitis. — Ed.] ◀

Danger of Accidental Person-to-Person Transmission of Creutzfeldt-Jakob Disease by Surgery.

Duffy et al. reported the first case of transmission of Creutzfeldt-Jakob disease (CJD) from man to man by corneal transplantation. C. Bernoulli, J. Siegfried, G. Baumgartner, F. Regli, T. Rabinowicz, D. C. Gajdusek and C. J. Gibbs, Jr.[7] report the cases of 2 patients who developed CJD about 2½ years after stereotactic EEG exploration, in which silver electrodes were used that had been previously implanted in a patient with proved CJD. The patients underwent excision of epileptic foci. The electrodes had been sterilized with 70% alcohol and formaldehyde vapor. The patients were aged 17 and 23 years, respectively. The source of contamination was a woman, aged 69, in whom the electrodes had been in place for 2 days. Her father had died after a rapidly progressive dementia. One of the 2 patients died and had preliminary autopsy findings characteristic of CJD.

Presumably these 2 patients were infected from electrodes contaminated by implantation in a CJD patient. The resistance of the CJD virus to 70% alcohol and formaldehyde was not clear at the time of the studies. Subsequently the electrodes were implanted in the frontal cortex of a young chimpanzee, and brain and spleen from the patient who died were inoculated into squirrel monkeys, capuchin monkeys and African green monkeys. These transmission studies will take at least a year.

► [Considering the ages of the patients (17 and 23 years, respectively), the rarity of this disease, the known possibility of transmission and the current knowledge that routine sterilization with alcohol and formaldehyde is inadequate for the inactivation of the Creutzfeldt-Jakob disease virus, surgical inoculation seems probable. — Ed.] ◄

Precautions in Medical Care of, and in Handling Materials from, Patients with Transmissible Virus Dementia (Creutzfeldt-Jakob Disease)

are outlined by D. Carleton Gajdusek, Clarence J. Gibbs, Jr., David M. Asher, Paul Brown, Arwin Diwan, Paul Hoffman, George Nemo, Robert Rohwer and Lon White[8] (Natl. Inst. of Health). Creutzfeldt-Jakob disease is a progressive, fatal disease of the central nervous system, affecting patients of both sexes in middle life. There is growing concern among medical and

(7) Lancet 1:478–479, Feb. 26, 1977.
(8) N. Engl. J. Med. 297:1253–1258, Dec. 8, 1977.

laboratory personnel about the potential hazard involved in caring for patients with presenile dementia and handling their tissues. The disease occurs throughout the world. Patients who have brain or eye operations may be iatrogenically infected. The natural modes of transmission of the agent of the disease are unknown. The virus has been found in nodes, liver, kidney, spleen, lung, cornea and cerebrospinal fluid as well as the brain and spinal cord. Several species of nonhuman primates are susceptible by various routes of inoculation.

A patient's blood or cerebrospinal fluid should be considered a potential source of infection. No special ward isolation procedures are warranted. Needle electrodes should be discarded or autoclaved, as should lumbar puncture needles. Tonometers used on demented patients should be decontaminated. Dentists should use the same precautions now used for known carriers of chronic hepatitis when treating confused or demented adults. Blood and tissues should not be taken from patients for clinical use. At surgery, all tissues must be considered potentially hazardous. The pathologist must also be concerned and should consider all tissues fully infectious, even after prolonged fixation in formalin and histologic processing. Morticians and mortuary workers should be warned of the hazards. Clinical laboratories must take care in handling blood and cerebrospinal fluid specimens.

▶ [The growing concern on the part of both medical and paramedical personnel about the infectiousness of Creutzfeldt-Jakob disease, and probably other dementias, has resulted in a need for more information and for advice about the necessary precautions. Doctor Gajdusek and his associates are the best possible source for answers to the many questions. It is comforting to know that although precautions are necessary, the epidemiologic evidence does not suggest that there is an unusual risk from patients with this disease. The precautions and procedures outlined seem reasonable and not excessive. – Ed.] ◄

Multiple Sclerosis

In Vitro Cell-Mediated Immunity of Cerebrospinal Fluid Lymphocytes to Myelin Basic Protein in Primary Demyelinating Diseases. Many workers believe that a cell-mediated immune response to central nervous system myelin components is a major pathogenic mechanism in multiple sclerosis, but efforts to demonstrate immune reactivity to neural antigens in lymphocytes of multiple sclerosis patients have given inconsistent results. Robert P. Lisak and Burton Zweiman[9] (Univ. of Pennsylvania), with the technical assistance of Kathie Manthorne and Marilyn Ludwick, compared the myelin-basic-protein-induced in vitro responses of cerebrospinal fluid lymphocytes to those of peripheral blood lymphocytes in 5 patients with clinically definite multiple sclerosis in acute exacerbation, 5 with progressive signs but no sudden change, 9 without signs of clinical activity for 2 months or longer, 6 with acute disseminated encephalomyelitis, 9 with other central nervous system diseases and 14 normal subjects (controls).

Basic protein-stimulated reactivity was significantly greater in the blood lymphocytes of patients with acute disseminated encephalomyelitis and progressive multiple sclerosis than in those of the normal subjects. The increase in progressive multiple sclerosis was due to an extremely high level in only 1 of 5 patients. Basic-protein-stimulated uptake by cerebrospinal fluid lymphocytes was significantly greater in the groups with acute disseminated encephalomyelitis, acute multiple sclerosis and progressive multiple sclerosis than in the groups with stable multiple sclerosis and other nervous system disease. The cerebrospinal fluid lymphocyte response to basic protein was greater than that in blood lymphocytes in the groups with acute and progressive multiple sclerosis but not in the group with acute disseminated encephalomyelitis.

---

(9) N. Engl. J. Med. 297:850–853, Oct. 20, 1977.

These findings suggest compartmentalized lymphocyte reactivity within the neuraxis in acute multiple sclerosis. The pathogenic implications of this are uncertain. The absence of such a response in stable multiple sclerosis rules against it as an immune marker in that disorder independent of a clinical expression of disease. It remains unclear whether cerebrospinal fluid lymphocyte immune reactivity to basic protein is pathogenic or a result of the demyelinating process.

▶ [These findings demonstrate that lymphocytic cells reactive to myelin basic protein are present in the cerebrospinal fluid during active demyelinating disease. These cells may be more reactive than peripheral blood lymphocytes. — Ed.] ◄

Antimyelin Antibody in Multiple Sclerosis: No Change during Immunosuppression. Azathioprine has failed to alter significantly the course of multiple sclerosis. In several diseases associated with anti-tissue antibodies, immunosuppression has depressed such antibody. L. D. Wilkerson, R. P. Lisak, B. Zweiman and D. H. Silberberg[1] (Univ. of Pennsylvania, Philadelphia) studied retrospectively the pattern of antimyelin antibody during treatment in the azathioprine-treated patients described by Silberberg et al. in 1973. Serums were taken before, during and after a trial of 2–4.5 mg azathioprine per kg daily from 13 patients who had multiple sclerosis. All patients but 1 completed at least 6 months of treatment. An average of 6 determinations of antimyelin antibody and serum IgG per patient were made.

The group mean titer of antimyelin antibody at various treatment intervals did not differ significantly from the pretreatment mean. The mean titer just before cessation of therapy did not differ significantly from that found 2 months later. Antimyelin antibody titers and isohemagglutinin titers were not related. Antibody titers tended to be elevated during times of increased disease activity in all patients but 2. The mean pretreatment serum IgG was 14.7 gm/l. No significant change was noted during treatment, and no consistent pattern was seen in individual patients. Serum IgG levels and antimyelin antibody titers were not correlated. In individual patients, sequential values of serum IgG often varied in the direction opposite to any change in antimyelin antibody titer.

(1)   J. Neurol. Neurosurg. Psychiatry 40:872–875, September, 1977.

Azathioprine therapy was not associated with significant changes in antimyelin antibody titers in this study, in apparent contrast to collagen vascular disease associated with anti-tissue antibody. No significant changes in levels of serum immunoglobulins were recorded.

▶ [In these patients with multiple sclerosis the administration of an immunosuppressive agent daily over a period of 6 months caused no significant change in antimyelin antibody titers, serum levels of immunoglobulins or the clinical status of the patients. This should discourage the widespread use of immunosuppressive agents in the treatment of this disease. – Ed.] ◀

Direct Leukocyte Migration Inhibition by Myelin Basic Protein in Exacerbations of Multiple Sclerosis. Delayed or cell-mediated hypersensitivity to central nervous system antigens has long been considered a pathogenetic factor in episodes of multiple sclerosis. William Sheremata, H. Triller, J. B. R. Cosgrove and E. H. Eylar[2] attempted to develop an easily reproducible means of measuring leukocyte migration using central nervous system antigen in order to evaluate clinical exacerbations of multiple sclerosis. Except for stroke patients, control subjects were matched for age and sex with 9 multiple sclerosis patients seen within 3 weeks of exacerbation and 16 seen 1–6 months after onset. Ten patients with stroke, 10 with Guillain-Barré syndrome and 13 normal subjects were also studied. The mean age of multiple sclerosis patients was 30 years. Human myelin basic protein was used as antigen in the leukocyte migration inhibition factor assay.

The multiple sclerosis group had a mean migration index of 88%, compared with a lower limit of normal of 86%. The mean migration index was 68% in the 1st week after onset, 73% in the 2d week and 90% in the 3d. The mean migration index of patients seen 1–6 months after an episode was 93%. Patients with Guillain-Barré syndrome had a mean migration index of 103% and the stroke patients, 107%. Six of 9 multiple sclerosis patients seen within 3 weeks of an exacerbation and 5 of 16 seen after 106 months had significant results.

If leukocyte migration inhibition factor is the factor that is elaborated before episodes of multiple sclerosis, this assay might be useful in anticipating attacks and in evaluating

(2) Can. Med. Assoc. J. 116:985–988, May 7, 1977.

therapeutic measures for preventing attacks. The present preliminary findings provide further evidence that cellular hypersensitization to a potent encephalitogenic agent is present during exacerbations of multiple sclerosis and suggest that it may, in combination with other unrecognized factors, be of pathogenetic significance.

► [These observations strengthen evidence that sensitization to this potent encephalitogenic agent occurs simultaneously with exacerbations of clinical disease. — Ed.] ◄

Antibodies to Oligodendroglia in Patients with Multiple Sclerosis. Several lines of evidence point to a possible role for autoimmunity in the pathogenesis of multiple sclerosis but it has not been definitely established as an autoimmune disease. Oded Abramsky, Robert P. Lisak, Donald H. Silberberg and David E. Pleasure[3] (Univ. of Pennsylvania), with the technical assistance of Joan George, used an indirect immunofluorescence technique to examine the possibility that antibodies against oligodendroglia are present in patients with multiple sclerosis. Serums were taken from 21 patients with clinically definite multiple sclerosis, 49 with other neurologic diseases and 14 normal subjects. Ten study patients had acute multiple sclerosis, 7 were stable and 4 had a chronic progressive course. Oligodendrocytes from calf cerebral white matter were used in the indirect immunofluorescence assay.

Serums of 19 patients with multiple sclerosis reacted with the surface membrane of isolated oligodendrocytes after they were absorbed with beef liver. One serum reacted equivocally. Positive responses were found in 3 of 5 patients with subacute sclerosing panencephalitis and 1 of 4 with acute disseminated encephalomyelitis. Serums from 14 multiple sclerosis patients reacted with the surface of oligodendroglial cells in sections of bovine white matter. One serum from a patient with subacute sclerosing panencephalitis reacted similarly. Binding of serums from multiple sclerosis patients to oligodendrocytes in suspension and in brain slices was prevented by prior absorption with either isolated oligodendrocytes or whole white matter. Pretreatment of isolated cells or brain sections with rabbit antioligoden-

(3) N. Engl. J. Med. 297:1207–1211, Dec. 1, 1977.

drocyte serum almost completely blocked the binding of positive human serums to oligodendroglia.

Antibodies to oligodendroglia were found in the serums of all but 2 patients with multiple sclerosis in this study, in various stages of the disease. The presence of these antibodies appears not to be simply a nonspecific result of oligodendrocyte destruction in central nervous system disease. Antibody-mediated damage to oligodendroglial cells may be important in the pathogenesis of multiple sclerosis.

▶ [These findings suggest that antibodies to oligodendroglia are distinct from the antibodies to myelin and that demyelination in multiple sclerosis could be a consequence of an immunopathologic reaction directed against oligodendroglia cells. — Ed.] ◀

Immunoglobulin-Containing Cells in Multiple Sclerosis Plaques. Immunoglobulin production in the central nervous system in multiple sclerosis (MS) appears to be abnormal, but the abnormality does not correlate with the clinical state. It is not clear whether the abnormality is a cause or a result of the disease. Margaret M. Esiri[4] (Radcliffe Infirm., Oxford) examined MS plaques by an immunoperoxidase technique to demonstrate immunoglobulin-containing cells. Autopsy material was obtained from 10 cases of MS. Sections of formalin-fixed, paraffin-embedded material from the brain and spinal cord were used. One hundred areas of normally myelinated (nonplaque) tissue were also examined. Examination was made of 33 recent, 32 moderately recent and 35 old plaques.

Areas of plaque contained significantly more Ig-containing cells than areas of nonplaque when cells stained for either light or heavy chains were compared. The largest number of immunoglobulin-containing cells was found in recent plaques; much smaller numbers were present in old plaques. All three plaque groups differed significantly from nonplaque tissue. Within plaques, 90% of cells containing heavy chains showed IgG. In normally myelinated tissue, 95% of cells with heavy chains contained IgG. More cells in plaques contained light chains than heavy chains; the difference was most striking for recent plaques. The chi-lambda ratio was significantly increased in moderately recent and recent

(4)   Lancet 2:478–480, Sept. 3, 1977.

plaques; in most recent plaques, more cells contained chi light chains than lambda light chains.

Each plaque in MS may be associated with local proliferation of a clone or small number of clones of immunoglobulin-producing cells, producing mainly IgG heavy chains with chi light chains, and occasionally with lambda light chains. The presence of immunoglobulin-containing cells appears to be closely associated with demyelination. There appears to be a local antigenic stimulus present within plaques. Further study of a larger number of plaques by this technique may help elucidate the pathogenesis of MS.

▶ [This study serves to confirm the theory earlier proposed by Tourtellotte that the immunoglobulin in the cerebrospinal fluid of patients with multiple sclerosis is manufactured in the plaques. — Ed.] ◀

Evaluation of Central Nervous System Vaccinia Antibody Synthesis in Multiple Sclerosis Patients. Workers have questioned whether elevated cerebrospinal fluid (CSF) viral antibody titers in some patients with multiple sclerosis (MS) are a result of antibody synthesis within the central nervous system or merely a leak in the blood-brain barrier. Joel A. Thompson, Lowell A. Glasgow and Patrick F. Bray[5] (Univ. of Utah) sought to determine whether elevated CSF vaccinia antibody titers reflect antibody synthesis within the central nervous system. Thirteen male and 7 female MS patients, with a mean age of 31.9 years, were studied, with 26 patients who had non-MS neurologic diseases and 28 normal controls. All had been vaccinated with vaccinia virus. A complement-dependent neutralization assay was used to measure antibody in serum and CSF specimens.

Mean serum antibody titers did not differ significantly in the three groups, but levels were elevated in the CSF of 60% of MS patients, compared with 7.7% of the other neurologic patients and 7.1% of the normal subjects. Nine MS patients showed a reduced serum-CSF vaccinia antibody ratio with no coincident reduction of the ratio for poliovirus I, suggesting central nervous system synthesis of vaccinia antibody. Only 1 normal subject had a reduced serum-CSF vaccinia antibody ratio, and the poliovirus I ratio was also reduced in this subject. Both ratio reductions in the neuro-

(5) Neurology (Minneap.) 27:227–229, March, 1977.

logic control group could be explained by leakage in the blood-brain barrier. The magnitude of CSF vaccinia antibody titers was unrelated to CSF IgG levels, duration of MS or clinical phase of the disease.

Viral antigens may play an important role, but the pathogenesis of MS is still obscure. A lacunar defect in cell-mediated immunity to certain viral antigens has been proposed, as has impairment of certain cell-mediated immune responses to specific viral agents by serum inhibitors.

► [It appears that vaccinial virus antigens may play an important role, either directly or indirectly, in the pathogenesis of multiple sclerosis. — Ed.] ◄

Evoked Potentials, Saccadic Velocities and Computerized Tomography in Diagnosis of Multiple Sclerosis. The diagnosis of multiple sclerosis (MS) may be difficult to establish in patients who present with neurologic dysfunction referable to only one central nervous system site and in those with atypical presentations or few neurologic signs. F. L. Mastaglia, J. L. Black. L. A. Cala and D. W. K. Collins[6] assessed the value of measuring visual and somatosensory evoked potentials and saccadic eye movement velocities and of computerized axial tomography (CAT) of the cranium and orbits in 102 unselected patients with clinically definite, probable or suspected MS. The 72 women and 30 men were aged 19–62 years. Mean durations of disease were 8.6 years in definite, 4.4 years in probable and 11.4 months in suspected cases. Visual evoked potentials generated by pattern reversal were recorded, and somatosensory evoked potentials were recorded from electrodes over C2 and over the hand area of the contralateral sensory cortex during median nerve stimulation. Computerized electro-oculography was carried out. A CAT study of the cranium was done in 62 patients, and the orbits were also studied in 36.

The visual evoked potential was abnormal in 80% of definite, 43% of probable or latent and 22% of suspected cases. The cervical somatosensory evoked potential was abnormal in 71%, 54% and 30% of cases, respectively, and the cortical potential in 50%, 40% and 18%. Saccadic velocities were abnormal in 64% of definite, 40% of probable and 33% of suspected cases. The CAT scan detected areas of reduced

(6) Br. Med. J. 1:1315–1317, May 21, 1977.

attenuation coefficients in the hemispheric white matter or in the cerebellum and brainstem in 61% of definite, 52% of probable or latent and 14% of suspected cases. Abnormalities in the optic nerves were identified in 11 cases. The rate of abnormalities was higher in patients studied by more than one technique, ranging up to 100% of patients with definite MS who had most of the studies.

These techniques are complementary and permit establishment of a more certain diagnosis of MS.

► [A large group of patients with suspected or established multiple sclerosis was studied by means of four ancillary techniques. Each of them proved to be valuable in detecting abnormalities, some of which were subclinical in many patients. These techniques have a complementary role in investigating suspected multiple sclerosis. — Ed.] ◄

Familial Multiple Sclerosis: Clinical, Histocompatibility and Viral Serologic Studies. Recently several workers have suggested that a gene predisposing to multiple sclerosis (MS) is located on chromosome 6 in the histocompatibility complex region. Roswell Eldridge, Henry McFarland, John Sever, Doris Sadowsky and Helen Krebs[7] (Natl. Inst. of Health) evaluated this suggestion in families with clinically well-defined cases of MS by analysis of the HLA A, B and D loci and viral antibody levels. Twenty-one affected members of 7 families included 12 clinically definite and 7 probable cases of MS. Seven of the original 14 presumptive MS families were eliminated when MS was not confirmed in a second close relative.

No segregation of HLA type was found between affected and unaffected subjects in the 7 families with confirmed MS. No consistent segregation was found in 28 other families described in the literature. The 7 families contained ten sibships in which there was useful genetic information for sibs and parents. The DW2 antigen was increased in frequency among affected members of the families, and the A3 B7 haplotype was more frequent in affected members of other families on which information has been reported. Unaffected members, however, also tended to have an increased frequency of these antigens. No relationship was found between HLA type and antimeasles antibody titers in the families studied.

The findings support other genetic evidence that there is

(7) Ann. Neurol. 3:72–80, January, 1978.

not a single, major gene mapping in the HLA complex that predisposes to MS. The response to measles, as measured by antibody level, is apparently not a critical genetically determined factor within the multifactorial process leading to MS. Identification of such a genetic factor may have to await demonstration of the antigenic stimulus leading to MS.

► [The response to measles, as measured by the antibody level, apparently is not a critical genetically determined factor within the multifactorial process that leads to multiple sclerosis. It may be that such a factor will not be identified until the antigenic stimulus leading to multiple sclerosis is demonstrated. — Ed.] ◄

Peripheral Nerve Abnormality in Multiple Sclerosis. Martin Pollock, Christopher Calder and Stephen Allpress[8] (Univ. of Otago, Dunedin, New Zealand) examined peripheral nerve biopsy specimens quantitatively from 10 minimally disabled patients with definite multiple sclerosis (MS). Fascicular sural nerve biopsy specimens were taken, and 100 single teased fibers were obtained from each nerve. Teased fiber internode lengths were measured, and photographs of transverse sections were used to estimate the number and diameter histogram of myelinated fibers. Only 1 patient had severe functional disability. Four were able to carry out normal activities without help. Conduction velocities and action potential amplitudes were normal except in 2 patients who had carpal tunnel syndrome. Six control sural nerves were also examined.

Abnormal teased fibers were found in 8 MS patients. The most common abnormality was that of internodes with at least a 50% reduction in myelin thickness. Four patients had thinly myelinated internodes associated with demyelinated internodes. Acute axon degeneration and excessively irregular myelin were infrequent findings. In 6 patients projections of myelin extended to overhang adjacent thinly myelinated internodes. There was no consistent increase in the percentage of abnormal fibers with longer histories of disease. Section of single fibers showed reduced myelin lamellae along thinly myelinated internodes and increased internode length of small MS fibers. The distribution of diameters of myelinated fibers was normal. Prominent collagen pockets and platelike processes of Schwann cells devoid of axons (Fig 27) were seen in MS nerves. Many fibers

(8)   Ann. Neurol. 2:41–48, July, 1977.

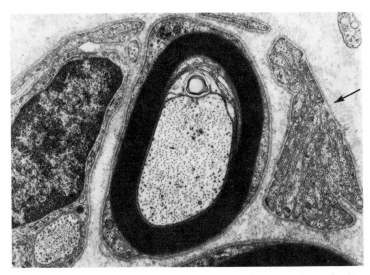

Fig 27.—Transverse section of sural nerve from MS patient shows platelike processes of Schwann cells devoid of axons (*arrow*). Myelinated nerve fiber has 36 myelin lamellae and axon area of 0.94 sq μ; reduced from ×26,400. (Courtesy of Pollock, M., et al.: Ann. Neurol. 2:41–48, July, 1977.)

appeared on electron micrographs to have reduced numbers of myelin lamellae. No onion bulb formations or abnormalities of axon organelles were observed.

Increased nerve fiber abnormalities were found in most MS patients in this study. The dominant finding was of sporadic internodes with reduced myelin thickness. It seems possible that a direct attack is made on both central and peripheral myelin in MS. A complement-dependent factor has been found in MS serum, which produces demyelination in vitro. Alternatively, peripheral myelin might be attacked indirectly in MS. Virus incorporation into oligodendrocytes and Schwann cells could alter surface antigenicity, and invaded cells might then be regarded as "nonself," leading to damaging allergic reactions. Schwann cell involvement in MS best explains the finding of multiple intercalated internodes.

▶ [Whereas it is quite generally stated that peripheral nerve involvement is not a part of multiple sclerosis, detailed history taking and neurologic examination may show evidence of such involvement in some patients.

This study demonstrates that peripheral myelin may be involved in this disease. — Ed.] ◄

Agarose Electrophoresis of Cerebrospinal Fluid in Multiple Sclerosis: Simplified Method for Demonstrating Cerebrospinal Fluid Oligoclonal Immunoglobulin Bands.

Oligoclonal bands of γ-globulins have been noted in the cerebrospinal fluid from patients with multiple sclerosis

Fig 28. — Agarose electrophoresis patterns for 3 patients: 1 with multiple sclerosis (*MS*), 1 a control with a primary brain tumor (*C*) and 1 with progressive rubella panencephalitis *(PRP)*. In each group, pattern *1* represents concentrated cerebrospinal fluid applied ×3 to the gel; pattern *2*, concentrated cerebrospinal fluid ×1; and pattern *3*, unconcentrated serum. Discrete oligoclonal bands of γ-globulins *(arrowheads)* have formed toward the cathode in cerebrospinal fluid from patients with MS and PRP. (Courtesy of Johnson, K. P., et al.: Neurology (Minneap.) 27: 273–277, March, 1977.)

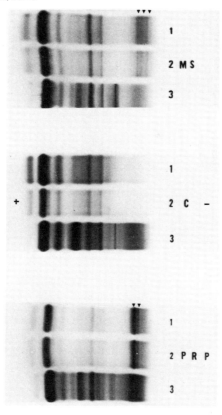

(MS) and other neurologic diseases. Kenneth P. Johnson, Sue Clear Arrigo, Barbara J. Nelson and Arthur Ginsberg[9] (San Francisco) describe a method of demonstrating oligoclonal bands in concentrated cerebrospinal fluid from patients with MS and other diseases by using easily obtained, well-standardized commercial reagents and apparatus.

Eight patients with definite and 8 with presumptive MS were studied, as were 3 with optic neuritis as the only sign of neurologic disease. Those with clinically definite disease had moderate disability. Seventeen patients with central nervous system disease other than MS were also evaluated. Five had persistent central nervous system inflammation.

The agarose electrophoretic patterns are shown in Figure 28. The γ-globulins of MS patients migrated as two to seven discrete populations, rather than as a broad homogeneous pattern without bands. The pattern of bands for each patient appeared to be unique but consistent. No common band was identified in all specimens. All 3 presumptive MS patients with elevated IgG levels exhibited oligoclonal bands. The 1 patient with optic neuritis and oligoclonal bands also had cerebrospinal fluid elevated IgG. Five control patients had oligoclonal bands; 2 had subacute sclerosing panencephalitis and 1 each had cryptococcic meningitis, treated central nervous system syphilis and progressive rubella panencephalitis. No patient with noninflammatory neurologic disorder had oligoclonal bands in the cerebrospinal fluid.

All patients with definite MS and most with presumptive MS in this study had oligoclonal bands in concentrated cerebrospinal fluid. The function of the discrete populations of γ-globulins demonstrated by oligoclonal banding is not known. It may become possible to analyze unconcentrated cerebrospinal fluid and to achieve further sensitivity in demonstrating oligoclonal bands.

▶ [Oligoclonal bands were seen in cerebrospinal fluid from all patients with clinically definite multiple sclerosis, even though some had normal cerebrospinal fluid γ-globulin levels, as well as in most patients with presumptive multiple sclerosis or other inflammatory conditions of the nervous system. — Ed.] ◀

Recovery of Paramyxovirus from Jejunum of Patients with Multiple Sclerosis (MS). Viral antigen, presumably measles virus, has been identified in epithelial and

(9) Neurology (Minneap.) 27:273–277, March, 1977.

lamina propria cells of the jejunum from patients with MS, but electron microscopy of the specimens failed to show viral particles. I. Prasad, J. D. Broome, L. P. Pertschuk, J. Gupta and A. W. Cook[1] (State Univ. of New York, Brooklyn) recovered paramyxovirus by co-cultivation or cell fusion techniques from jejunal biopsy specimens from 6 consecutive patients with MS, and identified the virus by immunofluorescence of antigen in infected HEp-2 and BSC-1 cells, by electron microscopy and by hemagglutination of rhesus monkey erythrocytes. Jejunal mucosal specimens were obtained by suction biopsy.

Frozen sections of all 6 specimens showed immune reactions and measles antigen in the lamina propria and the epithelium. Syncytium formation was not initially seen in fresh BSC-1 and HEp-2 cultures, but stronger infections

Fig 29.—Ultrastructure of viral particles in extracts of infected HEp-2 cells, showing outer viral envelope *(lower arrowhead)* and free nucleocapsids *(upper arrowhead)*; original magnification ×140,000. *Inset,* nucleocapsid fragment; original magnification ×320,000. (Courtesy of Prasad, I., et al.: Lancet 1:1117–1119, May 28, 1977.)

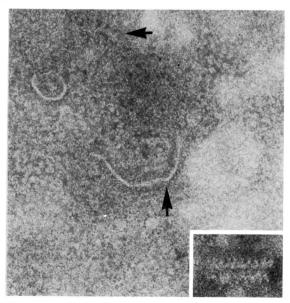

(1) Lancet 1:1117–1119, May 28, 1977.

were seen in all cases where cell fusion was induced by inactivated Sendai virus. A number of controls were used to insure that the immunofluorescence was not due to Sendai virus. Hemagglutination of rhesus monkey cells was produced by isolates from 3 of the 6 cases. In 2 cases this occurred in extracts of cells from the first passage, concentrated 10-fold. Electron microscopy showed a small number of virions 120–250 nm in diameter, and also free viral envelopes and fragmented nucleocapsids with a herringbone appearance (Fig 29). Other viral forms that resembled adenovirus and myxovirus were seen in much smaller numbers. Virus particles were not seen in cell extracts from HEp-2 cells exposed to inactivated Sendai virus by the fusion technique and cultured for 5 days.

Virus can be recovered relatively easily from the jejunum of patients with MS. The characteristics of the virus are those of a paramyxovirus. Antigenically, it appears to be measles. The relationship of the virus recovered to known measles viruses must be tested experimentally.

▶ [This report adds confirmation to a prior one by the same authors in which viral antigen (presumably measles) was identified by immunofluorescence in epithelial and lamina propria cells of the jejunum in 24 patients with multiple sclerosis. The reported findings have not, however, been confirmed by others, the specificity of the observations is open to some question and the relationship of the virus recovered to known measles virus has yet to be demonstrated. — Ed.] ◀

Jejunal Immunopathology in Amyotrophic Lateral Sclerosis and Multiple Sclerosis: Identification of Viral Antigens by Immunofluorescence. Measles virus antigen has been identified in jejunum of patients with multiple sclerosis (MS). L. P. Pertschuk, A. W. Cook, J. K. Gupta, J. D. Broome, J. C. Vuletin, D. S. Kim, D. J. Brigati, E. A. Rainford and F. Nidsgorski[2] (State Univ. of New York, Brooklyn) report the presence of an immunologic reaction in the jejunal mucosa of 7 patients with amyotrophic lateral sclerosis (ALS) and the identification by immunofluorescence of various viral antigens in 5 patients. Seven patients with ALS and 20 with MS were studied, as were 3 patients who had other neurologic diseases and 5 who did not have neurologic disease. Jejunal mucosa was also obtained from 21 freshly resected surgical and 6 autopsy specimens

(2) Lancet 1:1119–1123, May 28, 1977.

from patients who did not have neurologic disease. Frozen studies were processed by both direct and indirect immunofluorescence techniques.

No electron microscopic abnormalities were observed. Immunoglobulin deposits were seen in the epithelial basement membrane in 5 cases of ALS. A great increase in cells labeled with IgG was apparent. Complement was seen in lamina propria cells in all 7 cases. The number of IgM-bearing cells was reduced in several cases of MS, and immunoglobulin deposits were seen on the epithelial basement membrane in 14 of 20 specimens. Complement components were detected in lamina propria cells in 8 cases of MS. Poliovirus antigen was identified in 4 cases of ALS and was seen in about 5% of the lamina propria cells. Measles virus antigen was identified in 1 case. One case of ALS exhibited herpesvirus hominis antigen in the jejunum. All MS patients had measles virus antigen in the jejunum. Other viral antigens occasionally observed included adenovirus, parainfluenza types 1 and 3, and mumps antigens.

The association of jejunal viral infections with chronic neurologic disease may represent a causative role of viral infection, or the infection may be a marker of abnormal host immune mechanisms. It is possible that virus is present elsewhere in the body or that jejunal virus produces toxic or antigen products that are fixed in and lead to damage of the nervous system tissues.

▶ [This study gives further support to the accumulating data that suggest that amyotrophic lateral sclerosis as well as multiple sclerosis may be either directly or immunologically related to prior viral infection. As is true of immunofluorescence studies by the same investigators on jejunal biopsies of patients with multiple sclerosis, this work has not been confirmed by other researchers and the specificity of the immunofluorescence studies is open to question. — Ed.] ◀

Anesthesia in Multiple Sclerosis. The anesthesiologist who provides care to multiple sclerosis (MS) patients should use agents known to have little effect on the course of the disease. C. Bamford, W. Sibley and J. Laguna[3] (Univ. of Arizona) questioned 100 patients with MS about their experiences with anesthesia. Forty-two reported 88 general anesthetics, and hospital records were available in 33 instances. Eight patients reported 12 episodes of spinal and caudal

(3) Can. J. Neurol. Sci. 5:41–44, February, 1978.

anesthesia. Ninety-eight patients reported receiving multiple local anesthetics. An association between anesthesia and worsening of MS was considered to be significant if deterioration began within a month after the anesthetic.

One patient reported an attack of MS in the month after general anesthesia and surgery. One reported deterioration of MS before a pelvic procedure, which continued postoperatively at an increased rate. No anesthetic complications were observed in the course of exposure to 47 general anesthetics in conventional dosages. One of 3 patients who had spinal anesthesia for delivery noticed deterioration of MS in the next month. One patient had fluctuations in MS symptoms with wound infection after spinal anesthesia for a minor procedure. Four patients reported deterioration of MS within a month after a single local anesthetic. They had no complications of local anesthesia on other occasions. Two of 46 patients for whom dental records were available had deterioration of MS in the month after exposure to anesthetics. These patients received more than 150 local anesthetics.

This study provided no evidence that general anesthesia precipitates relapses of MS or increases the rate of progress of disability. Temporary fluctuations in MS symptoms can follow surgery because of the effects of fever and metabolic imbalance on nerve transmission. Spinal anesthesia should probably be avoided in MS until its safety has been convincingly established. Local anesthesia is well tolerated by MS patients.

▶ [Patients with multiple sclerosis, and their surgeons, often ask about the risk of surgery and the choice of method of anesthesia. Many neurologists feel that intraspinal injections of any type should not be given to patients with this disease and that the risk of exacerbation is increased by general anesthetics. This study, although not an all-encompassing one, indicates that local anesthesia is probably the procedure of choice. — Ed.]

Multiple Sclerosis among Orientals and Caucasians in Hawaii: Reappraisal. Previous studies suggested that multiple sclerosis (MS) might affect Orientals and Caucasians differently, with lower rates in Orientals. A high rate of optic nerve involvement has been described in case studies from Asian countries. Hiroshi Shibasaki, Michael M. Okihiro and Yoshigoro Kuroiwa[4] compared MS in Orientals and Caucasians seen in the practice of a single neurolo-

(4) Neurology (Minneap.) 28:113–118, February, 1978.

gist in Honolulu in 1970 – 75. Diagnostic criteria were the same as those used in a survey in Japan. Forty probable and 14 possible cases of MS were reviewed. Thirty-two Caucasians and 20 Orientals were evaluated.

Two Oriental patients and no Caucasians had the Devic syndrome. Mean age at onset and sex distribution were comparable in the two racial groups. Over half the Oriental patients and 20% of the Caucasians had reduced visual acuity at the onset of MS. Bilateral visual impairment and bilateral optic atrophy were more common in Orientals, and acute transverse myelopathy was much more frequent in Orientals than in Caucasians. Ataxia was more common in Caucasians. Remissions and exacerbations were similar in the two groups. No significant difference in motor disability was found. More Caucasians than Orientals had cerebellar symptoms. Optic-spinal-brain stem and optic-spinal forms of MS were more frequent in the Oriental patients.

Certain clinical differences in MS were found between Orientals and Caucasians in Hawaii in this study. A careful clinical study of Oriental MS patients born in the West is warranted.

► [While there are many similarities between multiple sclerosis in Orientals and multiple sclerosis in Europeans and Americans, there are quite different clinical and pathologic characteristics, and it is still to be proved that they are the same disease. Furthermore, we know much more about the clinical and pathologic findings of multiple sclerosis in the Japanese than we do in other Orientals, and perhaps it would be more accurate to consider only the Japanese in this study. – Ed.] ◄

Possible Association between House Pets and Multiple Sclerosis. Stuart D. Cook and Peter C. Dowling[5] encountered 3 sisters in whom multiple sclerosis (MS) developed in the same year and who lived together with an aged family dog, which had an acute encephalopathy. A fourth sister, a nonidentical twin, had left home and had no neurologic symptoms. A retrospective case-control study was carried out to determine whether close exposure to cats or dogs was temporally related to subsequent MS. Thirty-eight families with at least 2 members who had MS were studied and 29 were evaluable. These had at least 1 member with advanced MS, and all but 4 had another household resident with definite MS. Controls had grown up in the same envi-

(5)   Lancet 1:980 – 982, May 7, 1977.

ronment as the patients. Large groups of other controls were also used.

All but 3 of 29 patients with MS owned small dogs, compared with 16 of 29 controls, a significant difference. Twenty-six patients with MS and 14 matched controls had small indoor dogs. Inclusion of cats increased the difference; all but 1 of the MS patients owned either a small indoor dog or a cat, compared with 16 controls. The MS patients were more likely to have had pets within 5 and 10 years before onset of neurologic symptoms. A significantly increased incidence of small dog ownership was found in the MS group, compared with the larger control groups.

A notably high frequency of small pet dogs or cats was found in the households of familial MS patients before onset of symptoms in this survey. The incidence of intimate house pet exposure in the few years before onset of initial MS symptoms was extremely high. These findings require cautious interpretation.

▶ [This report has already received excessive lay publicity. The observations may be pertinent and important ones, but it often disturbs the physician-patient relationship when information about observations such as these first appear in the lay press. — Ed.] ◄

Further Evidence of a Possible Association between House Dogs and Multiple Sclerosis. Recently a possible association between exposure to household pets, especially small house dogs, and subsequent familial multiple sclerosis was reported. Stuart D. Cook, Benjamin H. Natelson, Barry E. Levin, Pamela S. Chavis and Peter C. Dowling[6] determined whether a similar relationship could be found in sporadic cases of multiple sclerosis. The records of 61 patients with the disease were reviewed, and 45 were confirmed by history or examination. Control subjects were matched for age, sex and race and generally for socioeconomic background. Study patients had been symptomatic for 14 years at the time of study.

No difference in overall dog ownership or in dog size was noted, but more multiple sclerosis patients than controls owned indoor dogs, including small indoor dogs, in the 5-year period before the onset of symptoms. Analysis of the 10-year period before symptom onset showed no differences in

(6) Ann. Neurol. 3:141–143, February, 1978.

ownership of indoor dogs. Six dogs of study patients had neurologic signs within 5 years before the onset of multiple sclerosis in their owners, compared with only one dog in the control group, a significant difference. No differences in cat ownership were observed and no difference in bird ownership was found. There was no difference in reports of previous tonsillectomy.

Dogs appear to be the principal pet involved in the association between house pets and the subsequent development of multiple sclerosis. Distemper virus is known to cause neurologic illness in affected dogs and can cause periventricular demyelination similar to that of multiple sclerosis. Studies in several geographic areas are needed before the importance of the present epidemiologic data can be determined.

▶ [These authors believe that this study gives further support to their hypothesis that small dogs serve as an animal vector in multiple sclerosis. In an editorial in *Annals of Neurology*, Kurland and Brian (Ann. Neurol. 3: 97, 1978) point out possible sources of error in a retrospective study of this type, and other investigators, including Proskanzer, Penney and Sheridan (Lancet 2:1204, 1977) failed to confirm the work of Cook and his associates. For the present, a skeptical perspective must be maintained and judgment must be used in the evaluation of these findings. — Ed.] ◀

Myasthenia Gravis

Myasthenia Gravis. *—Part 1.*—Daniel B. Drachman[7]
(Johns Hopkins Univ.) notes that myasthenia gravis is a
neuromuscular disorder characterized by weakness and fa-
tigability of voluntary muscles and due to faulty neuromuscular transmission as a result of a reduction of available
acetocholine receptors at neuromuscular junctions (Fig 30).
Ultrastructural studies have supported the concept of a
postsynaptic abnormality in this disease. The possibility
that myasthenia is an autoimmune disease has been proposed. Antireceptor antibody has been identified by several
different methods. The roles of myasthenic immunoglobulin
action on receptor degradation, blockade and synthesis
remain to be determined. It is not clear whether the immune
mechanisms of autoimmune attack on the acetylcholine receptors are invariable, or differ in individual patients. The
origin of the autoimmune response is not clear.

Part 2.—Drachman[8] states that muscle weakness in myasthenia gravis results from failure of neuromuscular transmission at many junctions, due to a reduction in available
acetylcholine receptors. Neuromuscular fatigue is the most
characteristic single feature of myasthenia gravis. Because
of progressive failure at the neuromuscular junctions, muscular contractions cannot be sustained or repeated. The concept of a humoral immune mechanism is strongly supported
by the fact that most patients have positive serum antibody
tests.

Recently treatment aimed at reducing the amount of serum antibody by thoracic duct drainage has been successful
in a limited number of myasthenic patients. Anticholinesterase agents continue to be the first line of treatment for
most patients with myasthenia gravis. Pyridostigmine is
the most widely used oral anticholinesterase drug. The most
widely accepted indication for thymectomy is the presence of

(7) N. Engl. J. Med. 298:136–142, Jan. 19, 1978.
(8) Ibid., pp. 186–193, Jan. 26, 1978.

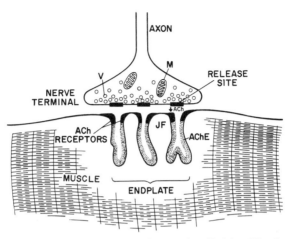

Fig 30. — Diagram of the neuromuscular junction. Vesicles *(V)* release their acetylcholine *(ACh)* contents at specialized release sites. After crossing the narrow synaptic space (path indicated by arrow), ACh reaches the ACh receptors, which are most densely situated at the peaks of the junctional folds *(JF)*. Acetylcholinesterase *(AChE)* in the clefts rapidly hydrolyzes the ACh. *M*, mitochondria. (Courtesy of Drachman, D. B.: N. Engl. J. Med. 298:136–142, Jan. 19, 1978.)

a thymoma. The prognostic implications of various factors such as age, sex, duration of disease and surgical technique involved are unclear. There is abundant evidence supporting the usefulness of adrenal corticosteroids in the treatment of myasthenia gravis. Steroid therapy may be considered whenever weakness is not satisfactorily controlled by anticholinesterase medication or thymectomy. Anticholinesterase medication is regulated as necessary during steroid therapy. The precise mechanism of action of steroids in myasthenia gravis has not been established. Immunosuppressive drugs have been used to some extent in myasthenic patients; the disadvantages of lowered resistance to infection and the risk of bone marrow depression limit their use.

► [This critical review article by a physician on the forefront of both research into and treatment of myasthenia gravis summarizes our current knowledge of the disease. — Ed.] ◄

Plasmapheresis and Immunosuppressive Drug Therapy in Myasthenia Gravis. Recent observations have strengthened the rationale for immunotherapy in myasthenia gravis. The results of thoracic duct drainage have suggested possible benefit from reducing serum antibody levels. Peter C. Dau, Jon M. Lindstrom, Christine K. Cassel, Eric H. Denys, Edward E. Shev and Lynn E. Spitler[9] (San Francisco) evaluated plasmapheresis and immunosuppressive drug therapy in 5 patients with symptoms of moderate to severe myasthenia gravis despite intensive conventional anticholinesterase drug therapy, prednisone therapy and thymectomy. The 4 women and 1 man were aged 29-56 years. Continuous-flow plasma exchange was carried out with an Aminco Celltrifuge to exchange 5% of the body weight of plasma with plasma substitutes. Patients received 60-100 mg prednisone, daily or on alternate days, and 2.5-3.5 mg azathioprine per kg daily from the 1st day of plasmapheresis.

All 5 patients improved remarkably during plasmapheresis. Four patients had major improvement after only 6 plasma exchanges. Peak clinical improvement has been maintained in each case, with immunosuppressive drug therapy either alone or with additional plasmaphereses at less frequent intervals. Mild hypoproteinemia developed during the plasma exchanges. An extremely steep fall in titers of antibody to acetylcholine receptor occurred during the first 3 plasmaphereses. γ-Globulin injections were given because of hypogammaglobulinemia that occurred during treatment. Three clinical relapses occurred during interruptions of plasmapheresis, each associated with a rise in titer of antibody to acetylcholine receptor.

Plasmapheresis combined with immunosuppressive drug therapy is effective in inducing rapid improvement in patients with myasthenia gravis who are resistant to thymectomy, prednisone therapy and optimal doses of drugs that facilitate neuromuscular transmission. Plasmapheresis might also be useful in myasthenic crisis, for improving respiratory function before thymectomy and to stabilize patients who worsen during the introduction of prednisone therapy. The present findings support participation of antibody to acetylcholine receptor in the pathophysiology of myasthenia gravis.

▶ [The results reported in this article suggest that plasmapheresis will find a place in the management of patients with myasthenia gravis. — Ed.]

(9) N. Engl. J. Med. 297:1134-1140, Nov. 24, 1977.

Function of Circulating Antibody to Acetylcholine Receptor in Myasthenia Gravis: Investigation by Plasma Exchange. Several lines of evidence point to a postsynaptic defect in myasthenia gravis. J. Newsom-Davis, A. J. Pinching, Angela Vincent and S. G. Wilson[1] (London) investigated the functional role of anti-acetylcholine receptor (anti-AChR) antibody in myasthenia gravis because of previous findings that plasma exchange, which reduces serum antibody levels, can cause a remission. Seven patients with acquired myasthenia gravis and increased anti-AChR antibody titers were studied, along with 1 having congenital myasthenia gravis whose anti-AChR titer was in the control range. Three patients had responded to plasma exchanges. Anticholinesterase medication was optimal throughout the study and all patients had had thymectomy. All but 1 were receiving prednisone; 3 patients also received cyclophosphamide. Up to nine daily plasma exchanges, usually of 2 L each, were undertaken for 10 – 12 days. Muscle extract was prepared from human calf muscle for assaying acetylcholine receptor and anti-AChR antibody.

Repeated plasma exchange led to a progressive fall in IgG and a parallel fall in anti-AChR antibody in the patients with acquired myasthenia gravis. All patients improved clinically after a minimum delay of 2 days. The delay between the initial fall in antibody titer and the earliest measured clinical improvement was 2 – 4 days. The anti-AChR antibody titers increased after completion of a series of exchanges, with a decline in clinical indices after a lag of 1 – 6 days. No clinical improvement occurred in the patient with congenital myasthenia gravis despite the usual decline in IgG during the period of exchange.

These results are consistent with the view that anti-AChR antibody is the principal factor interfering with neuromuscular transmission in acquired myasthenia gravis. Antibody levels may be a reliable index of disease activity in the individual patient and should provide an objective means of assessing the effectiveness of treatment of myasthenia gravis.

► [These findings are consistent with the view that anti-acetylcholine receptor antibody is the principal factor interfering with neuromuscular transmission in acquired myasthenia gravis. – Ed.] ◄

(1) Neurology (Minneap.) 28:266 – 272, March, 1978.

Rational Approach to Total Thymectomy in Treatment of Myasthenia Gravis. Alfred Jaretzki III, Morrison Bethea, Marianne Wolff, Marcelo R. Olarte, Robert E. Lovelace, Audrey S. Penn and Lewis Rowland[2] (Columbia Univ.) began performing total thymectomy in 1973 and operated on 22 patients with myasthenia gravis in 1973–76. Mean age was 29 years. Myasthenia gravis had been present for a mean of 2 years. All but 4 patients had moderate to severe generalized myasthenia gravis and were incapacitated in daily living and work. Three patients had mild generalized myasthenia gravis, and 1 had only ocular myasthenia. Most patients received anticholinesterase medication preoperatively, and 4 received steroids also. Four patients proved to have thymomas, 1 of which was malignant and had invaded the innominate vein. A cervical approach was used in 6 patients, 3 of whom required median sternotomy to complete the dissection. One partial median sternotomy was extended to obtain full exposure. Of 16 patients in whom complete median sternotomy was the primary approach, 9 required another cervical incision.

No deaths or phrenic nerve injuries occurred. Four patients who underwent median sternotomy required tracheostomy, 1 before and 3 after operation. The patients explored by median sternotomy were ventilated for an average of 6 days. No patient had evidence of hypoparathyroidism subsequently, though parathyroid tissue was removed from 5. Mean follow-up was 13 months. Three patients are in complete remission, 16 are improved and 3 are unchanged. Over 80% of patients had surgically significant variations in thymic anatomy in the neck, mediastinum or both. Ten patients had variations in the neck; 7 had abnormalities of the superior pole. Sixteen patients had notable variations in the mediastinum. Often these consisted of large volumes of thymic tissue and were multiple. Seventeen accessory lobes lay adjacent to or distant from the main lobes in 10 patients. Two patients had a microscopic focus of thymus in fat lying distant from gross thymic tissue.

The value of thymectomy in patients with myasthenia gravis appears to be established. Complete removal of all thymic tissue seems to be important. Wide exposure is nec-

(2) Ann. Thorac. Surg. 24:120–130, August, 1977.

essary, through a median sternotomy with an extended mediastinal dissection and a separate cervical incision and exploration. The increased morbidity is justified by the need for complete thymectomy.

▶ [The authors believe that wide exposure by means of median sternotomy with direct vision is required to remove all of the extracapsular thymus in many patients, and good cervical exposure is required to remove the anomalous tissue in the neck. — Ed.] ◀

Antimyasthenic Action of Corticosteroids. Recent reports have suggested that the beneficial effect of prednisone and related steroids in myasthenia gravis is a result of a direct pharmacologic action at the neuromuscular junction. William W. Hofmann[3] (Stanford Univ.) used the rat phrenic nerve-diaphragm preparation to evaluate the action of high concentrations of prednisolone (0.1 mM) on nerve backfiring, twitch tension, tetanus decay, various parameters of miniature end-plate potentials (MEPPs) and the number of transmitter units released in end-plate potentials (EPPs). Stimulation was with supramaximal pulses of 0.4 msec at frequencies of 0.5–200 Hz. Methylprednisolone sodium succinate was used in vitro and a sustained-release form of the compound for in vivo studies.

No repetitive activity was seen after steroid administration, and prednisolone usually reduced or abolished iterative firing when this was noted in the control state. Intramuscular methylprednisolone injections did not induce repetitive nerve firing. The time course and contraction strength of twitches were not increased in steroid-treated preparations, and tetanus decay was not greatly altered after steroid treatment in vivo. Maximum tetanus tension fell in proportion to the observed block in neuromuscular conduction. Studies of responses at single junctions showed no "veratrinic" action of prednisone. Inhibition of transmitter release in excess Mg^{2+} was not altered by exposure to prednisolone, but a slight rise in MEPP frequency was observed. Equilibration in prednisolone solution produced no evidence of decurarization after the induction of postsynaptic block.

The action of steroids in myasthenia cannot be said to be wholly or even substantially at the neuromuscular junction. It seems likely that prednisone and its congeners are of use

(3) Arch. Neurol. 34:356–360, June, 1977.

because they inhibit immune responses, but it rèmains to be determined whether the suppression affects thymus-modulated lymphocytes having a direct cytotoxic action at the end-plate or those synthesizing the circulating antireceptor antibody demonstrated in myasthenia gravis.

▶ [From the time that corticosteroids were first used in the therapy of myasthenia gravis, there has been controversy regarding both the value of and the rationale for their use. They may worsen the symptoms when first given, but seem to be extremely effective in some cases with prolonged use. This study shows that corticosteroids do not owe their therapeutic efficacy to action at the myoneural junction. The author concludes, therefore, that the clinical benefits from steroids are related to their systemic action and suggests that this action is due to their immunosuppressive effects. – Ed.] ◀

Effective Treatment of Infantile Myasthenia Gravis by Combined Prednisone and Thymectomy. Experience with thymectomy in children with myasthenia gravis is much more limited than that in adults. Harvey B. Sarnat, John D. McGarry and J. Eugene Lewis, Jr.[4] (St. Louis Univ.) describe 2 children in whom myasthenia gravis developed at ages 2 and 3 years, respectively, and in whom thymectomy, preceded by a 3-month course of prednisone, was followed by dramatic improvement.

CASE 1. – Boy, aged 2 years, had ptosis and impaired ocular movements. Improvement after prolonged treatment with cholinesterase inhibitors was minimal. There was no apparent involvement of limb muscles, but quadriceps biopsy showed lymphorrhages. A 3-month course of prednisone, 2 mg/kg on alternate days, was followed by thymectomy. Ptosis improved within a few days after operation and ocular movements were normal after 2 months. Prednisone was discontinued 7 months after operation. The child is in complete remission on prednisone and neostigmine therapy at age 3½ years.

CASE 2. – Girl, aged 3 years, with progressive generalized myasthenia, received prednisone and underwent thymectomy and was well 8 months postoperatively, except for minimal ptosis and mild eye muscle weakness. She is much more responsive to neostigmine than before thymectomy; prednisone has been discontinued.

Thymectomy is an effective treatment of myasthenia gravis in young children but should be reserved for children with progressive disease who do not respond satisfactorily to cholinesterase inhibitors. A short course of prednisone is

(4) Neurology (Minneap.) 27:550–553, June, 1977.

recommended before operation. A good response to steroids may allow thymectomy to be deferred until it may be better tolerated immunologically. A small maintenance dosage of prednisone may be needed for several months after thymectomy. Patients who undergo incomplete remission are more responsive to cholinesterase inhibitors after thymectomy.

▶ [The natural course of myasthenia gravis in children treated only with anticholinesterase drug therapy is usually protracted and unpredictable. Experience with thymectomy in young children is quite limited and the effectiveness of this procedure in infancy and early childhood is incompletely known. For that reason, this report is an important one. – Ed.] ◀

Malabsorption of Pyridostigmine in Patients with Myasthenia Gravis. Increasing drug requirements are often noted in myasthenic patients who are receiving oral anticholinesterase agents. Some patients become refractory to increasing doses and may even have a "cholinergic crisis," in which increasing doses result in worsening muscle weakness, including respiratory distress. Stanley L. Cohan, Kenneth L. Dretchen and Angela Neal[5] (Georgetown Univ.) studied 4 patients with myasthenia gravis who had less than satisfactory responses to oral pyridostigmine therapy. Pyridostigmine concentrations were measured by gas chromatographic and cholinesterase inhibition methods. Patients received 2 mg pyridostigmine intravenously, and venous blood was sampled at 1-minute intervals for 15 minutes. Four nonmyasthenic subjects and 9 patients with myasthenia gravis who responded well to pyridostigmine were also studied.

All myasthenia patients with unsatisfactory control had markedly lower serum pyridostigmine levels than those of control subjects and well-controlled myasthenic patients (Fig 31). One patient with gastrointestinal hypermotility had levels comparable with those of control and pyridostigmine-responsive subjects after receiving atropine intramuscularly and pyridostigmine orally; motor strength also improved transiently. Atropine was ineffective in 2 other patients. Serum drug levels and rates of disappearance after intravenous pyridostigmine were comparable in study and control subjects. All patients had improved muscle strength for up to 1 hour after pyridostigmine was administered intravenously.

(5)   Neurology (Minneap.) 27:299 – 301, March, 1977.

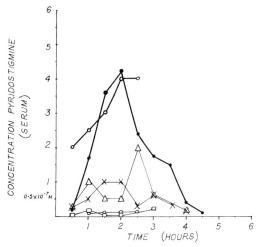

Fig 31.—Serum concentration of pyridostigmine after oral administration. *Solid circles*, 13 controls who each received 60 mg every 6 hours. *Open circles*, patient who received 105 mg every 4 hours before and after coadministration of 0.4 mg atropine intramuscularly. *Triangles*, patient who received 180 mg every 6 hours. *Squares*, patient who received 200 mg every 3 hours. (Courtesy of Cohan, S. L., et al.: Neurology (Minneap.) 27:299–301, March, 1977.)

Reduced absorption of oral anticholinesterase drugs by the gastrointestinal tract is an apparent additional cause of increased dose requirements in some patients with myasthenia gravis. Serum drug measurements are useful in determining the cause of poor clinical response in some myasthenic patients who are receiving pyridostigmine. Malabsorption may result from a drug-induced change in the gastrointestinal epithelia, either by induction of esterases that degrade the drug or because the drug damages the epithelium. Similar absorption problems might obtain for neostigmine. If adequate blood drug levels are not achieved, anticholinesterases should probably be abandoned in favor of another treatment, such as alternate-day steroid therapy.

► [This study demonstrates that failure to achieve adequate serum pyridostigmine levels in myasthenia gravis patients after oral administration is due to malabsorption rather than to increased rates of tissue uptake, degradation or excretion of the drug.—Ed.] ◄

New Myasthenic Syndrome with End-Plate Acetylcholinesterase Deficiency, Small Nerve Terminals and Reduced Acetylcholine Release. In myasthenia gravis the defect in neuromuscular transmission is associated with lack of postsynaptic acetylcholine receptor sites. In the Lambert-Eaton myasthenic syndrome, the quantum content of end-plate potentials is abnormally small at low frequencies of stimulation. Andrew G. Engel, Edward H. Lambert and Manuel R. Gomez[6] (Mayo Clinic and Found.) describe a third type of neuromuscular transmission defect in a patient whose symptoms began soon after birth.

Hindu boy, 16 (Fig 32), had eyelid ptosis at age 5 days, which temporarily disappeared after he slept. Prostigmin tests were negative. He walked alone at age 3 years, when lordosis was evident.

Fig 32. – Patient at age 16 years. Note ptosis, facial and cervical muscle weakness, reduced muscle bulk and scoliosis. (Courtesy of Engel, A. G., et al.: Ann. Neurol. 1:315–330, April, 1977.)

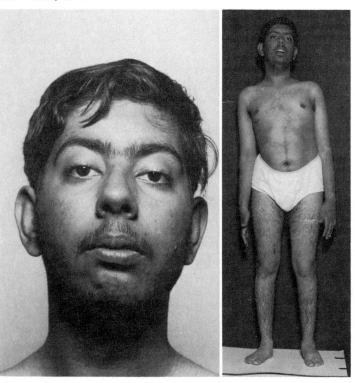

Generalized weakness was worsened by exertion. Treatment with pyridostigmine had no clinical effect. At age 11 he had an episode of respiratory failure with a common cold. At age 14 there was weakness of all external ocular muscles and of facial, cervical, trunk and limb muscles, greater proximally than distally in the extremities. Muscle tone was reduced and tendon reflexes were decreased. Two siblings were well. Electromyography showed a repetitive muscle action potential like that seen with excessive anticholinesterase medication, but the patient was taking no drugs. Moderate postactivation facilitation was followed by slight postactivation exhaustion. A Tensilon test did not alter the transmission defect. Treatment with guanidine was ineffective, but prednisone therapy was associated with subjective improvement. No change in the transmission defect was seen on electromyography.

In vitro microelectrode studies were carried out on intercostal muscle. The miniature end-plate potentials were of normal amplitude but reduced frequency and their duration and half-decay time were prolonged. The quantum content of the end-plate potentials was decreased due to a reduced store of quanta immediately available for release, but the probability of release was normal. A threefold or fourfold reduction in nerve terminal size and a reduction in postsynaptic membrane density were seen on electron microscopic study. The postsynaptic folds were focally degenerated, and many were distended by labyrinthine membranous networks that communicated with the synaptic space. Degenerating nuclei were found in the junctional sarcoplasm. Acetylcholinesterase (AChE) was absent from the motor endplates. Biochemical studies showed total absence of the endplate-specific 16S species of AChE and a marked reduction in total-muscle AChE.

The basic abnormality in this condition may be a congenital defect in the molecular assembly of AChE or in its attachment to the postsynaptic membrane. Further studies of the disorder might shed light on trophic interactions between nerve and muscle and the biologic significance of the different molecular forms of AChE.

► [This is a most interesting case report. Doctor Lambert and his associates are describing another myasthenic syndrome. It seems that a congenital defect in the molecular assembly of acetylcholinesterase or in its attachment to the postsynaptic membrane might represent the basic abnormality and determine the morphological and physiologic alterations. — Ed.] ◄

Myopathies

Muscular Dystrophy: Some Recent Developments in Research are reviewed by John N. Walton[7] (Univ. of Newcastle). Duchenne-type muscular dystrophy is a disease with a high mutation rate, which explains the frequent occurrence of isolated cases in families with no past history of the disease. Occasional female carriers of the gene have been found to exhibit minimal clinical abnormalities such as muscle weakness. Genetic counseling programs have proliferated in the past decade, but no specific genetic marker has been identified in amniotic cell culture, and no other means is available to determine whether a male fetus will have muscular dystrophy. Serum creatine kinase activity can be used for carrier detection, but it is elevated in only about two thirds of female carriers. Muscle biopsies may show some histologic abnormality in some carriers. Quantitative electromyography is a complex, time-consuming procedure not precise enough for general clinical application. Recently, morphological and biochemical abnormalities have been detected in red blood cells of carriers.

A neurogenic hypothesis of muscular dystrophy has assigned a primary pathogenic role to dysfunction of motor neurons. The electrophysiologic evidence for this hypothesis has recently been challenged. Schwann cell abnormality and amyelination have not been found in autopsy studies of Duchenne-type muscular dystrophy. Another hypothesis is that functional ischemia of skeletal muscle may be important in the pathogenesis of Duchenne dystrophy. Abnormalities of circulating erythrocytes may also be present in Duchenne dystrophy and in myotonic dystrophy. A striking early abnormality in the skeletal muscle in Duchenne dystrophy is hypercontraction or hyaline necrosis of isolated fibers or parts of them, possibly due to a localized inability of sarcomeres to relax. The central myofibrillar clumping may

(7) Isr. J. Med. Sci. 13:152–158, February, 1977.

result from a defect in the mitochondria, Z line or sarcoplasmic reticulum.

▶ [This article summarizes recent research in muscular dystrophy. Its author is one of the leaders in the field of muscle disease – and, for that matter, in the entire discipline of clinical neurology. – Ed.] ◀

Spectrum of Mild X-Linked Recessive Muscular Dystrophy. A number of families with an X-linked recessive form of muscular dystrophy that has a more benign and prolonged course than that of Duchenne-type muscular dystrophy have been described in the past decade. Steven P. Ringel, James E. Carroll and S. Clifford Schold[8] (Univ. of Colorado) investigated the spectrum of mild X-linked muscular dystrophy in 12 families, including 19 affected men. The criteria included survival past age 32 years or preserved walking past age 16 years in the patient or an affected male relative and a family pedigree compatible with X-linked recessive inheritance.

Age range was 6 – 43 years. Most patients had an onset after age 7 and walked beyond age 20 – 30 years. Common clinical features included mild hypertrophy of the calves, mild joint contractures and high-arched feet. Psychometric tests, ECGs and EEGs were usually normal. Many patients had significant lordosis and several, mild scoliosis. Pes cavus deformity was seen in many patients. Serum creatine phosphokinase levels were markedly elevated in all patients in whom they were determined; levels generally declined with age. All muscle biopsies showed increased variability in fiber size. Atrophy was more marked than hypertrophy, but all biopsy specimens contained both atrophic and hypertrophic fibers. Large, rounded, opaque fibers were present in over half the specimens. Fiber-type differentiation was good. Degenerative changes were present in all specimens, but necrosis and phagocytosis were usually mild. Numerous split fibers were seen. Proliferation of endomysial and perimysial connective tissue was present in all cases. There was no significant inflammatory response.

The spectrum of mild X-linked dystrophy includes families with more severe involvement and muscle biopsy changes resembling those of Duchenne-type muscular dystrophy and families with milder involvement and biopsies

(8)   Arch. Neurol. 34:408 – 416, July, 1977.

showing more features in common with limb girdle dystrophy. Within a given kindred the clinical picture is usually quite similar, permitting reasonable predictions of outcome for newly affected members within a kindred.

► [It has never been definitely established whether the more mild type of X-linked muscular dystrophy described by Becker is a homogeneous entity, distinct from the more severe Duchenne type. This may in part be due to the fact that most of the cases that have been reported deal only with single families. These investigators have studied 19 patients in 12 families. They express the belief that it is a distinct entity, variable in course and onset in different families, but homogeneous within each family. The prognosis is much better than that in Duchenne's muscular dystrophy. — Ed.] ◄

Prenatal Diagnosis of Duchenne's Muscular Dystrophy. Duchenne's muscular dystrophy is an X-linked recessive disorder that occurs almost exclusively in boys. The serum creatine phosphokinase (CPK) activity is increased early in life and is useful in establishing the diagnosis in infants before symptoms appear. Maurice J. Mahoney, Florence P. Haseltine, John C. Hobbins, Betty Q. Banker, C. Thomas Caskey and Mitchell S. Golbus[9] tested the hypothesis that the pathologic process leading to elevated CPK levels is present during fetal life by measuring CPK activity in fetal plasma, obtained in utero by placental sampling techniques. The findings in 16 control fetuses and 2 male fetuses at risk for Duchenne's dystrophy were reviewed. Sampling was by either fetoscopy or blind placental aspiration. Nine control pregnancies were being aborted, and 7 were at risk for a fetal hemoglobinopathy.

A fetus at risk, studied at 18 weeks' gestation, had an activity of 96 IU/L, compared with a control range of 0–150 IU/L in the fetuses not at risk for the disorder. The pregnancy continued and the infant was normal at birth. The second fetus at risk, studied at 20 weeks, had a significant elevation of CPK activity to 540 IU/L, and the fetal blood showed considerable hemolysis. Examination of fetal muscle after abortion showed characteristic features of Duchenne's dystrophy, including wide variation in fiber diameter and a reduction in the number of fibers per fasciculus.

These findings illustrate the potential usefulness of fetal plasma for prenatal diagnosis, and specifically of CPK activ-

(9) N. Engl. J. Med. 297:968–973, Nov. 3, 1977.

ity for the diagnosis of muscular dystrophy. It is likely that other diseases can be diagnosed by measuring plasma constituents and that therapeutic interventions in the fetus can be monitored in the same way.

► [These cases illustrate the potential usefulness of fetal plasma, and specifically of creatine phosphokinase activity, for the prenatal diagnosis of Duchenne's muscular dystrophy. — Ed.] ◄

Lactate Dehydrogenase Isoenzyme 5 in Detecting Carriers of Duchenne's Muscular Dystrophy. Until the inborn metabolic error responsible for Duchenne's muscular dystrophy is delineated biochemically, carrier detection must be indirect. Lactate dehydrogenase (LDH) measurements have been less useful than creatine phosphokinase (CPK) measurements in determination of carrier status. A. D. Roses, M. J. Roses, G. A. Nicholson and C. R. Roe[1] (Duke Univ.) evaluated serum LDH-5 measurements in screening for carriers of Duchenne's dystrophy. Zones of LDH activity in agar gels were revealed by the nitroblue tetrazolium staining technique. Mothers with a mean age of 34 years were tested; mean age of controls was 30 years.

Of 33 consecutive mothers of sons affected with Duchenne's muscular dystrophy, 12 had possible new mutations. Ten of these had at least one qualitatively increased LDH-5 interpretation, and 5 had quantitative elevations. Over half the LDH isoenzyme patterns in 25 mothers were qualitatively at least somewhat increased. Only 4 of 34 consecutive matched female controls had an increased LDH-5 pattern, and all were quantitatively within the control range. There were no differences in quantitative LDH-5 levels between known carriers and the possible new mutation group. Four of five mothers in the latter group with elevated LDH-5 levels had female relatives with quantitatively increased LDH-5 levels. Further, several female relatives had elevated CPK or serum glutamic oxaloacetic transaminase levels. Lactate dehydrogenase isoenzyme determinations identified several mothers who had normal creatine kinase levels. The combination of CPK and LDH-5 determinations, with extensive pedigree testing, identified 28 of 30 mothers as probable heterozygotes.

The findings support the view that cases of Duchenne's

(1) Neurology (Minneap.) 27:414–421, May, 1977.

dystrophy resulting from spontaneous mutation are less common than is currently believed. Determination of LDH-5 levels in mothers of patients with Duchenne's dystrophy is as sensitive a means of carrier detection as CPK analysis. The authors attempt to examine all female members in every pedigree with all available methods before prospective genetic counseling is undertaken. By identification of women at risk, prevention of most Duchenne's dystrophy births through prenatal detection methods becomes a reasonable goal.

► [These data support the suggestion that cases of Duchenne's muscular dystrophy as a result of spontaneous mutation are more uncommon than currently believed. – Ed.] ◄

Blood Vessel Structure in Duchenne's Muscular Dystrophy: I. Light and Electron Microscopic Observations in Resting Muscle. Numerous suggestions as to the pathogenesis of Duchenne's muscular dystrophy have been advanced. Recently, functional changes in the vascular bed have been implicated. Judith Koehler[2] (Stanford Univ.) examined muscle biopsy specimens from 8 patients with a clinical diagnosis of Duchenne's dystrophy. Light and electron microscopic studies were carried out, with particular attention paid to the capillary-venous bed.

The arterioles and metarterioles contained normal endothelium, as did the capillary bed for the most part. Pale endothelial cells were seen in 2–6% of vessels, but active degeneration was not seen. Fenestrated endothelial cells were seen in 1 patient. The capillary basement membranes were finely fibrillar and tended to be bilamellar or trilamellar. Encasement by collagen fibrils that merged into the capillary basement membrane was frequently observed and often resulted in separation of the vessel from the muscle fibers. Swirls of almost nodular proliferating collagen were seen occasionally, compressing the lumens of intact vascular structures. A Schwann cell appeared to be involved in 1 case, but these structures could have originated from vascular elements.

Lesions characteristic of vasoactive amine vascular injury are not present in Duchenne's dystrophy. The mild abnormalities observed in the vascular tree may be present in

(2) Neurology (Minneap.) 27:861 – 868, September, 1977.

other neuromuscular diseases. Further studies of functional microvascular abnormality and determinations of physiologic reactivity of the vascular bed are needed in patients with Duchenne's dystrophy. No present evidence supports a primary vascular abnormality in this disease.

▶ [The minimal abnormalities appear to be nonspecific and do not substantiate postulated vascular injury by vasoactive mediators or ischemia. No current evidence supports a primary vascular abnormality in Duchenne's dystrophy. — Ed.] ◀

Immunologic Myopathy: Linear IgG Deposition and Fulminant Terminal Episode. David M. Judge, Thomas J. McGlynn, Arthur B. Abt, John R. Luderer and Samuel P. Ward[3] (Pennsylvania State Univ.) report a new syndrome of primary long-standing muscular manifestations, and subsequent multisystem involvement leading to death, associated with linear IgG staining of muscle and kidney basement membranes.

Woman, 73, had microscopic hematuria, proteinuria, azotemia, recurrent hemoptysis and a 9-year history of muscle weakness. Initially she had noticed difficulty combing her hair and rising from a chair without help, which resolved spontaneously. Progressive limb weakness had recurred a year before admission. Vertical diplopia had been present for 3 years and left-sided ptosis for 1 year. A thyroidectomy had been done and a sympathectomy for Raynaud's phenomenon. Ocular movements were restricted on the left side and the left pupil was constricted, with lid ptosis. The proximal and distal limb muscles were markedly weak to resistance, especially on the right side. Truncal ataxia and dysmetria of the extremities were observed. Sensation was intact. Jaw jerk, snout and bilateral grasp reflexes were present. The signs waxed and waned over 13 days in the hospital. The right hemidiaphragm was paralyzed. An intravenous pyelogram was within normal limits.

Sore throat followed muscle and renal biopsies, with subsequent periorbital and tongue edema and laryngeal stridor. The right elbow and wrist became warm, swollen and painful. Intubation was necessary for 12 hours. A maculopapular rash developed on the arms and upper eyelids and progressed to necrotic papules. Joint aspirates contained many polymorphonuclear leukocytes. The skin lesions progressed despite intravenous corticosteroid therapy. The serum creatinine concentration increased, with progressive dyspnea and wheezing, supraventricular tachycardia and metabolic acidosis. The patient became hypotensive and died with refractory cardiac arrhythmias.

(3) Arch. Pathol. Lab. Med. 101:362–365, July, 1977.

The muscle biopsy showed widely varying fiber diameters and groups of atrophic fibers, some containing rod bodies. Intense linear staining for IgG was seen. The renal capillary basement membranes were thickened, and linear IgG staining was observed. The skin exhibited an acute necrotizing vasculitis with subepidermal bullae and extensive dermal necrosis. Autopsy showed rapidly progressive glomerulonephritis and acute vasculitis of the skin, lungs and spleen. Small foci of acute bronchopneumonia were observed. The central nervous system was unremarkable.

This patient's multisystem disease is suggestive of a variety of collagen vascular disorders. The muscle exhibited type 2 fiber atrophy. Whether the preterminal acceleration of disease represented the natural course or was due to allergy to contrast medium is unclear.

► [The data suggest the presence of an antibody to a basement membrane antigen shared by muscle and kidney. – Ed.] ◄

Myoglobinemia in Inflammatory Myopathies. The myoglobin assay has been useful not only in assessing the presence of muscle disease, but in alerting the physician to the risk of renal failure, which may complicate myoglobinuric states. Lawrence J. Kagen[4] (Cornell Univ. Med. College) reviewed experience with the myoglobin immunoassay in patients with myositis over a 5-year period. Patients with diagnoses of dermatomyositis, polymyositis or myopathy associated with other connective tissue diseases had myoglobin assayed in their serum or urine. Immunoassays were done both by immunodiffusion and complement fixation techniques; both methods were specific for myoglobin. Serum myoglobin was determined in 21 patients with dermatomyositis, 21 with polymyositis and 20 who had myopathy associated with other connective tissue disorders. Most patients in each group were women. Five patients had neoplasms.

Two thirds of patients with dermatomyositis and about half of those with polymyositis had myoglobinemia, as did 40% of those with myopathy associated with other connective tissue disorders. Of the last, 4 of 6 patients with scleroderma and 3 of 7 with systemic lupus had myoglobinemia. The frequency of myoglobinemia was not related to age or

(4)   J.A.M.A. 237:1448–1452, Apr. 4, 1977.

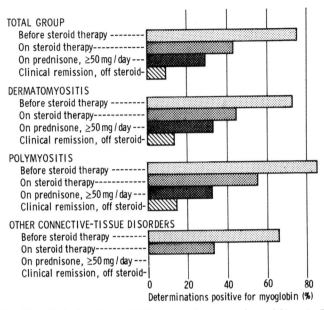

Fig 34. — Effect of corticosteroid therapy on frequency of myoglobinemia. Total group is sum of data from other three groups. Steroid therapy was discontinued in those patients in clinical remission. (Courtesy of Kagen, L. J.: J.A.M.A. 237:1448 – 1452, Apr. 4, 1977.)

sex. The relationship of myoglobinemia to steroid therapy is shown in Figure 34; it was most common in patients with active illness who had not yet received steroid therapy. Myoglobin was frequently present where there were marked elevations of serum glutamic-oxaloacetic transaminase, lactic dehydrogenase and creatine phosphokinase activities. Sequential studies of 6 patients showed a rapid reduction in serum myoglobin levels with treatment, usually before enzyme levels had returned to normal. In 1 patient with dermatomyositis followed for 30 months, myoglobinemia correlated with clinical exacerbations of rash and weakness more than did enzyme values.

Immunologic techniques for myoglobin may provide additional means of diagnosing and evaluating muscle disease and of suggesting possible risks that patients may encounter. Persistent myoglobinemic and myoglobinuric states have been associated with renal failure in patients with myositis.

▶ [Myoglobinemia correlated with clinically observed exacerbations of rash and weakness in patients with inflammatory myopathies to a greater degree than did enzyme elevations. — Ed.] ◀

Neurologic Complications of Systemic Disease

Neurologic Manifestations of Cogan's Syndrome are discussed by J. M. Bicknell and J. V. Holland[5] (Univ. of New Mexico). Cogan's syndrome is a multisystem inflammatory vascular disease characterized by nonsyphilitic interstitial keratitis and vestibuloauditory symptoms. Some 70 case reports have appeared over 30 years. Diverse, potentially serious neurologic problems may occur in patients with Cogan's syndrome. Review was made of data on 38 male and 41 female patients with a median age of 26. Sixty-eight had systemic problems and 44 had neurologic features.

The most common general abnormalities were fever, weight loss, leukocytosis and an elevated sedimentation rate. Aortic insufficiency was the most severe cardiovascular problem. Gastrointestinal problems included ulcers, melena and ileus. Musculoskeletal aches and pains, cutaneous nodules or rashes, adenopathy, hepatosplenomegaly and genitourinary disorders were also noted. A mild interstitial inflammation of the cornea often became apparent at about the same time as inner ear symptoms. One of the present patients had phrenic and long thoracic nerve paralysis and optic neuritis and ultimately had a picture of fluctuating cerebral, cerebellar and spinal cord lesions. A second patient presented with seizures, hyperreflexia, ataxia and severe organic mental syndrome with only minor systemic problems. Cases of seizures, peripheral neuritis, ophthalmoplegia and cerebrovascular syndromes have been described. In a number of patients, neurologic manifestations were part of a catastrophic multisystem process.

The success of treatment in Cogan's syndrome varies with the target organ or symptom. Acute systemic symptoms and ocular inflammation may respond to corticoids. Cardiac

(5) Neurology (Minneap.) 28:278–281, March, 1978.

valve replacement has corrected heart failure due to aortic valve incompetence. Ear problems have been inexorably progressive in most cases. Whether patients will respond to long-term, high-dose steroid or immunosuppressive drug therapy remains to be determined.

▶ [The presence of Cogan's syndrome must be considered when neurologic defects are accompanied by ocular, otologic and systemic manifestations. – Ed.] ◀

Cervical Myelopathy Associated with Rheumatoid Arthritis: Analysis of 32 Patients, with 2 Postmortem Cases. Kenneth K. Nakano, William C. Schoene, Richard A. Baker and David M. Dawson[6] reviewed data on 32 patients with neurologic disorder due to cervical dislocation from rheumatoid disease. Thirteen had typical anterior subluxation of C1 on C2. Two patients came to autopsy. The patients were among 1,100 seen in 1970 – 75 with rheumatoid arthritis. The most common finding was mild spastic quadriparesis, often more evident in the hands, with hyperreflexia and extensor plantar responses. Sensory symptoms were prominent. A sensory level was discernible in the upper cervical dermatomes in 64% of patients. Six patients had symptoms of medullary or pontine dysfunction, which usually were transient. Symptoms usually developed slowly, the myelopathy appearing in late middle age after an average of 18 years of disability from advanced generalized rheumatoid disase.

Twelve patients were managed surgically; half of these were treated in halo traction. Surgery consisted of posterior decompressive laminectomy, laminectomy plus fusion of C1, C2 or C3 to the occiput, or fusion without laminectomy. Patients having fusion and halo traction did best. Seven of 19 patients not having surgery showed progressive neurologic dysfunction and 2 died. The 2 autopsies showed maximal tissue damage limited to the anterior gray horns and some damage to the posterior gray horns and adjacent white matter of the lateral and posterior columns (Fig 35). Secondary tract degeneration was seen above and below the region of maximal damage. The surface of the spinal cord appeared relatively unaffected in these cases.

Distal branches of the anterior spinal artery may have

---

(6) Ann. Neurol. 3:144 – 151, February, 1978.

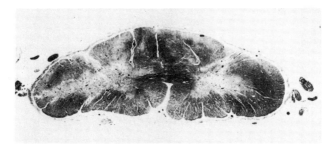

Fig 35.—Necrosis of the anterior horns and adjacent white matter in the lateral and posterior columns in compressed upper cervical spinal cord. Hematoxylin-eosin; reduced from ×7. (Courtesy of Nakano, K. K., et al.: Ann. Neurol. 3:144–151, February, 1978.)

been occluded by direct anteroposterior compression in these cases, thus reducing blood flow to the central gray matter and the adjacent white matter of the spinal cord which is supplied by the distal sulcal branches of the anterior spinal artery.

▶ [Involvement of the cervical spine is now recognized to be a relatively common complication of rheumatoid arthritis. This may lead to transverse myelitis and even death. Decompressive laminectomy and fusion of the cervical vertebrae may be necessary. – Ed.] ◀

Neurologic Manifestations in Sarcoidosis: Review of the Literature, with Report of 23 Cases. Peyton Delaney[7] (Georgetown Univ.) reviewed the neurologic findings in 7 of 77 patients seen in 1970–75 with sarcoidosis who had neurologic findings and in 16 other patients with neurologic sarcoidosis, including 13 with autopsy findings. Most patients in both groups were aged 20–40. The average duration of neurologic manifestations was 2.6 years. The racial distribution was predominantly black. Stigmas of sarcoid were usually present at the onset of neurologic symptoms and correlated well with the presence of disseminated granulomas in 13 of 14 autopsied cases. Neurologic dysfunction, however, was often the presenting or only clinical finding. The overall frequency of neurologic manifestations in reported cases is 5%.

Central nervous system involvement usually occurs in the early phase of the disease and peripheral nervous system

(7)   Ann. Intern. Med. 87:336–345, September, 1977.

and skeletal muscle involvement in the chronic stages. Sarcoid lesions have been described in every cranial nerve. The facial and optic nerves are most frequently involved. Encephalopathy may be due to both granulomas and metabolic dysfunction. Meningeal involvement is common. Seizures occur in 5–18% of patients with neurologic sarcoidosis. About 20 intracranial space-occupying lesions have been described. Six patients with progressive multifocal leukoencephalopathy have been described in sarcoidosis. The most common intracranial sites of involvement are the hypothalamus, third ventricular region and pituitary gland. The brain stem and cerebellum are seldom primarily involved. Transient ischemic attacks and strokes are rare, as is spinal cord involvement. The frequency of peripheral neuropathy is 15%. Myopathic involvement may be symptomatic or asymptomatic.

The diagnosis of neurologic sarcoidosis is sometimes one of exclusion. There is little evidence that serial brain scanning, biopsy specimens, cerebrospinal fluid examinations or electromyography are as useful as thorough neurologic evaluation at each follow-up visit.

► [A current review of the neurologic manifestations of sarcoidosis is timely because this disease is recognized and diagnosed more frequently now than it was 10 or 20 years ago and because it has been more than 10 years since an extensive neurologic review of sarcoidosis has been published. – Ed.] ◄

Cerebrospinal Fluid Sorbitol and Myoinositol in Diabetic Polyneuropathy. Increased sorbitol in the lens has been associated with diabetic cataract and an increase in peripheral nerves with neuropathy in diabetic rats. Increased sorbitol levels have been found in the cerebrospinal fluid (CSF) of human diabetics. Carita Servo, Lea Bergström and Rainer Fogelholm[8] (Univ. of Helsinki) correlated signs of diabetic polyneuropathy in 21 patients with CSF concentrations of sorbitol and myoinositol and with plasma glucose levels. Five diabetics with a normal nerve status were also evaluated; all 5 were receiving oral hypoglycemic drugs. Five patients with polyneuropathy were on insulin and 11 were on oral hypoglycemic agents; 1 had carbohydrate restriction. No patient was ketotic. The results were compared with the findings in 27 control subjects.

(8) Acta Med. Scand. 202:301–304, 1977.

Cerebrospinal fluid sorbitol levels were significantly increased in diabetics with elevated plasma glucose. Myoinositol levels were significantly reduced in the patients with polyneuropathy. Both alterations were present within 2 months after the onset of symptoms of diabetes. Patients with polyneuropathy on oral hypoglycemic drugs had reduced CSF myoinositol levels compared with those on insulin, but normal plasma glucose levels and CSF sorbitol levels not unlike controls. The 4 patients with the most severe electromyographic signs of polyneuropathy all had uncontrolled hyperglycemia and significantly altered polyol concentrations in the CSF. Only sensory neuropathy was present in 3 patients with normal plasma glucose levels, no glucosuria and a stable type of diabetes, despite a duration of diabetes of 2–22 years. These patients also had normal CSF myoinositol concentrations.

These findings are compatible with the theory that sorbitol is synthesized from glucose in nervous tissue and the synthesis is increased with hyperglycemia. The metabolic disturbance in diabetes apparently causes alterations in the central nervous system levels of sorbitol and myoinositol, which also alter polyol concentrations in the CSF. These changes can probably be avoided by adequate control of diabetes. The reduction in CSF myoinositol in diabetes may be associated with the development of neuropathy.

► [Alterations in the sorbitol pathway and in myoinositol metabolism have both been associated with complications of diabetes. In this study sorbitol concentrations in the cerebrospinal fluid were significantly increased in patients with elevated plasma glucose concentrations. The myoinositol concentrations in the cerebrospinal fluid were significantly decreased in patients with polyneuropathy compared with controls. Both alterations in polyol concentration were present within 2 months of the onset of the polyneuropathy and apparently play a part in its pathogenesis. These alterations can possibly be avoided with adequate control of the diabetes. — Ed.] ◄

Cardiorespiratory Arrest and Diabetic Autonomic Neuropathy. Unexplained cardiac arrests have been reported in 2 diabetics with severe autonomic neuropathy. M. McB. Page and P. J. Watkins[9] (King's College Hosp., London) report 12 arrests seen over 5 years in 8 diabetics with severe autonomic neuropathy. The 6 women and 2 men were aged 31–41 years and had had diabetes for 14–32 years. All

(9) Lancet 1:14–16, Jan. 7, 1978.

had diabetic complications, including peripheral neuropathy. All but 1 had clinical features of autonomic neuropathy, most commonly postural hypotension, diarrhea and gustatory sweating. All the cardiorespiratory arrests occurred in the hospital. Three occurred during surgery, 2 during general anesthesia. One attack followed recovery from hypoglycemic coma. All patients but 1 responded rapidly to external cardiac massage and assisted respiration. No patient was hypoglycemic at the time of the arrest. One patient had temporary sinus bradycardia followed by asystole after the attack and died a week later of irreversible brain damage.

It seems probable that many if not all of these arrests were primarily of respiratory origin. It is unlikely that if asystole or ventricular fibrillation were responsible, normal rhythm would regularly have been established by the time ECG monitoring was begun. Probably normal respiratory reflexes are often impaired in diabetic autonomic neuropathy. Reduced sensitivity to hypoxia could result from impairment of afferent impulses from the carotid body and aortic arch chemoreceptors, transmitted by the glossopharyngeal and vagus nerves, respectively. It has been difficult to isolate precipitating causes in these cases, but patients with diabetic autonomic neuropathy may be particularly susceptible to drugs with respiratory depressant effects. Continuous cardiac monitoring and intensive postoperative supervision are recommended. Four of the patients have died subsequently, 2 without apparent cause even at autopsy. It appears that cardiorespiratory arrest is a specific feature of diabetic autonomic neuropathy and probably contributes to the mortality in this condition.

▶ [Autonomic neuropathy is an important complication of diabetes mellitus, especially in young patients. Cardiorespiratory arrest appears to be a specific feature of diabetic autonomic neuropathy and may contribute to the mortality in this disorder. – Ed.] ◀

Syndrome of Diabetic Amyotrophy. S. Chokroverty, M. G. Reyes, F. A. Rubino and H. Tonaki[1] obtained evidence that diabetic amyotrophy is a distinct clinical entity, most likely due to involvement of the intramuscular branches of the proximal crural nerves and secondary to a metabolic cause rather than to diabetic microangiopathy.

(1)   Ann. Neurol. 2:181 – 194, September, 1977.

Studies were performed in 12 men with a mean age of 57 years who had diabetic amyotrophy. All had difficulty climbing stairs, and all but 1 reported pain in the low back or thigh. Only 1 had evidence of diabetic retinopathy. The illness had progressed slowly over weeks to months. All patients improved on appropriate therapy for diabetes during follow-up for 1 – 36 months. Six had marked and 3 had moderate functional improvement. Bilateral electromyographic studies were carried out, and biopsy specimens were obtained from the vastus medialis muscles on one side in the region of the motor points.

Electromyograms of the pelvifemoral muscles showed changes of chronic neuropathic involvement, including fibrillations at rest, reduced interference and firing patterns, and excessive polyphasic potentials. Conduction velocities in the tibial and peroneal nerves were slightly to moderately reduced. Muscle biopsy specimens showed small or large groups of atrophic angular type I and type II fibers and atrophic single fibers. Targets were seen in type I fibers. Phosphorylase reaction was absent in the atrophic fibers. All but 2 patients had evidence of mixed fiber atrophy. Fine structural studies showed myofibrillar degeneration, subsarcolemmal accumulation of lipofuscin bodies, and packed tubular aggregates in the subsarcolemmal region of type II fibers. Motor point biopsy specimens showed many enlarged, complex, degenerated subneural apparatuses, beaded and thickened terminal axons, double end-plates and occasional ultraterminal fibers.

Apparently, diabetic amyotrophy is due to a proximal intramuscular crural neuropathy, which in some cases may resemble a nonischemic mononeuropathy multiplex. Its pathogenesis is unclear. The response to control of hyperglycemia and the findings of tubular aggregates and mitochondrial abnormalities indicate a metabolic cause for diabetic amyotrophy.

▶ [An editorial immediately preceding this article in *Annals of Neurology* ends with a paragraph stating, "The purpose of this editorial is to suggest that diabetic amyotrophy is neither a distinct clinical entity nor a well-defined term" (Asbury, A. N.: Ann. Neurol. 2:179, 1977). The original abstract of this article ends with the statement, "We conclude that diabetic amyotrophy is a distinct clinical entity and is secondary to metabolic derangement rather than diabetic microangiopathy." Most neurologists feel that so-called diabetic amyotrophy is a manifestation of asymmetric proximal diabetic neuropathy or mononeuropathy multiplex, and it has also been called a subacute proximal diabetic neuropathy (Williams, I. R., and Mayer, R. F.: Neurology (Minneap.) 26:108, 1976). Garland, who with Taverner described the syndrome in 1953 and gave it the name "diabetic amyotrophy," stated in 1960 that the underlying pathology of the syndrome had not yet been established and that the scanty evidence was conflicting. He stated further that the lesion responsible might be at any place from the anterior horn cell to the muscle end-plate or at several sites (Garland, H.: Proc. R. Soc. Med. 53:137, 1960). — Ed.] ◄

Pellagra: Analysis of 18 Patients and Review of the Literature. Pellagra is curable, but if untreated it results in irreversible neurologic damage and death. Jerry L. Spivak and David L. Jackson[2] (Johns Hopkins Univ.) reviewed the findings in 18 patients seen in 1970–74 with pellagra. The 11 men and 7 women had a mean age of 44 years. All but 2 patients were alcoholics, and 5 had chronic pancreatitis. Two had had subtotal gastrectomy for ulcer disease. One was receiving intravenous alimentation when pellagra developed. Most patients were seen in the summer and fall. Marked weight loss was common and preceded onset of overt manifestations of pellagra. All patients had dermatitis, but only 1 presented with an acute erythematous rash of early pellagra. Six patients had reached a phase of hyperpigmentation and desquamation. Seven patients had loose or frequent stools. Two developed intestinal obstruction. Nine patients had abnormalities in higher integrative functions; in 5 this was limited to disorientation and impaired recent memory. Dementia developed in 2 hospitalized patients from failure to correct the niacin deficiency.

Anemia was present in all patients but 2, but it was usually mild. Nine patients were hyperuricemic and only 2 of these were azotemic. Hypokalemia, hypomagnesemia and hypocalcemia were frequent, but no episodes of tetany occurred. The serum thyroxine concentration was reduced in 5 of the 9 patients evaluated. Fourteen patients were febrile. Excessive alcohol consumption was implicated in 15 cases.

Failure to recognize the central nervous system manifestations of niacin deficiency can be avoided if attention is paid to the EEG. Five patients, all of them demented, exhibited a diffuse increase in slow wave activity. Most patients respond promptly to treatment with a rapid change in affect

(2) Johns Hopkins Med. J. 140:295–309, June, 1977.

and mentation, followed by improvement in the diarrhea and dermatitis. The EEG can also serve as a therapeutic guide. The events leading to the malnourished state must be determined and measures taken to prevent recurrences.

► [Endemic pellagra was eradicated in the United States many years ago, but sporadic cases still occur. It should be recognized early because it is a curable disorder, but one that, if untreated, may result in irreversible neurologic damage. After the problem has been resolved, it is incumbent upon the physician to determine the events leading to the malnourished state and to institute measures to prevent repetition. — Ed.] ◄

Some Features of the Neuromuscular Complications of Pulmonary Carcinoma. Heikki Terävänen and Andreo Larsen[3] (Univ. of Helsinki) studied the records of 33 consecutive patients with pulmonary carcinoma for myopathy and peripheral neuropathy. The 26 men and 7 women had a mean age of 60.9. Fourteen patients had epidermoid, 9 had anaplastic and 7 had alveolar carcinoma. Nine patients with noncarcinomatous lung disease, with a mean age of 35.3, were also evaluated. No patient from whom a biopsy specimen was obtained or who was studied with use of intracellular microelectrodes received cytotoxic drugs. Nerve conduction velocity was determined in 19 patients with pulmonary carcinoma and in 6 control patients. Intercostal muscles from 13 carcinoma patients and 5 control patients were studied with use of intracellular microelectrodes.

Fifteen study and 8 control patients had normal neurologic findings. No patient had atrophy. Four of the 16 study patients with clinical neuropathy had received cytotoxic drugs and 1 was diabetic. The study patients with clinical neuropathy had reduced conduction velocities in the sural nerve. Sensory conduction velocities were subnormal in 6 of 7 study patients with and 4 of 12 without clinical neuropathy. Muscle biopsy specimens showed no significant differences between the study and control patients (Fig 36) on light microscopy. Resting membrane potentials were similar in the two groups, but the mean frequency of miniature end-plate potentials in normal bathing solution containing 5 mM K^+ was higher in the study patients. Mean miniature end-plate potential amplitudes were similar. Muscles from study patients had a reduced ability to increase transmitter release in presynaptic depolarization performed with bath-

(3) Ann. Neurol. 2:495–502, December, 1977.

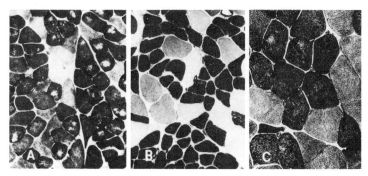

Fig 36. – Photomicrograph from transversely sectioned external intercostal muscles. **A,** biopsy specimen from a man, aged 44, in the control group with a clinical diagnosis of bronchiectasis illustrates the maximum number of irregularities in the NADH-diaphorase distribution observed in the present study; reduced from ×100. **B,** section incubated with ATPase (preincubation at pH 4.2) from a man, aged 63, with epidermoid carcinoma of the lung. There was only modest type grouping (bottom of picture) and some fiber size variation; reduced from ×100. **C,** section incubated with NADH-diaphorase from a woman, aged 62, with anaplastic pulmonary carcinoma. One small, angulated, atrophic fiber with intense NADH-diaphorase activity is present among fibers of normal size and internal structure; reduced from ×180. (Courtesy of Teräväinen, H., and Larsen, A.: Ann. Neurol. 2:495–502, December, 1977.)

ing solution containing 20 mM K^+. The quantum content calculated was less in 1 carcinoma patient than in 2 control patients.

Patients with pulmonary carcinoma have an increased tendency to acquire peripheral sensory or combined sensorimotor neuropathy and a reduced ability to release acetylcholine from the presynaptic nerve ending of the motor endplate. Impaired acetylcholine release indicates that these patients may have a variable predisposition to acquire clinically evident myasthenia.

▶ [Despite a rather extensive literature on the remote effects of carcinoma, there have been few physiologic and pathologic studies to confirm the presence of such effects. This study shows that there are changes in both function and structure of nerves and muscle in patients with pulmonary carcinoma. – Ed.] ◀

Sleep Apnea Syndrome in a Patient with Shy-Drager Syndrome is described by Kenneth L. Lehrman, Christian Guilleminault, John S. Schroeder, Ara Tilkian and Lysia N. Forno[4] (Stanford Univ.). Hemodynamic studies were carried

(4) Arch. Intern. Med. 138:206–209, February, 1978.

out in a patient with the unique combination of sleep apnea syndrome and Shy-Drager syndrome.

Man, 59, had had progressive urinary incontinence, impotence and perianal numbness for 5 years. He had noticed increasing light-headedness on standing or exercise and had two episodes of orthostatic syncope. Mineralocorticoid therapy had become less effective. Periodic respiration was noted during sleep, with periods of apnea. The slightly obese man exhibited orthostatic hypotension with no rise in pulse rate. Conjunctival methacholine gave no response. Digital blood flow was considerably reduced and sweat testing resulted in hyperthermia. Possible unilateral vocal cord paresis was observed. Mild distal airway obstruction responded to bronchodilators. An 8-hour ambulatory ECG study showed minimal variation in heart rate and infrequent premature ventricular contractions. Cyclical variation in heart rate was associated with apneic episodes during sleep.

Resting hemodynamics were normal but there was a minimal heart rate response to all interventions except atropine administration. An exaggerated hypertensive response occurred with left ventricular failure with all pressor agents. The Valsalva response was abnormal. During sleep, respiratory effort increased substan-

Fig 37.— **A,** rostral pons. Gliosis in midline tegmentum in superior central nucleus and nucleus of dorsal raphe. Fourth ventricle is seen in upper right corner. Holzer stain; reduced from ×63. **B,** rostral pons from man, aged 57, with mild idiopathic parkinsonism. No gliosis present. Holzer stain; reduced from ×63. (Courtesy of Lehrman, K. L., et al.: Arch. Intern. Med. 138:206–209, February, 1978; copyright 1978, American Medical Association.)

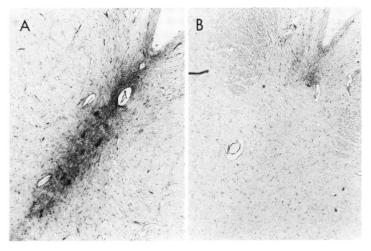

tially and periods of transient pulmonary hypertension were noted. The average duration of apneic episodes was 18.5 seconds, representing 54.5% of sleep time without air exchange. A permanent tracheostomy was done and cyproheptadine given, but the patient died in his sleep about 2 weeks after discharge.

Autopsy showed changes consistent with idiopathic orthostatic hypotension, including nerve cell loss in the thoracolumbar intermediolateral column, dorsal motor vagus nucleus and vestibular nuclei, with marked gliosis in midline raphe nuclei throughout the brain stem (Fig 37). Only gliosis of the solitary tract was observed in the pontine or medullary respiratory areas. Sympathetic ganglia were normal except for frequent vacuolation adjacent to nerve cells.

Multiple areas of degeneration were found in central nervous system areas outside the medullary respiratory centers in this patient, suggesting their importance in the respiratory abnormalities in sleep apnea syndrome.

► [The autopsy evidence of lesions in regions associated with the sleep mechanisms suggests an important role in the sleep apnea syndrome for lesions in areas outside the medullary respiratory center. — Ed.] ◄

Pathogenesis of Central Nervous System Infiltration in Acute Leukemia. The origin of leukemic cells infiltrating the leptomeninges has been controversial. One hypothesis suggests that leukemic cells arise locally in the central nervous system, and another suggests that infiltrates come directly from the blood, either by diapedesis or in association with petechial hemorrhages. Biagio Azzarelli and Uros Roessmann[5] (Case Western Reserve Univ.) compared the pattern of dural infiltration and its frequency with involvement of the subarachnoid space in 31 autopsy cases, 17 of acute myeloblastic and 14 of acute lymphocytic leukemia. In 23 cases sections from the dura included the sagittal sinus. Aggregates with substantial numbers of fresh red blood cells admixed with leukemic cells were not considered to be true infiltrates.

Infiltrates were found in the dura in 93% of cases, in the arachnoid in 71%, as perivascular cuffing in 54% and in brain parenchyma in 16%. In 9 cases dural infiltration was the sole manifestation of the disease. In only 3 cases was there isolated involvement of the arachnoid. Parenchymal involvement was seen only when there was massive infiltra-

(5)   Arch. Pathol. Lab. Med. 101:203–205, April, 1977.

Fig 38. – Acute lymphocytic leukemic infiltrate pervading entire dural thickness. Hematoxylin-eosin; reduced from ×40. (Courtesy of Azzarelli, B., and Roessmann, U.: Arch. Pathol. Lab. Med. 101:203–205, April, 1977; copyright 1977, American Medical Association.)

tion of the Virchow-Robin space. Rupture of the pia-glia was occasionally observed. A focal aggregate of leukemic cells surrounded veins in the dura in 22 cases; the entire vessel wall was often heavily infiltrated. In 5 cases the entire dura was permeated with dense collections of leukemic cells (Fig 38). Leukemic aggregates were present in the epidural space in 12 cases. No infiltration of arachnoid granulations was seen in cases of leptomeningeal invasion.

Perivenular infiltration in the dura was the most common finding in this study. The pattern of central nervous system involvement in acute leukemia appears to follow an anatomical gradient, starting in the marrow and ending in brain tissue. The frequency and density of infiltrates decrease from dura to brain parenchyma. The pia-glia is the only real anatomical barrier. Probably leukemic cells infiltrate directly from the skull bones into brain parenchyma via the perivenous adventitial tissue connecting the dura and subarachnoid space.

► [The anatomical evidence supports the concept that leukemic cells infiltrate the central nervous system by way of perivenous adventitial tissue connecting the dura mater and subarachnoid space. It is suggested that this pathway leads directly from the bones of the skull into the brain parenchyma. — Ed.] ◄

Neurologic Complications of Acute Myelomonoblastic Leukemia of Four Years' Duration. James O. Ballard, Javad Towfighi, Robert W. Brennan, Shazadi Saleem and M. Elaine Eyster[6] (Pennsylvania State Univ.) describe an adult with the acute myelomonoblastic subtype of acute nonlymphoblastic leukemia who survived 53 months with prophylactic treatment of the central nervous system.

Woman, 24, with fatigue and easy bruising for 1 month, was anemic and had about 50% blasts with a white blood cell count of 46,000/cu mm. A marrow aspirate confirmed myelomonoblastic-type acute leukemia. A complete marrow remission was obtained with cytosine arabinoside and 6-thioguanine, lasting 4 years before papilledema and right limb weakness developed. A brain scan showed increased uptake in the left posterior parietal lobe, where EEG slowing was evident, and angiography showed a large avascular frontoparietal mass. The bone marrow was normal. Symptoms resolved on dexamethasone therapy, but recurred several months later, with a generalized seizure, and evidence of a right parietal lesion was obtained. Intrathecal cytosine arabinoside therapy and whole brain irradiation were followed by rapid, complete improvement. Subsequently irradiation of the sacral spine relieved low back pain. Paresis of the right leg and absence of the right ankle jerk persisted. Right eye pain and impaired vision ensued, with a progressive 3d nerve palsy. Orbital radiotherapy produced improvement. Reinduction chemotherapy was unsuccessful the next year, and complete right-sided blindness preceded the patient's death, about 4½ years after diagnosis.

Autopsy showed hemorrhagic vesiculobullous lesions in the left trigeminal distribution and lumbar and sacral dermatomes. Cowdry type A inclusions were found in the skin lesions and in erosions of the lower esophagus, and herpes-like particles were seen in the nuclei of degenerating skin squamous cells. The viscera were virtually free from leukemic infiltration. A $3 \times 3 \times 4$-cm right frontoparietal tumor consisted of sheets of immature cells (Fig 39) with

(6) Neurology (Minneap.) 28:174–178, February, 1978.

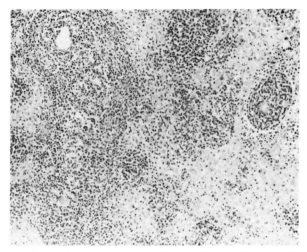

Fig 39. – Section from margin of cerebral tumor. Tumor cells have perivascular location in periphery (*right*); original magnification ×70. (Courtesy of Ballard, J. O., et al.: Neurology (Minneap.) 28:174–178, February, 1978.)

adjacent leukemic infiltration of the falx cerebri. The leptomeninges and lower cranial and all spinal nerve roots and ganglia were infiltrated by tumor cells. The optic nerves showed large areas of axon loss and demyelination in their intracranial portions. Inclusions were present in glial cells in involved areas, and herpes-like virus particles were seen intranuclearly in the optic nerves and left trigeminal ganglion.

Progressive neuropathy is the most common neural disorder in acute nonlymphoblastic leukemia. An intracerebral myeloblastic tumor was found in this patient. Her long survival permitted proliferation of leukemic cells in multiple areas of the central nervous system. The need for early central nervous system prophylaxis may become evident as longer remissions of acute nonlymphoblastic leukemia are obtained.

► [The prophylactic treatment of the central nervous system during remission of acute nonlymphoblastic leukemia may prove to be of benefit to patients with this disorder. – Ed.] ◄

Giant Cell Arteritis with Normal Sedimentation Rate. The erythrocyte sedimentation rate (ESR) is helpful in the diagnosis of giant cell arteritis, because it is almost always elevated during active stages of the disease, but a normal ESR does not unequivocally rule out giant cell arteritis. Tulay Kansu, James J. Corbett, Peter Savino and Norman J. Schatz[7] (Philadelphia) observed a normal ESR in 2 biopsy-proved cases of giant cell arteritis.

CASE 1. — Man, 73, who presented with reduced vision in the right eye and severe blurring on the left side, after 3 months of headaches, had an ESR of 13 mm/hour and subsequent values of 14 – 18 mm during treatment. Temporal artery biopsy 10 days after the start of steroid therapy was diagnostic of giant cell arteritis. The patient improved subjectively but had no improvement in visual function.

CASE 2. — Woman, 79, with sudden loss of vision on the right side and periorbital pain, had an ESR of 22 mm/hour and a repeat value of 30 mm/hour. Systemic steroid therapy did not lead to a return of vision in the right eye. Platelet counts were low and idiopathic thrombocytopenic purpura was diagnosed 9 months later.

Isolated cases of biopsy-proved giant cell arteritis with a normal ESR have been reported previously. Patients with ischemic optic neuropathy or retinal artery occlusion must receive large doses of systemic corticosteroids immediately. Anticipated temporal artery biopsy is no reason to delay treatment. A normal ESR in a patient with other suggestive clinical signs does not rule out giant cell arteritis.

▶ [Because of the potentially dangerous consequences of untreated giant cell arteritis, early therapy based on clinical diagnostic criteria is urged even though the erythrocyte sedimentation rate may be normal. — Ed.] ◀

Giant Cell Granulomatous Angiitis of Central Nervous System. Giant cell granulomatous angiitis is a rare noninfective inflammatory disease of the blood vessels. It has a predilection for the central nervous system, to which it may be almost entirely confined; however, it may also involve the large extracerebral vessels of the head and neck or other organs. K. Jellinger[8] (Vienna) reports 5 autopsy cases of giant cell granulomatous angiitis of the central nervous system in 3 men and 2 women, aged 42 – 71 years. Two patients died in weeks; the other 3 had recurrent illness for 16 months to 5 years. Clinical features included mental changes associated with hemiparesis or tetraparesis, extrapyramidal signs, visual disorders with optic atrophy, and

(7) Arch. Neurol. 34:624–625, October, 1977.
(8) J. Neurol. 215:175–190, 1977.

brain stem syndromes with final coma. The cerebrospinal fluid typically exhibited mild lymphocytosis and increased protein and γ-globulin levels.

The findings in a woman, aged 52, who 5 years earlier developed hemiparesis and visual disorder are shown in Figure 40. Autopsies showed generalized giant cell angiitis with aortitis in 2 patients and lesions confined to the central nervous system vasculature, affecting all types and sizes of vessels, in 3. The latter cases showed predominance of the disease for small leptomeningeal and intracerebral or spinal vessels. Disseminated microinfarctions of the brain and spinal cord were present in 2 cases. Larger recent and old infarcts were also observed. The earliest signs of the vasculitis were swelling and hyperplasia of the endothelium and lymphocytic infiltration of the adventitia. Fibrinoid changes and vessel wall necrosis appeared in the tunica media, with

Fig 40. – Right middle cerebral artery with incomplete occlusion of lumen, abundant fibrous tissue, partial destruction of internal elastic lamina and sparse lymphoid infiltration with absence of giant cells. Van Gieson; original magnification ×30. (Courtesy of Jellinger, K.: J. Neurol. 215:175–190, 1977; Berlin-Heidelberg-New York: Springer.)

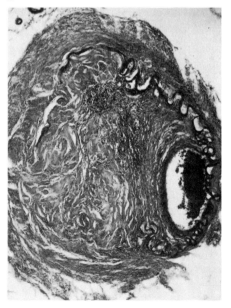

fragmentation of the internal elastic lamina, but caseous necrosis was not observed. The subarachnoid space contained moderate lymphomonocytic infiltrates in the adventitia of affected pial vessels.

Granulomatous angiitis of the central nervous system is considered to be a local variant of giant cell vasculitis, not a separate nosologic entity. The disease is perhaps best regarded as an immune complex disorder, although viral infection is also a consideration. Use of immunosuppressive agents and steroids might be indicated in suspected cases of giant cell angiitis of the central nervous system.

▶ [Most clinical neurologists would alter the term "might be indicated," as used above, to "is indicated." Temporal arteritis is a form of giant cell arteritis. At least one of these patients had a diagnostic temporal artery biopsy and all had elevated sedimentation rates. Steroid therapy is essential in giant cell arteritis, and with it ocular and cerebral complications may be avoided in many cases. — Ed.] ◀

Hemorrhagic Complications of Cerebral Arteritis. Intracranial hemorrhage due to cerebral arteritis is uncommon and not well known. Keith R. Edwards[9] (Univ. of Vermont) reports 2 cases that demonstrate the most serious such complications of cerebral arteritis: subarachnoid hemorrhage and intracerebral hematoma.

Woman, 21, had sudden occipital headache immediately after an intravenous injection of methamphetamine. She had a history of oral and intravenous amphetamine abuse and had had headaches and nausea after intravenous injections. On this occasion she had used far more than the usual amount of amphetamine. Confusion developed after a day at home and she was delirious and disoriented at the hospital. Gross hematuria and hematemesis developed the next day, and she was found to be lethargic and disoriented, with hyperreflexia and moderate nuchal rigidity. The cerebrospinal fluid pressure was 240 mm H_2O and the fluid was grossly bloody, with a xanthochromic supernatant. The protein concentration was 146 mg/100 ml. Angiography showed areas of segmental narrowing of many medium-sized arteries, with maximum involvement in the middle and anterior cerebral distributions (Fig 41). Several anterior branches of the left operculofrontal arteries were included. The patient improved on supportive care and was discharged after 3 weeks in a normal general medical and neurologic status.

The other patient had ulcerative colitis and developed an

(9)   Arch. Neurol. 34:549–552, September, 1977.

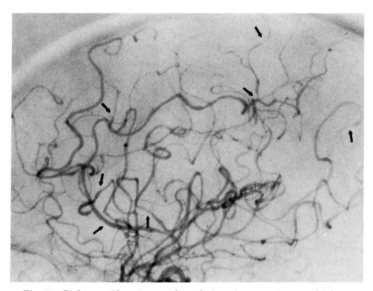

Fig 41. — Right carotid angiogram, lateral view. Arrows point to multiple areas of segmental narrowing and ectasia (subtraction technique). (Courtesy of Edwards, K. R.: Arch. Neurol. 34:549 – 552, September, 1977; copyright 1977, American Medical Association.)

intracerebral hematoma; diffuse arteritis was demonstrated by carotid angiography. This patient presented with focal seizures, hemiparesis, aphasia and an abnormal EEG. The hematoma may have been related to the use of heparin for treatment of thrombophlebitis.

There are several reports of intracranial hemorrhage in amphetamine abuse. Intracranial hemorrhage associated with collagen vascular diseases is infrequent, but available data may not reflect the true incidence of spontaneous intracranial hemorrhage in this setting. The diagnosis requires a high degree of suspicion and cerebral angiography. Rapid intervention with corticosteroids may be beneficial.

► [Although cerebral arteritis is relatively uncommon, it may be a cause of intracranial hemorrhage. It should always be suspected as a cause of subarachnoid hemorrhage or intracerebral hematoma, especially in patients with evidence of cerebral disease. — Ed.] ◄

Idiopathic Regressing Arteriopathy. Bahram Mokri, O. Wayne Houser and Thoralf M. Sundt, Jr.[1] (Mayo Clinic

(1)   Ann. Neurol. 2:466 – 472, December, 1977.

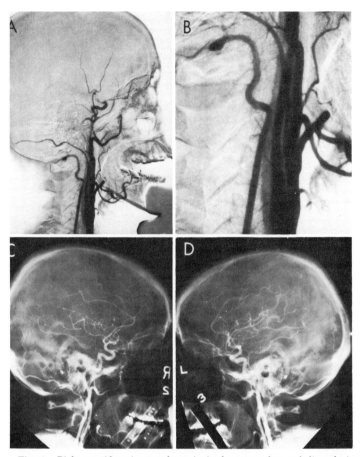

Fig 42. — Right carotid angiogram shows, in **A**, almost complete embolic occlusion of the supraclinoid segment and marked stenosis of the intracanalicular segment of the internal carotid artery, most likely due to arterial dissection. **B**, intimal irregularities of the cervical segment of the internal carotid artery are well seen. Notice visualization of the right vertebral artery due to reflux of contrast medium from the carotid into the innominate artery and to the right subclavian artery as a result of obstruction in the distal internal carotid artery. **C** and **D**, right and left carotid angiograms, respectively, 8 months later; carotid arteries are normal. (Courtesy of Mokri, B., et al.: Ann. Neurol. 2:466–472, December, 1977.)

and Found.) recently encountered 3 relatively young patients with an unusual nonatheromatous occlusive cervicocephalic arterial disease, angiographically similar to fibromuscular dysplasia. The disorder does not seem to be a simple spontaneous arterial dissection. Clinically and radiographically, the condition seems to be reversible.

Woman, 36, had a brief syncopal episode without injury, followed in a few hours by left hemiparesis and a steady left frontotemporal headache. Fibromuscular dysplasia of the right internal carotid artery was diagnosed at angiography elsewhere. Birth control pills, used for 8 years, were discontinued. The hemiparesis improved but persistent left orbital-periorbital pain was reported 7 months later. A mild left spastic hemiparesis was present. A computerized axial tomography scan showed a cystic lesion in the right posterofrontal region. Studies for collagen vascular disease and inflammatory disease were negative. Review of the previous angiograms showed stenosis of a long segment of the cervical part of the internal carotid artery (Fig 42, A and B). Repeat angiography, done 9 months after the first study, showed no abnormalities (Fig 42, C and D). The patient has had steady but slowly decreasing pain in the left orbital-periorbital region.

These patients presented with unilateral headache or focal head, neck or mastoid pain at a relatively young age. The angiographic changes resolved partially or completely. The angiograms showed intimal irregularities and multiple-vessel involvement, with a tendency to arterial dissection and aneurysm formation. Intracranial arteries were spared. This entity has been termed "idiopathic regressing arteriopathy," pending histopathologic studies. The arterial abnormalities were never typical of fibromuscular dysplasia.

▶ [The authors have chosen a rather inept title for the syndrome they have described. According to *Webster's Third New International Dictionary,* "regression" means a trend "toward a lower or less perfect state," or a progressive decline. The vasculitis regressed but the patients all improved, and their angiograms showed lessening or disappearance of abnormal features. — Ed.] ◀

Abnormality of a Thiamine-Requiring Enzyme in Patients with Wernicke-Korsakoff Syndrome. John P. Blass and Gary E. Gibson[2] (Univ. of California, Los Angeles) report the finding of abnormalities of a thiamine-dependent enzyme in 4 patients with the Wernicke-Korsakoff syn-

(2) N. Engl. J. Med. 297:1367 – 1370, Dec. 22, 1977.

drome. They were the first patients with the syndrome studied and had clinical abnormalities characteristic of the syndrome. All had a history of alcohol abuse and chronic malnutrition, were admitted with acute Wernicke's syndrome, responded promptly to thiamine and had a documented residual confabulatory psychosis. Skin cells from a biopsy specimen were cultured in modified minimal essential medium supplemented with heat-inactivated fetal calf serum. Transketolase activity was measured by double-beam spectrophotometry. Control cell lines were obtained from 4 clinically normal subjects and 2 patients with Friedreich's ataxia.

Transketolase in fibroblasts from study patients bound thiamine pyrophosphate less avidly than did that in control cell lines. The apparent mean K_m values for thiamine pyrophosphate was 195 μM for transketolase in patient cell extracts and 16 μM in 6 control lines. The abnormality persisted through serial passages in tissue culture in cells grown in medium containing excess thiamine and no ethanol, indicating that the aberration is genetic rather than dietary.

These findings indicate an abnormality in a thiamine-dependent enzyme, transketolase, in patients with the Wernicke-Korsakoff syndrome. Reduced transketolase activity may be involved in the pathogenesis of at least this form of thiamine deficiency. The abnormality would presumably be clinically unimportant if the diet were adequate. Interaction between abnormalities in a specific enzyme protein and a specific environmental stress in patients who acquire "Korsakoff's psychosis" may prove to be a model for the relationship between genetic and environmental factors in more common psychoses.

► [Patients who develop the Wernicke-Korsakoff syndrome have been shown to have a serious inborn enzymatic defect — an abnormality of transketolase, a thiamine-requiring enzyme. This abnormality would presumably be clinically unimportant if the diet were adequate, but when it is thiamine deficient and excessive alcohol is ingested, the Wernicke-Korsakoff syndrome develops. — Ed.] ◄

Diagnosis of Alcohol Ingestion in Mild Head Injuries. Alcoholic intoxication and concussion have many features in common. The doctor in an accident-and-emergency department would wish to know about the alcoholic state of a patient with head injury to make a correct diagnosis, mon-

itor the level of consciousness and guard against accumulation of water by brain cells in a patient with a high blood
alcohol content. Legal testimony also requires knowledge of
the alcoholic state of a patient. William H. Rutherford[3]
(Belfast, Northern Ireland) evaluated the effects of alcohol
ingestion as part of a study on the aftereffects of mild head
injuries with concussion. Clinical and laboratory findings in
114 patients with head injuries were reviewed.

Forty-eight of the 114 patients had positive blood alcohol
tests. Three patients with negative tests were judged clinically to have alcohol in their blood, for an error rate of 4.5%.
A total of 14 errors was made (12.3%) overall, or 8.3% if
blood alcohol concentrations of 1–99 mg/dl are excluded.

Over 40% of patients in this series with mild head injuries
had positive blood alcohol tests. The problem of diagnosis is
of more than academic importance. Some errors resulted
from doctors discounting the importance of signs that they
observed and recorded. Until further study shows that clinical diagnosis can be made more accurate, there is a strong
case for a laboratory test for blood alcohol. It is debatable
whether a test of serum osmolality has any advantage over
a blood alcohol test. Both readings might be of advantage for
seriously injured patients. A paper dipstick test would probably be adequate in many cases, with more accurate laboratory confirmation the next morning.

► [For correct treatment of a confused patient who has had a head injury,
a laboratory test giving immediate quantitative information about recent
alcohol ingestion is needed. – Ed.] ◄

**Brain Damage in Chronic Alcoholism: Neuropatho-
logic, Neuroradiologic and Psychologic Review** is presented by M. A. Ron[4] (London). Alcohol abuse and its consequences are among the more serious and frequent of the
problems facing medical and social agencies. A number of
recognized neuropsychiatric conditions follow alcohol withdrawal or are associated with nutritional deficiencies, but
the possibility that less clinically obvious forms of brain
damage occur in chronic alcoholics is more controversial.

The presence of cerebral atrophy in some patients is clear,
but it is difficult to extrapolate these neuropathologic find-

(3) Lancet 1:1021–1023, May 14, 1977.
(4) Psychol. Med. 7:103–112, February, 1977.

ings to the alcoholic population as a whole. Neuroradiologic evidence of cerebral atrophy has emerged repeatedly in chronic alcoholics, but it is unclear how frequent these changes may be in an unselected series. No significant difference in IQ has been found between large groups of chronic alcoholics and the normal population. A specific pattern of deficits is observed on special testing. Impairment of ability to perform complex psychomotor tasks and impairment of some functions usually attributed to the frontal lobes are evident. The deficits can be found in subjects of above-average IQ. A long-term follow-up of chronic alcoholics who continue drinking over many years would be needed to determine whether brain damage due to alcoholism is progressive.

Studies on a large, representative group of alcoholics are necessary to minimize sampling bias. Assessments must be extremely comprehensive and include the collection of historical and clinical data, psychologic testing with carefully selected instruments, and the use of appropriate neuroradiologic techniques. Such a cohort must be assessed repeatedly over a period of years. Autopsy studies should be done whenever possible, although their value is likely to remain limited. Present evidence seems to be sufficient to justify alerting the clinician to the possibility of brain damage in a proportion of his alcoholic patients.

▶ [Whereas it is often assumed that diffuse brain damage occurs in chronic alcoholism, there have been few definitive studies to verify this. This article reviews the current neuropathologic, neuroradiologic and psychologic data on chronic alcoholism and stresses the need for more detailed objective study of this problem. — Ed.] ◀

Clinical Manifestations of Chronic Thiamine Deficiency in Rhesus Monkey. Both Oriental beriberi and the Wernicke-Korsakoff syndrome are attributed largely to nutritional thiamine deficiency. Marek-Marsel Mesulam, Gary W. Van Hoesen and Nelson Butters[5] (Boston) report observations on 4 rhesus monkeys subjected to recurrent episodes of rigorous thiamine deficiency for periods of up to 350 days. Four control animals received weekly thiamine injections. Thiamine was given intramuscularly to all animals when death seemed imminent, and another episode of deficiency was then begun.

(5) Neurology (Minneap.) 27:239–245, March, 1977.

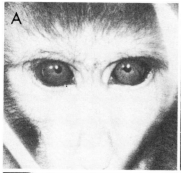
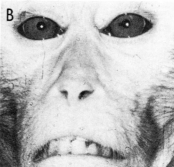
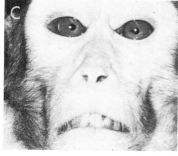

Fig 43. – Bilateral abducens pareses. A, convergent strabismus. B, ice water in right ear elicits expected adduction of left eye, but right eye fails to abduct. C, ice water in left ear demonstrates failure of abduction of left eye. (Courtesy of Mesulam, M.-M., et al.: Neurology (Minneap.) 27:239–245, March, 1977.)

The study animals exhibited anorexia, apathy, weakness of the leg muscles, nystagmus, abducens weakness, heart failure and truncal and limb ataxia. Loss of reflexes, abnormality of sensation and peripheral edema were not observed. Most signs were rapidly reversed by thiamine administration. Maximal clinical deterioration occurred after 39–105 days of the thiamine-deficient diet. Anorexia and apathy were the earliest signs, the latter heralding a phase of rapid deterioration. All study animals exhibited ataxia and abnormal ocular movements (Fig 43). The first sign of recovery was amelioration of apathy and anorexia. The clinical impression of thiamine deficiency was nearly always corroborated by blood transketolase determinations. No control animals showed any abnormal clinical features.

The clinical picture in these animals is remarkably similar to that of Wernicke's encephalopathy in both alcoholic and starved subjects. The paradigm of recurrent thiamine-deficient episodes resembles the nutritional pattern of many

habitual alcoholics. Genetic differences may be largely responsible for the manifestation of thiamine deficiency as
Oriental beriberi and as the Wernicke-Korsakoff syndrome.
Eventually the early identification of vulnerable persons
may lead to the adoption of preventive measures.

► [In Orientals the major manifestations of thiamine deficiency are those
of beriberi, whereas in Occidental populations the usual picture is that of
the Wernicke-Korsakoff syndrome. This study of thiamine deficiency in
rhesus monkeys shows that these laboratory animals develop some manifestations of both the syndromes, but not the complete picture of either.
Genetic factors may be responsible for determining the type of manifestations that occur in human beings. — Ed.] ◄

Neuropathies

Lead Neuropathy in Adults and Children. Robert G. Feldman, Margaret K. Hayes, Robert Younes and Franklin D. Aldrich[6] found in field studies of steel burner workers and of children in a housing project that measurement of motor nerve conduction velocity (MNCV) may serve as a factor in the diagnosis of otherwise unrecognized toxic effects of lead. The adult patients studied worked in high-risk environments and had had increased body burdens of lead for 4–20 years. Blood concentrations were generally above 80 μg/100 ml. The neuropathy was principally motor oriented. The mean peroneal MNCV in 6 cases was 41.4 m per second, significantly different from the adult control mean of 54.1 m per second. Four patients had an MNCV less than 2 SD below the control mean.

A field study was done on workers exposed to lead oxide fumes when they were dismantling a lead-painted elevated train track network. There were no abnormal physical findings. Both burner and nonburner workers had reduced MNCV values. Free erythrocyte protoporphyrin levels were elevated. The concentration of lead in respired air was high. The response to chelation therapy confirmed the diagnosis. The mean MNCV in 26 housing project children was 46.7 m per second, significantly below the mean for unexposed children. Ten children had values 1 SD or more below the control mean. Seven children were chelated with edetate disodium calcium. A possible relationship was found between MNCV slowing and amount of lead excreted in the urine after provocation.

The toxic effects of lead have both central and peripheral nervous system manifestations. Both segmental demyelination and axon degeneration have been demonstrated in the peripheral nerves of guinea pigs with chronic lead ingestion. Accumulation of exuded protein-rich material in the endo-

(6) Arch. Neurol. 34:481–488, August, 1977.

neural compartment could produce Schwann cell damage by pressure or indirectly by ischemia. Measurements of MNCV may help in diagnosis of otherwise unrecognized toxic effects of lead.

► [It appears that all parts of the nervous system may be affected in lead intoxication, regardless of the age of the patient or the source of environmental hazard. — Ed.] ◄

Alcoholic Neuropathy: Clinical, Electrophysiologic and Biopsy Findings. F. Behse and F. Buchthal[7] (Copenhagen) reviewed the findings in 37 patients who had alcoholic neuropathy with or without overt nutritional deficiency and compared them with those of 6 nonalcoholic postgastrectomy patients who had neuropathy associated with nutritional deficiency. Most study patients took beer at a level of about 100 ml ethanol daily. Fourteen alcoholics had overt evidence of nutritional deficiency. Six had marked weight loss, and 6 had signs of malabsorption secondary to chronic pancreatitis or gastrectomy. Two had hepatic cirrhosis, associated in 1 with thiamine deficiency. Sural nerve biopsy specimens obtained from 42 patients and teased fibers from 23 nerves were evaluated.

Major involvement, with severe leg muscle weakness and reduced sensation in the feet, was present in 19 alcoholic patients. Eleven had weakness in distal upper extremity muscles. Eighteen patients had mild involvement. Neuropathy had been present for over a year in two thirds of the patients. Muscle weakness improved substantially on thiamine therapy in 6 of 9 cases. Sensory potential amplitudes were reduced in alcoholic neuropathy. Conduction abnormality was confined to the nerves of the leg in 7 patients. Sensory and motor conduction was markedly slowed in the leg nerves in all nonalcoholic patients. Biopsy specimens in alcoholics showed a reduction in myelinated fibers and myelin clumps from degenerated fibers in those patients with and those without nutritional deficiency. Three specimens from postgastrectomy patients showed marked fiber loss. Essentially all examined muscles of alcoholic patients showed electromyographic signs of denervation or reinnervation. All muscles in postgastrectomy patients showed these signs.

Primary segmental demyelination is not the underlying

---

(7)　Ann. Neurol. 2:95–110, August, 1977.

abnormality in alcoholic neuropathy; a toxic action of alcohol on peripheral nerve is more likely. Teased fibers from postgastrectomy patients with malnutrition exhibit segmental demyelination. Malnutrition and low blood vitamin B levels do not appear to be necessary for the development of neuropathy in alcoholics.

► [The authors interpret their data as showing evidence that alcoholic neuropathy is not due to vitamin deficiency or malnutrition and suggesting that alcohol has a toxic action on the peripheral nerves. This certainly is in contrast to the more or less universally held opinion that alcoholic neuropathy is a deficiency disease. These conclusions need further confirmation. — Ed.] ◄

Subacute Sensory Neuropathy: Remote Effect of Carcinoma. Mark S. Horwich, Lucy Cho, Robert S. Porro and Jerome B. Posner[8] describe 7 new patients with subacute sensory neuropathy seen at Memorial Hospital for Cancer and Allied Diseases, New York, and review the findings in 29 previously reported cases. Subacute severe sensory loss is usually associated with relatively good motor power, a high cerebrospinal fluid protein level, and inflammation and widespread degeneration of dorsal root ganglia in these cases. With rare exceptions the condition is associated with an underlying neoplasm. All 7 current patients were women; their average age was 51 years. Only 5 had proved cancer. Lung carcinoma was present in 1 case and in 24 of the 29 previously reported cases.

Initially, pain, paresthesias, dysesthesias and numbness occur in the extremities, usually distally, and spread proximally over a period of weeks. Unsteadiness of gait is prominent and disabling. Hypotonia and muscle wasting are frequent findings, but weakness is never as severe as the sensory symptoms. Occasionally signs of more diffuse nervous system involvement are present.

The cerebrospinal fluid protein has been elevated in most cases, and several patients had mild lymphocytosis. The EEG was abnormal in 4 current cases, showing bilateral slowing without a distinctive pattern. On electromyography, spontaneous activity suggesting a neurogenic disorder is unusual. Four previous patients had circulating antineuronal antibodies. No virus has been isolated. Various treatments have failed to reverse the syndrome. Remov-

(8)   Ann. Neurol. 2:7 – 19, July, 1977.

al or destruction of neoplastic tissue in 3 of the present cases was not followed by neurologic improvement. The neuro-pathologic findings include degeneration of dorsal root ganglia, posterior roots and peripheral sensory nerves and the posterior white columns of the spinal cord. Minimal neurogenic muscle atrophy is observed.

The primary pathologic process appears to be in the dorsal root ganglion, with secondary degeneration producing proximal and distal nerve changes. The cause of this sensory neuropathy is unknown. Antibrain antibodies were not found in the 2 current patients evaluated.

► [Subacute sensory neuropathy is a rare condition. When the diagnosis is made, one should always consider the possibility that it may be a remote effect of carcinoma. – Ed.] ◄

Acute Peripheral Facial Palsy: Part of a Cranial Polyneuropathy? Increasing evidence points to viral infection as a cause of acute peripheral facial palsy (APFP). Gisle Djupesland, Miklos Degré, Ragnar Stien and Sverre Skrede[9] (Rikshosp., Oslo) investigated the possible involvement of other cranial nerves in APFP in 18 consecutive patients, 16 of them evaluable. The 11 female and 5 male patients were aged 12 – 61 years. All were initially seen within a week after onset of palsy. Ten patients accepted hospitalization for cerebrospinal fluid (CSF) examination.

Other cranial nerves often exhibited impaired function. Ten patients had trigeminal dysfunction on the same side as the facial palsy. The 2d cranial nerve was affected in 5 patients. Six had a transitory sensorineural hearing loss on the affected side; 2 had herpes zoster oticus. Transitory stapedius paralysis was found in 4 of these patients. Seven patients had difficulties with equilibrium and posture, impaired fine movements, and nystagmus. Definite ipsilateral palatal paresis was present in 1 patient. Six patients, besides the 2 with herpes zoster oticus, had significant changes in viral antibody titers; varicella-zoster virus was implicated in 3 of these and cytomegalovirus in 2. No viral isolations were made. The CSF total protein and γ-globulin levels were significantly increased. The sedimentation rate and immunoglobulin levels were abnormal in a few patients.

It is concluded that in most patients APFP is part of a

(9) Arch. Otolaryngol. 103:641 – 644, November, 1977.

cranial polyneuropathy. "Monosymptomatic" peripheral facial palsy was present in only 2 patients in this series. The viral and laboratory studies further indicate that acute cranial polyneuropathy may be caused by a viral infection, possibly at a proximal or even brain stem level of the involved nerves.

► [From this study, as well as those of Adour and others, it appears that many, if not all, cases of acute peripheral facial palsy are part of a cranial polyneuritis (Adour, K. K.: Arch. Otolaryngol. 102:262, 1976). — Ed.] ◄

Vascular Disease of the Nervous System

Carotid and Vertebral-Basilar Transient Ischemic Attacks: Effect of Anticoagulants, Hypertension and Cardiac Disorders on Survival and Stroke Occurrence – Population Study. Jack P. Whisnant, Niall E. F. Cartlidge and Lila R. Elveback[1] (Mayo Clinic and Found.) followed 199 patients from the time of their first carotid or vertebral-basilar transient ischemic attack in 1955 – 69. The index carotid symptoms included motor or sensory symptoms limited to one side of the body, aphasia or dysphasia, and retinal ischemia (amaurosis fugax). Vertebral-basilar features included bilateral motor or sensory symptoms, or both, ataxia of gait or clumsiness of the extremities on both sides, diplopia, dysphagia and bilateral homonymous hemianopia. Vertigo alone was not an indication of transient ischemic attack. The aim of oral anticoagulation was to maintain the prothrombin time at about two times the control value. Study was made of 122 patients with carotid and 64 with vertebral-basilar transient ischemic attacks.

Survival was significantly lower than expected for untreated patients at 1 and 5 years. Patients with carotid transient ischemic attack who did not receive anticoagulants had significantly lower than expected survival through 5 years of observation. Treated patients and both treated and untreated groups with vertebral-basilar transient ischemic attack had no significant differences from expected survival. Both treated and untreated patients had higher stroke rates than expected for age and sex. Anticoagulated patients had a significantly lower risk of stroke at 3 months. Intracranial hemorrhage was more frequent in anticoagulated patients, especially those aged 55 – 74. Almost all hemorrhages occurred after a year or more of anticoagulation in patients

---

(1) Ann. Neurol. 3:107 – 115, February, 1978.

over age 65. Stroke was more frequent in patients with high diastolic blood pressure. Survival and stroke were not related to previous myocardial infarction, angina, valvular heart disease, cardiac arrhythmia or congestive heart failure.

The only factors influencing stroke occurrence in this series of patients with carotid and vertebral-basilar transient ischemic attack were diastolic blood pressure and anticoagulant therapy.

▶ [It appears from this study that diastolic blood pressure levels and anticoagulant therapy are the only factors that influence stroke recurrence. Previous myocardial infarction, angina pectoris, valvular heart disease, cardiac arrhythmia and congestive heart failure, either individually or combined, did not influence patient survival or the recurrence of stroke. — Ed.] ◀

Supraorbital Photoplethysmography: Simple, Accurate Screening for Carotid Occlusive Disease. The risks and discomfort of contrast angiography prevent its use in routine screening for carotid occlusive disease. Ophthalmodynamometry and ultrasound study require considerable attention to technique for maximal accuracy. Thermography and ocular plethysmography require expensive equipment and the latter requires topical anesthesia of the eye. Robert W. Barnes, James M. Clayton, George E. Bone, Earlene E. Slaymaker and John Reinertson[2] (Univ. of Iowa) have used a simpler technique of supraorbital photoplethysmography (PPG) to record abnormal flow dynamics in the frontal and supraorbital arteries, which are terminal branches of the ophthalmic artery on the forehead. Seventy-eight consecutive patients undergoing contrast angiography for suspected cerebrovascular disease were used to evaluate this modality. The PPG consists of a transducer with power source and a strip-chart recorder. Patients are studied while they are supine during a series of maneuvers to compress major external carotid branches and each common carotid artery.

Attenuation of the PPG tracing is significant if the supraorbital pulsation decreases by more than one third of the resting amplitude on temporal artery compression or by over 15% on infraorbital or facial artery compression. The PPG correctly identified all stenoses of 50% or greater and all occlusions of the extracranial internal carotid artery.

(2) J. Surg. Res. 22:319–327, April, 1977.

There were no false negative results. The study indicated 10 of 44 lesser stenoses. The supraorbital PPG was normal in 68 of 76 patients with angiographically normal carotid arteries. When 10 arteries with an abnormal PPG and stenosis of less than 50% were omitted, the specificity of the study in excluding significant carotid disease was 92.7%. Two of 8 false positive studies were associated with proved retinal artery occlusions and 2 others with anomalous sources of supraorbital artery flow. Two other patients had had forehead lacerations. The ipsilateral temporal artery was the primary source of collateral circulation in over two thirds of truly abnormal studies.

Supraorbital photoplethysmography is a simple, noninvasive means of detecting significant obstruction of the extracranial internal carotid artery. The study may be definitive in many situations in which detection of a hemodynamically significant lesion is of prime importance in patient management. It is also useful in screening high-risk patients for asymptomatic carotid disease and in screening patients with a neurologic deficit after carotid endarterectomy for occlusion of the vessel that was operated on. The results must be interpreted cautiously in patients with cerebrovascular ischemia.

▶ [This technique, which requires no ocular anesthesia or risk of ocular injury, may prove to be a useful noninvasive technique to screen patients for significant carotid artery occlusive disease. — Ed.] ◀

Carotid Stenosis and Coexisting Ipsilateral Intracranial Aneurysm: Problem in Management. Harold P. Adams, Jr.[3] (Univ. of Iowa) describes a patient treated surgically for carotid stenosis who later died of subarachnoid hemorrhage from rupture of an asymptomatic ipsilateral cerebral aneurysm.

Woman, 84, seen for an episode of right amaurosis fugax and transient left hemiparesis, had normal neurologic findings. An arch aortogram showed marked irregularity of the right carotid bifurcation and origin of the internal carotid and marked stenosis of the left carotid bifurcation. Severe stenosis of the left subclavian and vertebral and brachiocephalic arteries was also found. A 5×10-mm left internal carotid-posterior communicating junctional aneurysm was observed. Expressive aphasia followed angiography. A plaque was removed at left carotid endarterectomy. The

(3)   Arch. Neurol. 34:515–516, August, 1977.

lumen had not been entirely compromised. The aphasia gradually resolved postoperatively, but the patient was found comatose 7 months later and died on the day of admission.

Autopsy showed a ruptured aneurysm arising from the junction of the left posterior communicating and internal carotid arteries. A small unruptured aneurysm was found arising about 0.5 cm proximal to the middle cerebral trifurcation on the right side. Moderate atherosclerosis affected the circle of Willis. A small cystic infarction in the left parieto-occipital junction was thought to be at least 2 months old.

The altered hemodynamics created by endarterectomy must be considered in the decision to treat a higher asymptomatic aneurysm ipsilateral to a carotid stenosis. Routine angiographic follow-up may not be adequate. A more aggressive approach to the aneurysm may be warranted in this setting.

► [When carotid stenosis and an ipsilateral cerebral aneurysm coexist, repair of the former may result in an increase in blood flow that may result in rupture of the higher aneurysm. – Ed.] ◄

Vertebral Artery Occlusion Complicating Yoga Exercises.

Yoga exercises are popular as a form of recreation and a mode of relaxation and infrequently may result in medical and neurologic complications. Steven H. Hanus, Terri D. Homer and Donald H. Harter[4] (Northwestern Univ.) report data on a patient who sustained vertebral artery occlusion with a marked neurologic deficit shortly after performing yoga exercises that involved neck manipulation.

Man, 25, had suddenly had paresthesias of the left side of the face 2 hours after performing yoga exercises; he had done such exercises each day for 18 months. Blurred vision and vertigo had developed, followed by inability to walk without help and dysphagia. In one exercise he had kept the head hyperrotated and extended to the left and then to the right for 3 minutes, followed by 5 minutes of inverted standing with the neck maximally flexed against the floor. Ecchymoses were seen over the spinous processes of C5 – 7. The patient could not walk even with help and exhibited rotatory nystagmus, hypalgesia and hypesthesia of the left side of the face, palatal deviation to the right and weakness and tremor of the left extremities. Pain sensation was impaired on the right side of the body. The signs were compatible with a left lateral medullary lesion. Angiography showed occlusion of the left vertebral artery at the C2 – C3 level and filling of the distal left vertebral ar-

(4)   Arch. Neurol. 34:574–575, September, 1977.

tery from the right side, with delayed emptying. A left Horner's syndrome developed and the patient remained extremely ataxic. He could walk with a cane 2 months after the onset, but continued to have marked difficulty performing fine movements with the left hand.

Only 1 other case of vertebral artery compromise due to yoga exercises is known. Neither patient had preexisting cerebrovascular disease or bony abnormalities of the cervical spine. The vertebral artery apparently can be compromised in normal subjects by neck movements that exceed physiologic tolerance. Yoga exercises should be considered as a possible precipitating event in patients with acute vertebral artery occlusion and medullary or cerebellar infarction.

▶ [It is apparent that yoga exercises are a potential cause of medullary and cerebellar infarction. – Ed.] ◀

Relationship of Arterial Hypertension to Intracranial Aneurysms. William F. McCormick and Elisabeth J. Schmalstieg[5] (Univ. of Texas, Galveston) analyzed the findings in 250 patients with proved intracranial saccular aneurysms: 100 autopsy patients had proved ruptured aneurysms, 100 autopsy patients had incidental unruptured aneurysms and 50 clinical patients had angiographically proved aneurysms. A total of 500 nonaneurysm adult autopsy cases, closely matched with the aneurysm patients for age, sex and race, served as controls.

Most patients who died with proved ruptured aneurysm were aged 45 – 55 years; the average age at death was 49 years. The average age at autopsy of patients with unruptured aneurysms was 61.9 years. Systemic hypertension was present in 37% of the patients with ruptured aneurysms and 43% of those with incidental aneurysms. The average age of the former patients was 55.2 years, compared with 45.3 years for normotensive autopsied patients with ruptured aneurysms. One fourth of all aneurysm patients had two or more aneurysms. The prevalence of hypertension in the nonaneurysm control group was 43.6%; average age in this group was 53.3 years. One hundred consecutive nonaneurysm patients with various central nervous system diseases had an average age of 47.7 years; 30% were hypertensive.

(5) Arch. Neurol. 34:285 – 287, May, 1977.

Fifty consecutive patients with angiographically proved saccular aneurysms had an average age of 47.8 years; 36% were hypertensive. There was no notable age difference between those with hypertension and the others.

A notable excess of hypertension has not been found in aneurysm patients. Present data do not support the view that hypertension is a major factor in the genesis of intracranial saccular aneurysms or the major factor in their rupture. Saccular aneurysms can and do rupture in the absence of fixed arterial hypertension, but transient elevations of blood pressure may play a role in aneurysm rupture. This role, however, is not all-important, because most aneurysms never rupture.

► [The authors conclude that there is no evident association between hypertension and multiplicity of aneurysms, the age at which aneurysms first become manifest clinically or their rupture. All available data indicate that saccular aneurysms can arise in the absence of fixed arterial hypertension and that they can also rupture in the absence of fixed hypertension. – Ed.] ◄

Importance of Holter Monitoring in Patients with Periodic Cerebral Symptoms. Transient cardiac arrhythmias may reduce cerebral blood flow and result in transient cerebral symptoms. Sterling Jonas, Irv Klein and Jacob Dimant[6] (New York) report the findings in 358 consecutive patients with intermittent dizziness or blackout who were referred for Holter monitoring in an 18-month period in 1974–75. None showed evidence of a pertinent arrhythmia on examination or a 1-minute resting ECG. The 188 women and 170 men had an average age of 67.2 years. None had a pacemaker present or had focal neurologic abnormalities. Monitoring was for 12 hours in 102 cases and for 24 hours in 256 cases.

Correlative arrhythmias were seen in 8.9% of patients, short-duration predisposing arrhythmias in 11.2% and high-frequency ectopic beats in 24.6%. Arrhythmias known to be related to dizziness or syncope were seen in 32 patients, the most common being sustained bradycardia. Fourteen patients had symptoms during the arrhythmia, and 8 others had the arrhythmia during sleep. Arrhythmias not ordinarily related to dizziness or syncope were demonstrated in 36.9% of the patients. No arrhythmias were demon-

(6) Ann. Neurol. 1:470–474, May, 1977.

strated in 18.4% of the patients. An increase in incidence of pertinent arrhythmias from 13.8% to 22.7% was seen with 24-hour compared to 12-hour monitoring.

Nearly 10% of patients with dizziness or blackout in this series exhibited arrhythmias known to correlate with cerebral symptoms on Holter monitoring. Nearly all patients in whom intermittent arrhythmias precipitated symptoms had many predisposing arrhythmias of short duration during the asymptomatic period. A specific arrhythmia at a given rate does not consistently result in cerebral symptoms, but symptoms in the presence of a normal tape recording would tend to rule out cardiac arrhythmia as a cause.

► [The importance of cerebral monitoring in patients with periodic cerebral symptoms has been emphasized in the past and reference to it has been made in previous editions of this YEAR BOOK. In the present study, however, it was brought out that the finding of pertinent arrhythmias increased from 13.8% to 22.7% when the duration of the monitoring was increased from 12 to 24 hours. — Ed.] ◄

Long-Term Prognosis in Untreated Cerebral Aneurysms: I. Incidence of Late Hemorrhage in Cerebral Aneurysm; Ten-Year Evaluation of 364 Patients. H. Richard Winn, Alan E. Richardson and John A. Jane[7] followed 364 patients for up to 21 years after subarachnoid hemorrhage from an aneurysm in the posterior communicating artery (PCA) or anterior communicating artery (ACA). They received no surgical treatment. Each patient had a single cerebral aneurysm. An ACA aneurysm was present in 71% and a PCA aneurysm in 29%. Most patients were considered to be surgical candidates but were allotted to nonsurgical treatment in an aneurysm trial. A total of 213 survivors were examined at 6 months and followed yearly. Forty-nine are still being followed through the first 10 years.

Of the 213 6-month survivors, 61 went on to have a late hemorrhage, 54 within the first 10 years. Peak incidence of rebleeding centered around year 3. Eleven patients with late hemorrhage died before hospitalization. Most hospital deaths occurred in the 1st week. Twenty-seven of 41 patients with ACA aneurysms and 10 of 20 with PCA aneurysms died. In the PCA group, the only factor related to rebleeding was blood pressure. Discriminant scores for PCA

(7) Ann. Neurol. 1:358–370, April, 1977.

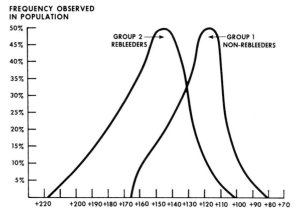

Fig 44.—Discriminant scores for PCA aneurysm patients: rebleeders versus non-rebleeders. Equation for discriminant score: $D_s = -22$ (1 for male, 0 for female) + 0.9 (systolic blood pressure) −0.069 (diastolic blood pressure). (Courtesy of Winn, H. R., et al.: Ann. Neurol. 1:358–370, April, 1977.)

Fig 45.—Relation between age and time to rebleeding. Patients over age 40 years took 4.4 years to rebleed, whereas those under age 40 years rebled at 9.8 years (P < 0.001 by t test). (Courtesy of Winn, H. R., et al.: Ann. Neurol. 1:358–370, April, 1977.)

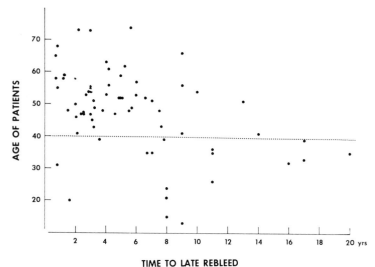

patients are shown in Figure 44 and the relation of age to time of rebleeding in Figure 45. All 17 patients who rebled and who had angiography at the time of hemorrhage, 1–9 years after initial bleeding, showed aneurysmal enlargement.

If the propensity to rebleed could be accurately predicted, the efficacy of treatment for cerebral aneurysms could be assessed more adequately. The evidence of a constant yearly rebleeding rate of at least 3% emphasizes the chronicity of this process. Assessment of treatment for cerebral aneurysms must therefore no longer deal merely with short-term prognosis.

▶ [This is really a remarkable study. Three hundred sixty-four patients with aneurysms that were not operated on have been studied for up to 21 years. There has long been debate, still unresolved, concerning medical versus surgical therapy for subarachnoid hemorrhage. The results of this study show that the prognosis in such patients is definitely better than it has been considered to be. Assessment of treatment for cerebral aneurysms, therefore, must no longer deal merely with the short-term prognosis. — Ed.] ◀

Miscellaneous Neurologic Disorders

Azorean Disease of the Nervous System. A degenerative disorder of the nervous system has been described in three families descended from immigrants from the Portuguese Azores. Two of the families reside in Massachusetts. Flaviu C. A. Romanul, Hilton L. Fowler, Joao Radvany, Robert G. Feldman and Murray Feingold[8] (Boston) studied 4 members of another Massachusetts family of the same origin with a degenerative nervous system disease; autopsies were done in 2 cases.

Man, 33, had difficulty walking and in the next years had progressive loss of strength, muscle wasting and difficulty swallowing. He became unable to walk at age 58, when speech was slow and dysarthric and nystagmus was present. A masklike facies and a limb tremor at rest were noted. Muscle tone was reduced and fasciculations were present in all muscles. Deep tendon reflexes and plantar responses were absent. Perception of all stimuli was reduced in the distal lower extremities. The cerebrospinal fluid was normal. The patient remained bedridden and died at age 61.

Autopsy showed an old myocardial infarction and acute bronchopneumonia. Brain sections showed striking depigmentation of the substantia nigra. Severe neuronal loss and gliosis were noted in the anterior horns and Clarke's column of the spinal cord. Mild pallor in the pyramidal tracts was detected in the lumbosacral segments (Fig 46). Neuron loss and gliosis in the brain stem were most marked in the vestibular nuclei and the substantia nigra. The cerebellar white matter showed marked gliosis, but the cortex was unremarkable. The basal ganglia and thalamus were normal, as was the cerebral cortex.

The 2 autopsy cases exhibited degeneration of neurons at many levels. The lower motor neurons, vestibular nuclei, neurons afferent to the cerebellum and extrapyramidal paths were chiefly affected. The clinical picture showed considerable variation in the 4 patients. Good clinicopathologic

---

(8) N. Engl. J. Med. 296:1505–1508, June 30, 1977.

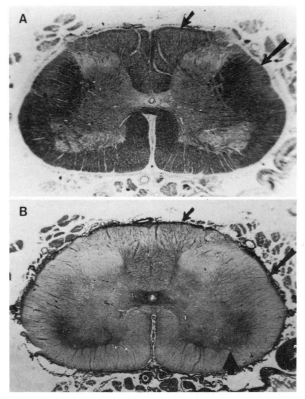

Fig 46. — Section of the lumbar spinal cord, **A,** shows loss of myelinated fibers in the fasciculus gracilis (*short arrow*) and pyramidal tract (*long arrow*); luxol fast blue myelin stain. **B,** same level of the cerebrospinal cord shows gliosis in the fasciculus gracilis (*small arrow*), pyramidal tract (*long arrow*) and anterior horn (*thick arrow*); Holzer stain. (Courtesy of Romanul, F. C. A., et al.: N. Engl. J. Med. 296:1505 – 1508, June 30, 1977.)

correlation was possible in these cases. The disease has an autosomal dominant inheritance pattern.

The other families with autosomal dominant inheritance of progressive ataxia have been reported as having "Machado disease," "nigrospinodentatal degeneration with nuclear ophthalmoplegia" and "autosomal dominant striatonigral degeneration." These and the present kindred are all descendants of persons born in the Azores around the middle of the 19th century. The term "Azorean disease" is proposed for this disease.

▶ [Comparison of the disease in this family with the findings reported in three families of similar Azorean ancestry, previously thought to have different disorders, suggested they may all represent a single genetic entity with variable expression. — Ed.] ◄

Electroencephalographic Prediction of Anoxic Brain Damage after Resuscitation from Cardiac Arrest in Patients with Acute Myocardial Infarction. M. Møller, B. Holm, E. Sindrup and B. Lyager Nielsen[9] (Odense, Denmark) examined the EEG as a predictor of short-term prognosis in 185 adult patients with acute myocardial infarction and an episode of clinical cardiac arrest in the coronary care unit. Men predominated 4:1. Average patient age was 63 years. Patients with ventricular arrhythmias were usually treated with lidocaine. Those with resistant cases were managed with procainamide, phenytoin, and β-blocking agents.

Eighteen of the 89 surviving patients had signs of anoxic brain damage. Ninety-six patients died, 76 of cerebral anoxia. Only 2 of 72 patients in whom the first EEG was classed as grade III–V (five-grade scale) survived; both records were obtained within a few hours after the cardiac arrest. No patient with a grade I EEG died of cerebral anoxia. Grade III EEGs showed continuous delta activity with little other activity, continuous spike activity, episodic reductions in voltage or a complete isoelectric period lasting less than 1 second. In grade IV records there were longer isoelectric intervals. There was a marked prognostic demarcation between grade I and grade II EEGs and grade III–V records. All grades of anoxic brain damage were seen in grades I and II, though no patient with a grade I record died of anoxic brain damage. Continued coma for over 24 hours after cardiac arrest did not necessarily indicate a fatal outcome. Nineteen patients recovered consciousness more than 24 hours after the arrest, and 6 survived without sequelae. Only 2 of 42 serially studied patients showed a shift from grades III–V to grades I and II.

Evaluation of a single EEG recorded 24 hours or more after a cardiac arrest in an infarction patient is of considerable

(9)   Acta Med. Scand. 203:31–37, 1978.

prognostic value. If a grade III–V EEG is recorded within 24 hours after cardiac arrest, the study should be repeated 1 or 2 days later.

▶ [It is not possible to predict on the basis of a single EEG the extent of anoxic brain damage after resuscitation following cardiac arrest. – Ed.] ◀

Neurologic Status and Prognosis after Cardiopulmonary Arrest: I. Retrospective Study. Treatment of the comatose survivor of cardiopulmonary resuscitation poses difficult ethical decisions regarding life-support measures when the prognosis for survival and final neurologic function are uncertain. Bruce D. Snyder, Manuel Ramirez-Lassepas and Dolores M. Lippert[1] (Univ. of Minnesota) conducted a retrospective survey of survivors of cardiorespiratory arrest. Data on patients aged 14 and over who sustained arrest in a 2-year period in 1973–74 were reviewed. Twenty-one patients were functional (group F), whereas 13 were neurologically impaired (group I), with severe dementia or a persistent comatose vegative state, and were totally dependent on nursing personnel for care. Seventeen group F patients were followed for a mean of 18 months.

The groups were comparable in sex, location of cardiorespiratory arrest, and diagnosis of the cause for the arrest. Ventricular fibrillation was the most common prearrest arrhythmia. Over one fourth of group F patients breathed spontaneously after cardiopulmonary resuscitation, whereas 84% of group I patients did not. Nine group F patients and only 1 in group I were arousable immediately after resuscitation, a significant difference. Nine group I patients were in deep coma after resuscitation, whereas only 1 in group F was in deep coma. The number of patients who recovered from coma to a normal mental status declined steadily as the duration of coma increased. Only 55% of patients initially in coma were discharged. Seizure activity persisted longer in group I patients. Only 2 group I patients survived hospitalization, and both were severely demented and died later. Two group F patients died in the hospital of recurrent arrhythmia. Fourteen of the 19 who were discharged are independent in activities of daily living.

Patients may not respond to voice for hours after cardiopulmonary resuscitation, yet still do well. The absence of

(1) Neurology (Minneap.) 27:807–811, September, 1977.

all motor responsiveness or of respiratory effort, and the combined absence of pupillary light reflexes and oculocephalic responses, are strongly indicative of a poor outcome. These data are preliminary and cannot provide an indication for terminating life support in a specific instance.

▶ [Prolonged coma, motor unresponsiveness, absent pupillary light reflexes and absent oculocephalic responses were closely associated with poor prognosis for recovery of neurologic functioning after cardiopulmonary arrest. — Ed.] ◀

Prospective Study of Nontraumatic Coma: Methods and Results in 310 Patients. Coma occurring in the course of an illness traditionally implies a poor prognosis, but few data define this precisely. D. Bates, J. J. Caronna, N. E. F. Cartlidge, R. P. Knill-Jones, D. E. Levy, D. A. Shaw and F. Plum[2] compared the neurologic findings and outcome in the first 310 patients in a prospective cooperative study of coma not due to trauma or drugs. Of the patients, 158 were in the United Kingdom and 152 in the United States. Coma was defined as sleeplike, unarousable unresponsiveness without evidence of psychologic awareness of self or environment. All patients were followed for at least 1 month. The age and sex distributions are shown in Figure 47. Mean patient age

Fig 47.—Numbers and ages of men and women making up series. (Courtesy of Bates, D., et al.: Ann. Neurol. 2:211–220, September, 1977.)

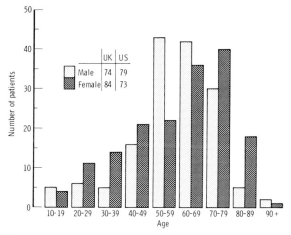

was 58 years. Most patients under age 65 were men; women constituted most of those over age 65 years. Most American patients had hypoxia-ischemia; most British patients had cerebrovascular disease.

The outcome differed little among the various diagnostic categories. An independent existence was achieved within a month by 16% of patients. Severe disability or a vegetative state developed in 25% of patients who were comatose for 6 hours and in 79% of those still in coma after 1 week. Patients who obeyed commands or moved their limbs appropriately in response to noxious stimuli had a better chance of regaining independent existence. Orienting eye movements, normal responses to oculocephalic or oculovestibular stimulation and normal muscle tone were also favorable signs. The chance of regaining independence was less for patients who, after 1 day, either had extensor responses of the limbs or failed to move them in response to noxious stimuli or who lacked eye opening, pupillary reactions, corneal responses or any eye movement in response to oculovestibular or oculocephalic stimulation. No clinical signs were found that reliably predicted the outcome of coma in all patients. Little functional improvement occurred after 1 month. Of 24 survivors at 6 months who were followed for a year, 21 were unchanged.

Whatever its origin, coma indicates a serious disturbance of brain function. Unless it is caused by exogenous and thus controllable poisons, the probability of recovery is poor. Systematic, repeated clinical observations are useful in coma. Better prediction of the outcome of coma will provide a means of judging the effects of future treatments.

► [The numbers of patients in this series who had particular signs of neurologic dysfunction are too small for use in confident prediction of outcome of coma, but they do suggest that careful clinical analysis of comatose patients may aid the clinician to prognosticate the probable future course of a comatose patient, and thus to judge the need for and results of further therapy. — Ed.] ◄

Pure Spastic Paralysis of Corticospinal Origin. The nosology of slowly progressive nonfamilial pure corticospinal disorders remains uncertain. C. M. Fisher[3] (Massachusetts Genl. Hosp.) encountered 6 patients in recent

(3) Can. J. Neurol. Sci. 4:251–258, November, 1977.

years with an unusual neurologic illness in which an extensive spastic paralysis slowly involved the legs, arms, face and tongue, without obvious involvement of any system other than the corticospinal tracts and without a family history of a similar condition. In the only neuropathologic study the clinical course was complicated by a stroke.

Man, 67, experienced leg stiffness, poor balance and difficulty walking and began using crutches within 10 months. After 17 months the arms became progressively weaker. The thighs and legs ached. A myelogram made after 15 months was negative. At the onset of symptoms an acute low backache had occurred while lifting. There was a past history of migraine headaches and a suprapubic prostatectomy. Severe spastic paraplegia was present 20 months after the onset. The arms were slow and weak. The tendon reflexes were abnormally brisk and the plantar responses were extensor. Sensation was normal. After $2\frac{1}{2}$ years a severe left hemiplegia with dysarthria developed. After a period of improvement the quadriparesis gradually worsened, with continuing low backache. Face and tongue movements were slow, and there were spasms of inappropriate laughing and crying. The cerebrospinal fluid was under a pressure of 123 mm and contained 38 mg protein per 100 ml. A ^{64}Cu scan was negative. An EEG was normal. The patient died of a myocardial infarction at age 72, 5 years after the onset of the neurologic symptoms. Intelligence had been preserved.

An old infarct was present in the right basis pontis, consisting of a series of old small cavitating infarcts in the right paramedian area. Large fibers were greatly reduced in the pyramids; gliofibrillar material was not increased. The lateral corticospinal tracts of the entire cord were pale. The anterior horn cells and anterior rootlets appeared normal.

Three men and 3 women aged 50–69 years were affected. All the women presented with dysarthria, whereas the men had limb involvement before dysarthria. The tempo of progression was variable. The final picture consisted of spastic quadriparesis, hyperactive reflexes, severe dysarthria and moderate dysphagia. All patients had periods of laughing and crying. There was no sensory loss or cerebellar involvement. The illness appears not to have been fatal. A patient with chronic progressive spastic quadriplegia was also studied, as was a patient with pure spastic paraparesis of short duration.

Chronic bilateral pure motor hemiplegia, chronic pure motor quadriplegia and primary lateral sclerosis appear to form a natural spectrum of pure corticospinal disease. Their possible relationship to amyotrophic lateral sclerosis is of theoretical interest.

▶ [Progressive spastic paraparesis (primary lateral sclerosis) has long been a clinical enigma. When one is confronted with a case, all possible etiologies must be considered, but usually no etiologic diagnosis is made. This article is an interesting discussion of the syndrome, but really adds nothing to our knowledge of it. — Ed.] ◀

Syndrome of Normal-Pressure Hydrocephalus: Possible Relation to Hypertensive and Arteriosclerotic Vasculopathy. Normal-pressure hydrocephalus is now considered to be a potentially reversible form of dementia. In autopsy cases the pathologic changes have been variable. A. Koto, G. Rosenberg, L. H. Zingesser, D. Horoupian and R. Katzman[4] (Albert Einstein College of Medicine) observed a patient who improved dramatically after a ventriculopleural shunt was inserted, but whose brain showed severe hypertensive and arteriosclerotic cerebrovascular disease and an advanced lacunar state.

Man, 67, was hypertensive and had had gait difficulty, mild dementia and urinary incontinence for 1 year. He had a long history of alcohol abuse but had worked steadily to age 65. The gait disturbance had progressed despite levodopa therapy. Blood pressure was 175/100 mm Hg. Speech was slow and difficulty with timed tests was apparent. There was a snout reflex and the patient walked slowly and sometimes could not initiate walking. Reflexes were symmetrically hyperactive and a tonic foot grasp was present bilaterally. Muscle tone was mildly increased. The cerebrospinal fluid homovanillic acid level was elevated and responded submaximally to probenecid. An air study showed marked dilatation of the lateral and 3d ventricles. Cisternography with ^{111}In showed activity in the ventricles at 48 hours. A right ventriculopleural shunt was carried out, with dramatic improvement in gait and disappearance of incontinence within 2 weeks and improved IQ scores. Later the patient's condition deteriorated despite a functioning shunt. Pulmonary embolism developed and he died.

Autopsy showed a large thromboembolus in the main pulmonary trunk. The shunt was in place and patent. There was evidence of old subdural hematomas bilaterally. Moderate to severe atherosclerosis was evident. Lacunae were present in the basal ganglia and white matter, some containing gliotic trabeculae and foamy macrophages. Many small intraparenchymal arteries were hypertrophied and hyalinosed, with occasional fibrinoid necrosis (Fig 48).

(4)   J. Neurol. Neurosurg. Psychiatry 40:73 – 79, January, 1977.

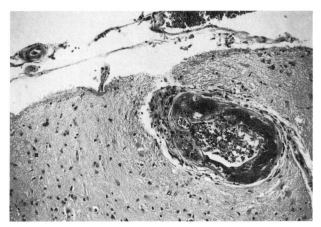

Fig 48.—Cortical blood vessel in frontal lobe, showing fibrinoid necrosis. Note also absence of meningeal fibrosis. Hematoxylin-eosin; reduced from ×110. (Courtesy of Koto, A., et al.: J. Neurol. Neurosurg. Psychiatry 40:73–79, January, 1977.)

This case fulfilled accepted criteria for normal-pressure hydrocephalus. Autopsy showed severe hypertensive and arteriosclerotic vasculopathy with many lacunar infarcts of various ages, mostly in the basal ganglia, thalami and periventricular white matter. Review of the literature indicated a high incidence of hypertensive or arteriosclerotic cerebrovascular disease or both in patients with idiopathic normal-pressure hydrocephalus. Cerebral blood flow is reduced in normal-pressure hydrocephalus and increases after shunting. Cerebral vasculopathy apparently can be another cause of normal-pressure hydrocephalus.

► [Normal-pressure hydrocephalus is a syndrome seen most frequently in aging persons. These authors suggest that vascular changes may play an important role in the pathophysiology in some cases of the syndrome.—Ed.] ◄

Traumatic Locked-in Syndrome. Although quadriplegics with bulbar and facial paralysis are paralyzed and may appear comatose, they are fully conscious and often can communicate with residual eye and lid movement. Lesions are usually found in the ventral pons. Most cases are due to thrombotic or embolic occlusion of the basilar artery. Richard H. Britt, Maie Kaarsoo Herrick and Richard D. Hamilton[5] report the first pathologically examined case of

(5) Ann. Neurol. 1:590–592, June, 1977.

locked-in syndrome due to direct trauma at the ventral pontomedullary junction.

Man, 21, whose car struck a pole, was ventilated in the emergency room and was found to have flaccid quadriplegia and decerebrate posturing on painful stimulation. Skull and cervical spine films showed no fracture. Spontaneous respirations developed in the next 24 hours, as did spontaneous eye movements. Bilateral 6th nerve palsies were present. By day 5 the patient responded with eye blinks to incoming information. Facial movement was weak bilaterally at 5 weeks. The patient understood speech but was aphonic. Complete spastic quadriplegia was present. There was a questionable left hemisensory deficit to pinprick and no light touch or positional sensation. The patient died of tracheal hemorrhage from erosion through the innominate artery 14 weeks after injury.

Autopsy showed bilateral cavitation of the lateral aspects of the medulla and complete destruction of the pyramids in the upper medulla (Fig 49). The destructive changes stopped at the midoli-

Fig 49. — Microscopic changes seen in brain stem. Levels **A–F** are shown on lateral view of brain stem in inset. Three grades of histologic change are depicted: darkest shading represents cavitation; stippled areas adjacent to cavitation represent glial scars with total loss of normal nerve components; fine-dot pattern in all sections represents variable mild to moderate loss of neurons or gliosis; crosshatched areas are regions of secondary tract degeneration. Patient's right is to viewer's left. (Courtesy of Britt, R. H., et al.: Ann. Neurol. 1:590–592, June, 1977.)

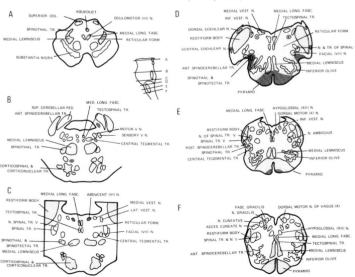

vary level. Destruction of tissue was total, with cavitation and marginal gliosis in the pyramidal tracts and arcuate nuclei. Secondary degeneration of interrupted tracts and variable neuron loss in the brain stem were also observed. The 6th cranial nerves were almost devoid of myelin and axons.

This case fulfills the criteria of the locked-in syndrome. Cavitary necrosis of the ventral pontomedullary junction and bilateral disruption of the 6th cranial nerves were present. The damage was due primarily to mechanical stretching that occurred during sudden hyperextension injury. Relative sparing of the pontine and midbrain tegmentum with preservation of the reticular activating system accounted for the maintenance of adequate, regular respiratory rhythm and a state of wakefulness.

► [This is said to be the first report of a locked-in syndrome resulting from trauma. A severe hyperextension injury caused damage to many levels of the brain stem. – Ed.] ◄

Nonhypoxemic Hazards of Prolonged Myoclonus. Death during status epilepticus or prolonged myoclonus is often unexplained, although hypoxia is often assumed to play a role, but recent experimental studies have shown that prolonged muscular contraction contributes to mortality through causing hyperkalemia, hyperthermia, lactic acidosis and hypotension. J. William Langston, Donald R. Ricci and Carol Portlock[6] (Stanford Univ.) documented these life-threatening disorders in a nonhypoxemic patient with prolonged myoclonus, who responded rapidly to the pharmacologic induction of total muscular paralysis.

Woman, 55, admitted for the treatment of cutaneous zoster, had been treated for nodular lymphocytic, poorly differentiated lymphoma (stage IVB) for 6 years. She had a history of hypertension and chronic pyelonephritis. Nuchal rigidity, fever and vomiting developed after a week in the hospital, and moderate neutropenia was found. The cerebrospinal fluid exhibited monocytic pleocytosis and increased protein. The blood urea nitrogen level was 58 mg/100 ml. Intravenous and intrathecal antibiotics did not prevent the appearance of bilateral extensor plantar responses and right knee clonus, as well as bursts of generalized myoclonus not responsive to large doses of phenobarbital and diazepam or to intravenous phenytoin. Myoclonus occurred at 5- to 10-minute intervals. The serum potassium level and body temperature rose sharply as the

(6) Neurology (Minneap.) 27:542– 545, June, 1977.

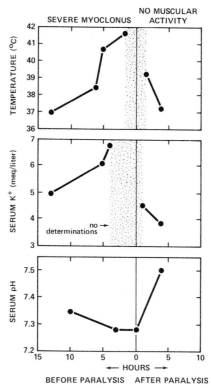

Fig 50. — Temperature, serum potassium and arterial pH before and immediately after induction of paralysis. (Courtesy of Langston, J. W., et al.: Neurology (Minneap.) 27:542–545, June, 1977.)

arterial pH fell (Fig 50). The blood lactic acid level was 6.5 mEq/L. After curarization with ventilatory assistance, the temperature fell and the acidosis resolved. The patient was paralyzed for 30 hours with pancuronium. The myoclonus abated spontaneously 4 days after its onset. The serum muscle enzymes returned to normal in the next 2 weeks. A cerebellar disorder emerged that resolved after phenytoin was stopped. Final neurologic examination was entirely normal.

Paralysis was induced as an emergency measure in this patient, because continuing muscle contraction appeared to be primarily responsible for the evolving hyperkalemia, hyperthermia, hypotension and lactic acidosis. Otherwise the patient might well have died of an arrhythmia or cardio-vascular collapse.

► [Induced neuromuscular blockade may be indicated when the system-ic effects of pathologically contracting muscle become life threatening. — Ed.] ◄

Spinal Myoclonus is often restricted to one somatic re-gion, is due to pathology at the involved level of the cord and is extremely resistant to treatment. It has been associated with tumor, infection, trauma and degenerative processes. Spinal myoclonus, though often increased by fatigue and stress, is usually unaffected by sensory stimuli or activity. Margaret M. Hoehn and Michael Cherington[7] (Univ. of Col-orado, Denver) describe 4 patients in whom spinal myoclo-nus was successfully treated with either tetrabenazine or clonazepam.

Woman, 50, had had jerks of the lower abdominal muscles for 11 years. Electromyography showed periodic rhythmic motor unit ac-tion potentials in the paraspinal muscles at this level, at a rate of 20 – 30 per minute. The EEG and cerebrospinal fluid were normal. Air myelography showed a small atrophic cord between T6 and T10, with a sagittal dimension of 6 – 9 mm, compared with 9.5 mm in the T2 – T4 region. The myoclonus was unresponsive to haloperi-dol, benztropine, thioridazine, diazepam, deanol, reserpine and phenytoin. On treatment with tetrabenazine at a dosage of 50 mg, increased by 50 mg every 2 days, the contractions ceased by the 6th day, when the dose was 150 mg. On three occasions when placebo was substituted, the myoclonus recurred on the 3d day; it disap-peared within 24 hours of the reinstitution of tetrabenazine. The response to clonazepam in 2 trials was similar; a dose of 1.5 mg dai-ly was effective. Presently the patient is taking a maintenance dose of 1 mg clonazepam daily.

Animal studies support the view that the spinal cord can initiate and maintain myoclonus. Tetrabenazine is a rapidly metabolized benzoquinolizine related to reserpine, which acts centrally to deplete stores of dopamine, norepinephrine and serotonin. Clonazepam is a benzodiazepine derivative. Three of the present patients responded dramatically to clonazepam. A combination of the two drugs in low doses was satisfactory in 2 patients who had adverse reactions to the individual agents.

► [Spinal myoclonus is a rare condition. Its diagnosis, as is true of the diagnosis of other varieties of myoclonus, is purely a clinical one, and

(7) Neurology (Minneap.) 27:942 – 946, October, 1977.

there often is lack of unanimity on the part of neurologists regarding the diagnosis in individual cases. These patients, however, appear to have been well-studied clinically, and the therapeutic trials were adequately controlled. Further study of the effect of these drugs in similar cases is indicated. — Ed.] ◄

Spinal Syphilis: Problem of Fluorescent Treponemal Antibody in the Cerebrospinal Fluid. Spinal syndromes due to syphilis, including tabes dorsalis, have become uncommon. A review of 241 cases of neurosyphilis by Hooshmand et al. (1972) included only 9 cases of spinal syphilis, all mimicking cervical spondylosis. Joseph F. John, Jr., and Albert C. Cuetter[8] (Moncrief Army Hosp., Fort Jackson, S. C.) describe 3 patients with presumptive nontabetic spinal syphilis at various cord levels who had positive treponemal serologic tests on the cerebrospinal fluid (CSF). All presented with paraparesis or paraplegia and sensory findings of various degrees. Two exhibited a definite sensory level to pinprick. No impairment of brain function was seen. One patient had an acute ventral medullary syndrome, 1 had progressive combined disease of the posterior and lateral columns and 1 had an acute complete cord transection. No patient had evidence of lower motor neuron disease. The CSF protein concentration was mildly elevated in 2 cases. The cellular response was absent or minimal, although all patients had serum and CSF reactive for treponemal antibody.

Spinal syphilis produces diverse neurologic syndromes. Compression of the cord, occlusion of spinal arteries with secondary infarction or necrosis or cavitation of the cord may result in every possible combination of long tract or local damage or both. The manifestations include syphilitic meningomyelitis, spinal vascular syphilis and hypertrophic pachymeningitis, which produces root syndromes and often spinal block. Cases of late symptomatic syphilis in previously treated patients continue to be reported. The possibility of syphilis should be considered in patients with obscure spinal syndromes. Failure to improve after penicillin therapy cannot be used to reject the diagnosis of neurosyphilis.

► [This article should serve as a reminder to physicians that cases of late syphilis continue to occur and may be manifested as obscure spinal syn-

(8)   South. Med. J. 70:309–311, 315, March, 1977.

dromes. These may be misdiagnosed unless the possibility of syphilis is constantly kept in mind. — Ed.] ◀

Postganglionic Cholinergic Dysautonomia. Only 9 cases of pure dysautonomia have been reported. In 3 cases the disorder was restricted to the postganglionic cholinergic fibers of both the sympathetic and parasympathetic systems. Sami I. Harik, Mustapha H. Ghandour, Fuad S. Farah and Adel K. Afifi[9] (American Univ. of Beirut) describe a fourth patient with profound postganglionic cholinergic dysautonomia, who made a slow, incomplete recovery spontaneously. Immunofluorescence histologic studies suggested an autoimmune origin of the illness.

Boy, 9 had headaches with blurred near vision a month before admission, followed by vomiting, obstipation and urinary retention. Residual contrast material was present in the abdomen from a barium enema done a week earlier; the material had not passed beyond the proximal duodenum during an upper gastrointestinal series. A duodenojejunostomy brought no improvement. Contrast material remained in the bladder after voiding despite the absence of obstruction. The pupils were noted to be maximally dilated and fixed. The supine blood pressure was 140/110 mm Hg. No pathologic reflexes were elicited. An EEG showed bilateral diffuse delta-wave activity. A brain scan and right carotid angiogram were negative. Carbachol injections led to severe abdominal cramps and defecation and urination, but neostigmine had no effect. Prednisone therapy for 2 weeks did not produce improvement. Bladder and bowel function improved gradually without specific therapy, and a repeat EEG was normal. The patient was attending school 18 months after discharge, but had recovered incompletely.

The pupils of this patient responded briskly to 1 drop of 0.25% pilocarpine solution. Carotid sinus massage failed to alter the heart rate or blood pressure, and norepinephrine infusion was also ineffective. A Schirmer test did not produce lacrimation, and salivary and sweating responses were subnormal. The intradermal histamine reaction was normal. Electromyography and motor nerve conduction studies gave normal findings. Immunoglobulin G was demonstrated in a skin biopsy on fluorescence study; indirect tests were negative. A sural nerve biopsy was normal. A muscle biopsy showed excessive lipid accumulation. Botulinum toxins were not demonstrated in the patient's serum.

(9)   Ann. Neurol. 1:393 – 396, April, 1977.

These patients have a subacute onset of marked, generalized failure of postganglionic cholinergic activity with a normal mental state and normal motor and sensory functions. The course of the illness is chronic. The clinical features suggest atropine-like poisoning, but botulinum toxin poisoning has been excluded. The EEG abnormalities and lack of antidiuretic hormone secretion may be due to involvement of cholinergic neurons within the central nervous system that share antigenic similarities to the postganglionic autonomic neurons.

▶ [Dysautonomia is a rare condition. This article illustrates that therapeutic measures may help alleviate the symptoms and that spontaneous recovery may occur. — Ed.] ◀

Alpha-Pattern Coma: 24 Cases with 9 Survivors. Alpha-pattern coma denotes the association of a comatose state with EEG activity that consists primarily of alpha-frequency rhythms that do not respond normally to visual or painful stimulation. Often such activity is of low amplitude, of diffuse distribution and predominant in the frontocentral regions. In the past 3 years, Alan B. Grindal, Cary Suter and A. Julio Martinez[1] (Med. College of Virginia) encountered 24 patients who had alpha-pattern coma. All but 3 patients with suspected brain stem infarction were comatose at the time of the initial EEG, and none of these was fully alert. Nine patients survived, 3 with no deficit, and 2 others were improving neurologically when they died in cardiopulmonary arrest. All survivors showed clinical improvement within a week of the initial EEG. Eleven patients initially had disordered brain stem reflexes, and only 2 of these survived, compared with 7 of 13 who had intact reflexes. The presence of spontaneous respirations on initial evaluation also favored survival.

Alpha-pattern coma was present initially in all but 5 cases. The alpha activity predominated in the anterior regions in 11 cases and posteriorly in 4. In patients with cardiopulmonary or respiratory arrest, alpha-pattern coma did not persist more than 4 – 5 days before slower activities in the theta and delta ranges appeared. This occurred both in survivors and nonsurvivors. In the 4 autopsies, gross pathologic changes in the central nervous system were unremark-

(1) Ann. Neurol. 1:371 – 377, April, 1977.

able. The degree of histopathologic changes varied with the severity of the anoxic episode and the survival time.

Diffuse anoxic changes were present in the cortex, thalamus, basal ganglia and brain stem in these cases after cardiopulmonary arrest. Autopsies were not obtained in patients with primary brain stem infarction. One patient who took an overdose of Doriden manifested typical alpha-pattern coma despite the absence of respiratory arrest. The pathophysiology underlying alpha-pattern coma remains to be elucidated.

► [These data would indicate that the pathophysiologic mechanisms underlying this disorder remain to be elucidated. – Ed.] ◄

Spinocerebellar Ataxia and HLA Linkage: Risk Prediction by HLA Typing. Yakura et al. suggested that the ataxia gene locus related to the inherited spinocerebellar ataxias might be on the 6th human chromosome near the histocompatibility (HLA) loci. John F. Jackson, Robert D. Currier, Paul I. Terasaki and Newton E. Morton[2] performed HLA typing and linkage analysis on 19 members of a kindred, in which spinocerebellar ataxia was segregating in an autosomal dominant pattern, to determine the possibility of genetic linkage of the ataxia with the HLA loci. The pedi-

Fig 51.—Partial pedigree of kindred with autosomal dominant spinocerebellar ataxia, showing HLA types. The HLA-A and HLA-B types are shown in haplotype form separated by horizontal lines. Parentheses indicate HLA types not tested, but deduced from typing of other members of kindred. (Courtesy of Jackson, J. F., et al.: N. Engl. J. Med. 296:1138–1141, May 19, 1977.)

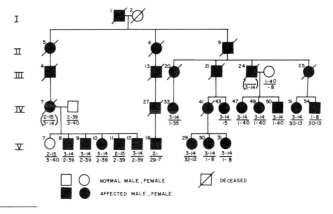

(2) N. Engl. J. Med. 296:1138–1141, May 19, 1977.

gree is shown in Figure 51. The HLA typing was done by peripheral blood lymphocyte microcytotoxicity techniques and tested for 16 HLA-A antigens and 18 HLA-B antigens.

The ataxia locus was on chromosome 6 at 12-centimorgan distance from the HLA complex with a lod score of 3.15. The lod score is the logarithm of the relative odds that the findings are due to linkage, compared with chance. Odds exceeding 1400:1 favor linkage over a chance finding. The presence of the ataxia gene in members of this kindred at risk can be predicted with about 90% accuracy by HLA typing in informative matings. It is not yet known on which side of HLA the locus resides. Linkage appears to be closer in male than in female subjects, as has been reported for other linkage groups in human beings.

With the rapid accumulation of information on the human gene map, the clinical application of linkage data will become pertinent in diagnosis and counseling in many diseases. It should be particularly helpful in inherited diseases with a late age of onset, beyond the time when childbearing usually occurs, such as spinocerebellar ataxia and other neurologic disorders.

► [These investigators have demonstrated that the presence of the ataxia gene can be predicted with about 90% accuracy by means of HLA typing and linkage analysis—Ed.] ◄

Diagnosis of Neurologic Disease

Cranial Computerized Tomography: Radiologic-Pathologic Correlation. Albert V. Messina[3] (New York Hosp.-Cornell Univ. Med. Center) determined the accuracy of computerized tomography (CT) of the head in demonstrating various lesions of the brain and related structures in 123 patients during 1974–75 who had CT within 2 months of death. Additional contrast enhancement was used in about half the patients studied with the 80×80-matrix display and in about 80% of those studied using the 160×160-matrix display. A bolus injection of iothalamate meglumine was given immediately before the scan.

Patients who had scans within 2 weeks of death on the 160-matrix EMI head scanner had a false negative rate of 11%. About one third of all lesions 1 cm or more in size were not demonstrated. False negative results were obtained in 27% of patients studied with the original 80×80-matrix display. Scan accuracy was slightly better with longer intervals between scanning and death. About 60% of all lesions were metastases. A total of 60 lesions that were 1 cm or more in greatest dimension were not identified on the CT scans. Improvement with the 160×160-matrix display, although modest, was obvious. Diffuse microscopic cerebral disease may cause no density changes detectable by CT scanning within the brain substance.

This study is based on a small selected patient population: patients with known cancer, usually terminal, and most certain to have multiple small lesions, as well as a selected group of referral patients, usually with difficult diagnostic problems. Though not infallible, CT scanning appears to be the most sensitive neuroradiologic diagnostic tool available.

► [Computerized tomography appears to be the most sensitive neuroradiologic diagnostic tool available, but certainly it is not infallible. In this study nearly one third of the lesions 1 cm or more in diameter were not demonstrated.

(3)   Arch. Neurol. 34:602–607, October, 1977.

A recent report from Vanderbilt University (Wells, C. E., and Duncan, G. W.: Am. J. Psychiatry 134:811, 1977) also warns of the danger of over-reliance on computerized cranial tomography. In this article 2 patients are described who were incorrectly diagnosed by highly trained physicians as having progressive dementia despite relatively minor changes in the tomography scan and conflicting clinical and laboratory data. They stress that the diagnosis of dementia cannot be established on the basis of any single feature (history, mental status, psychologic testing, EEG or computerized tomography scan). — Ed.] ◄

Evaluation of Recent Cerebral Infarction by Computerized Tomography. Computerized tomographic (CT) scans of recent cerebral infarctions are not consistent in pattern, so that diagnosis by CT scanning is problematic. Joseph C. Masdeu, Berhooz Azar-Kia and Frank A. Rubino[4] (Loyola Univ., Maywood, Ill.) studied 20 cases of well-substantiated cerebral infarction by serial CT scanning. The patients were men with a sudden, persistent neurologic deficit and a lesion that clinically involved a substantial amount of brain tissue. Scans were done before and after infusion of 300 ml of 30% diatrizoate meglumine. The first scan was done an average of 2 weeks after onset of the deficit. Seven-

Fig 52 (left). — Right hemispheric infarction producing partial obliteration of right lateral ventricle and shift of midline structures.

Fig 53 (right). — Absence of mass effect 1 month later.

(Courtesy of Masdeu, J.C., et al.: Arch. Neurol. 34:417–421, July, 1977; copyright 1977, American Medical Association.)

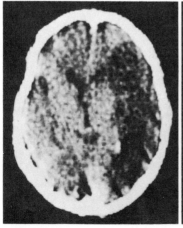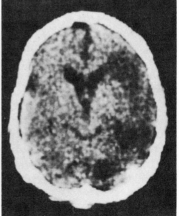

ty-two double-scan studies were carried out. Mean observation time was 3 months. Eleven patients had angiography. Autopsy findings in 2 patients correlated well with the CT patterns.

A mass effect (Fig 52) was present in 70% of patients scanned within a week after stroke, but it disappeared fairly rapidly (Fig 53), being seen in only 29% of patients by the end of the 3d week. No patient had a mass effect by week 8. Nearly two thirds of patients had enhancement in their post-infusion scans within 2 weeks after stroke. After 4 weeks only 38% of infarcts showed enhancement. The infarct in 1 patient continued to enhance 6 months after the stroke. Most often the area of lucency or the perinecrotic area was enhanced. Contrast enhancement was most helpful in evaluation of infarcts that had subtle findings on preinfusion scans. Abnormal radionuclide uptake usually outlasted contrast enhancement on CT scanning. The distribution of abnormal radionuclide uptake matched well the areas of contrast enhancement. Two hemorrhagic infarctions were recognized. Electroencephalograms showed a clear-cut focal abnormality in 3 patients with normal initial CT scans.

Probably a combination of arteriocapillary dilatation, alteration of the endothelial membrane and possibly capillary proliferation explains the presence of contrast enhancement in cerebral infarction. Follow-up CT scans may be necessary for conclusive diagnosis of recent cerebral infarction, and clinical correlation is of the utmost importance.

▶ [The timing of performance of computerized tomography in relation to the onset of the neurologic deficit is an important factor to consider when evaluating cerebral infarction by this technique. — Ed.] ◀

Cranial CT Appearance of Acute Multiple Sclerosis. John F. Aita, Donald R. Bennett (Univ. of Nebraska), Robert E. Anderson and Fred Ziter[5] (Univ. of Utah) report on 3 cases of acute multiple sclerosis in which computerized tomography (CT) studies showed contrast-enhanced lesions in the periventricular and deep white matter of the cerebral hemispheres.

Woman, 27, was admitted the day after an acute onset of aphasia, 15 months after the occurrence of left leg weakness and numbness in the left arm and left side of the face. Subsequent admissions were for exacerbations, mainly of the left-sided findings. Bladder

(5) Neurology (Minneap.) 28:251–255, March, 1978.

incontinence, dysarthria, diplopia, migratory paresthesias and blurred vision had developed. An enhanced CT scan 11 months before had shown no abnormalities. Examination showed a conductive aphasia, difficulty with short-term memory, moderate weakness and ataxia of the left limbs and minimal central paresis of the right side of the face. Reflexes on the left side were hyperactive and a left Babinski sign was evident. An EEG showed a left frontal delta wave focus and a brain scan showed increased activity in the right parietal region. A subsequent CT scan without enhancement was normal, but with iodine a 2-cm area of enhancement was seen in the deep part of the right parietal lobe (Fig 54). Four-vessel angiography and cervical myelography were normal. The language disorder improved over the next month, but increased disequilibrium and mental slowing then developed. Bilateral corticobulbar and spinal findings predominated. A repeat CT scan

Fig 54.—A and B, initial 13-mm scans without and with iodine, respectively, demonstrating a right parietal white matter enhanced lesion. C and D, 13-mm sections with contrast obtained 9 weeks after A and B, showing isodense resolution of the enhanced lesion and the development of one, or possibly two, left periventricular low-density abnormalities. (Courtesy of Aita, J. F., et al.: Neurology (Minneap.) 28:251–255, March, 1978.)

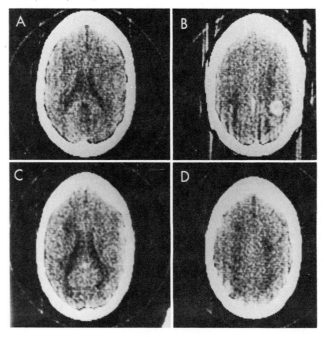

showed isodense resolution of the previous enhanced lesion and the development of one or possibly two left periventricular low-density lesions. Left retrobulbar neuritis subsequently developed. Corticotropin and steroids have given varying benefit.

These 3 young women with acute bouts of multiple sclerosis had contrast-enhanced lesions in the periventricular and deep white matter. The scan changes did not always correlate anatomically with the clinical features. The lesions did not have mass effect and were not noted on angiographic study. The lesions evolved to areas of density similar to the surrounding white matter, or to low-density lesions. New enhanced lesions and low-density areas appeared when the patients were symptomatic. Both contrast-enhanced and low-density lesions may be found on cranial CT in multiple sclerosis. These lesions are more easily seen in 8-mm than in 13-mm CT sections.

▶ [Enhanced cranial computerized tomography may be helpful in diagnosing acute multiple sclerosis and in following the course of the white matter lesions. – Ed.] ◀

Plaque of Multiple Sclerosis Seen on Computerized Transaxial Tomogram. No neuroradiologic procedure is thought to provide evidence for the diagnosis of multiple sclerosis. Monroe Cole and Ronald J. Ross[6] (Case Western Reserve Univ.) report the finding of contrast-enhanced lesions that occurred at different times and neurologic sites in a patient with multiple sclerosis.

Woman, 18, had vertical diplopia for 2 weeks and had had intermittent diplopia 6 months previously. She was noted to have skew deviation, vertical diplopia on right, left and upward gaze, and rotatory nystagmus on right and left lateral gaze. Neurologic examination was otherwise negative. A brain scan was normal. Computerized transaxial tomography (CT) showed a zone of reduced density 1.2 cm wide adjacent to the left frontal horn of the ventricle, before and after the injection of iothalamate sodium. A doughnut-shaped area of increased density 1.6 cm in diameter was seen in the right centrum semiovale after the injection of contrast material. Diplopia was not reported a month after the onset, but it could be elicited by use of a red glass; nystagmus was absent. A scotoma was present 12–18 degrees above fixation in the right eye. Repeat CT scanning showed a 2×1.5-cm area of reduced density above the left anterior horn of the ventricle. Contrast enhancement was seen in this area after iothalamate injection.

(6) Neurology (Minneap.) 27:890–891, September, 1977.

The clinical findings in this case indicated a posterior fossa lesion, but the CT scan showed left and right frontal lesions. The clinical course and cerebrospinal fluid findings were consistent with multiple sclerosis, and the bilateral hemispheric lesions seen on CT scanning supported the diagnosis. The spectrum of CT scan lesions in multiple sclerosis is not yet known. Inflammatory acute lesions may pick up contrast medium, but it is not clear whether or not all acute plaques are enhanced by contrast material.

► [It is too early to say whether or not computerized cranial tomographic scanning will definitely aid in the diagnosis of multiple sclerosis. It is significant, however, that in this case, with the use of contrast-enhanced tomograms, lesions were seen that appeared at different times and neurologic sites in a patient with multiple sclerosis. Demyelinating lesions have also been delineated by computerized tomography in children with other types of demyelinating disease, such as the leukodystrophies (Robertson, W. C., Jr., et al.: Neurology (Minneap.) 27:838, 1977). — Ed.] ◄

Three-Dimensional Computerized Tomographic Scans of Brain: New Approach to Intracranial Diagnosis. Most techniques of coronal and sagittal reconstruction

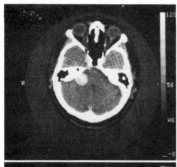

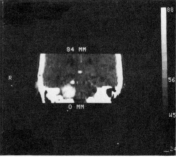

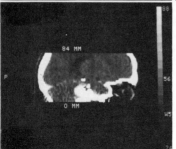

Fig 55 (above left). — Computerized tomographic image of 3-mm slice, showing typical 8th nerve tumor.

Fig 56 (above). — Reconstruction of coronal image from same data.

Fig 57 (left). — Reconstruction of sagittal image from same data.

(Courtesy of Rosenbaum, H. E.: Arch. Neurol. 34:386 – 387, June, 1977; copyright 1977, American Medical Association.)

of computerized tomographic (CT) images of brain involve
successive overlapping of the field of scanning, because of
the large beam width required by most available units to
obtain sufficient photons for adequate statistical quality of
the image. A higher radiation dose and a need to rescan the
patient result. Herbert E. Rosenbaum[7] (Washington Univ.)
had used an Artronix scanner, which provides slices 3 mm
thick of adequate statistical quality (Fig 55). Routinely 32
such slices are made, each taking 12 seconds. Coronal and
sagittal reconstruction from the same data as were obtained
in the initial horizontal scan (Figs 56 and 57) is then possible without rescanning of the patient. The radiation dose is
3.7 rad. Any part of the cranial cavity can be reconstructed.

Sagittal and coronal reconstruction is useful in demonstrating spatial relations between lesions and anatomical
landmarks in particular areas, such as the suprasellar region, posterior fossa and corpus callosum. It is particularly
useful for preoperative localization. The method is also
useful in demonstrating aneurysms and their points of
origin from vessels in the region of the circle of Willis.

► [A new method for displaying computerized tomographic cross sections of the brain in the coronal and sagittal planes is described. This
technique should be of particular importance in the diagnosis of potentially surgical lesions. — Ed.] ◄

**Multiple Sclerosis: Diagnostic Usefulness of Cere-
brospinal Fluid** is discussed by Kenneth P. Johnson and
Barbara J. Nelson[8] (Univ. of California, San Francisco).
The diagnosis of multiple sclerosis is often difficult to make
especially in early, atypical or progressive cases. The cerebrospinal fluid (CSF) is altered in nearly all cases. A modest
increase in mononuclear cells may occur but CSF cytology
has not been a clinically useful test. Total CSF protein elevations are infrequent and nonspecific. The CSF γ-globulin
fraction is increased in about two thirds of patients. Both
the CSF IgG-albumin index and the demonstration of oligoclonal IgG bands in concentrated CSF on agarose electrophoresis have been used diagnostically. Cerebrospinal fluid
IgG is conveniently quantitated by any of a variety of techniques. Oligoclonal IgG bands have been found in about 90%
of patients with clinically definite multiple sclerosis. This

(7) Arch. Neurol. 34:386 – 387, June, 1977.

(8) Ann. Neurol. 2:425 – 431, November, 1977.

finding is not, however, specific for multiple sclerosis. The function of these restricted populations of IgG is largely unknown. The kappa-lambda ratio of IgG light chains is elevated in multiple sclerosis CSF. Antibodies against specific viral antigens have been identified in the CSF in multiple sclerosis.

The CSF IgG or albumin level can be fairly accurately measured with the use of an immunodiffusion kit. The determination of CSF IgG percentage, the IgG-albumin index and oligoclonal IgG bands can show abnormalities in most patients. Each of these tests may aid in detecting CSF changes in a single specimen. Measurement of IgG bands appears to be the most convenient test and the one most likely to reveal abnormalities. When a central nervous system demyelinative or chronic infectious process is a possibility, failure to demonstrate specific abnormalities in the CSF necessitates a much wider-reaching diagnostic evaluation.

► [With the newer techniques now available in clinical diagnostic laboratories, it can be shown that the cerebrospinal fluid is abnormal in more than 90% of the clinically definite cases of multiple sclerosis. The finding of the abnormalities in the cerebrospinal fluid may be a major aid in diagnosis. — Ed.] ◄

Rapid Fluorometric Assay for Cerebrospinal Fluid Immunoglobulin G. Joseph Menonna, Deena Galantowicz, Peter Dowling and Stuart Cook[9] compared a new quantitative immunofluorometric technique for measuring cerebrospinal fluid (CSF) IgG to reference values obtained by two established methods, the immunoprecipitation and the radial immunodiffusion techniques. Cerebrospinal fluid samples with a wide range of known IgG levels as determined by immunoprecipitation were used in the study. Prototype immunoglobulin fluorescent assay kits were used in which Microbead reagent, a solid bead to which monospecific antibody to human IgG has been linked, reacts to bind CSF IgG.

Fifty-nine CSF samples with IgG values found in close agreement with results of the immuno precipitation assay and the low-level immunodiffusion technique were assayed by the fluorometric technique. Good correlation was obtained between the fluorometric and the reference values obtained by the radial immunodiffusion method (Fig 58).

(9) Neurology (Minneap.) 27:481–483, May, 1977.

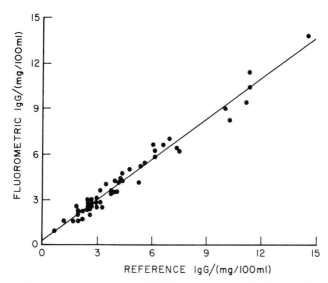

Fig 58. – Linear regression curve of CSF IgG values obtained by fluorometric assay compared with reference method, radial immunodiffusion, showing good correlation between the new method and reference values (correlation coefficient, r = 0.98). (Courtesy of Menonna, J., et al.: Neurology (Minneap.) 27:481–483, May, 1977.)

The fluorometric method was found to be quite reproducible. The coefficient of variation was 5.7%.

This technique is a rapid one requiring minimal volume. Over 40 samples can be conveniently processed in a single run. The assay has an extremely wide range of sensitivity. It should be possible to devise assays for other trace CSF components present in far less quantity than IgG, such as IgM. The value of CSF IgM measurement as a marker of disease activity in patients with multiple sclerosis should be resolvable by use of the fluorometric technique.

▶ [The fluorometric method is rapid, reproducible and easy to perform. Its suitability for laboratories engaged in the measurement of cerebrospinal fluid IgG appears promising. – Ed.] ◀

Treatment of Neurologic Disease

Acute Overdosage with Benzodiazepine Derivatives. Benzodiazepine drugs are used extensively as sedative, hypnotic and antianxiety agents and are being increasingly implicated in cases of deliberate or accidental overdosage. David J. Greenblatt, Marcia D. Allen, Barbara J. Noel and Richard I. Shader[1] (Boston) reviewed the records of patients seen in 1962–75 with benzodiazepine overdosage. Among 773 admissions for overdosage with a psychotherapeutic drug, 99 involving 93 patients implicated a benzodiazepine derivative. Diazepam was involved in 52 instances and chlordiazepoxide in 48. The 60 female and 33 male patients had respective mean ages of 35 and 33. None of the patients died. In only 12 cases was a benzodiazepine the only drug taken.

Only 1 of 12 patients taking only a benzodiazepine reached stage 3 coma and none required assisted ventilation. Seven of 12 patients taking nonbarbiturate sedative-hypnotics as well reached grade 3 or 4 coma and 3 required ventilatory assistance. Twenty-one patients took benzodiazepines with other psychotropic drugs, often with ethanol as well. Eleven reached grade 3 or 4 coma and 9 required ventilatory assistance. Of 31 patients taking benzodiazepines with barbiturates, with or without alcohol, over two-thirds reached grade 3 or 4 coma and half required ventilatory assistance. In most of these cases the dose of benzodiazepine was not excessive, but the barbiturate dosage was often extremely high.

Self-poisoning with multiple drugs is more common than overdosage with a single drug. Serious intoxication is considerably more frequent when benzodiazepines are taken with other drugs than when they are ingested alone. Benzodiazepines apparently may produce fatal intoxication, though no deaths occurred in the present series.

► [Ingestion of benzodiazepines together with other drugs appears to be

(1) Clin. Pharmacol. Ther. 21:497–514, April, 1977.

much more common than benzodiazepine ingestion alone as a cause of drug intoxication. The severity of intoxication in such cases of multiple-drug ingestion depends largely on the type and quantity of the agents other than benzodiazepine taken. — Ed.] ◄

Oral Choline Administration to Patients with Tardive Dyskinesia. Choline administration to rats and human subjects leads to an increased choline concentration in cerebrospinal fluid, suggesting that choline might be useful in treatment of patients with diseases such as tardive dyskinesia, which presumably result from deficient central cholinergic tone. John H. Growdon, Madelyn J. Hirsch, Richard J. Wurtman and William Wiener[2] evaluated choline therapy in a double-blind, crossover study of 20 patients with tardive dyskinesia. All had received phenothiazines or haloperidol and had stable, chronic buccal-lingual-masticatory dyskinesia. Thirteen were still taking these drugs. Anticholinergic agents were discontinued during the study. Choline chloride was given orally in dosages of 150 mg/kg daily for 1 week and 200 mg/kg daily in the 2d week. The placebo was sucrose octa-acetate. A crossover was made after a 10-day rest interval.

The mean plasma choline value 1 hour after a dose was 33.5 nM/ml in the 2d week of therapy, a 170% increase. Dyskinetic movements lessened in 9 patients during choline therapy; 5 patients improved greatly. Tongue movements decreased markedly in 2 patients with more severe dyskinesia but increased markedly in 1 patient. No serious side effects were observed. All effects were dose related and subsided when the dosage of choline was reduced.

Choreic movements decreased in nearly half the patients in this study on choline therapy. Oral doses of choline can be useful in neurologic diseases in which an increase in acetylcholine release is desired. Lecithin administration also elevates blood choline values in human subjects, but its ability to suppress buccal-lingual-masticatory movements in patients with tardive dyskinesia remains to be tested.

► [The actual period of observation in this group of patients was too brief for adequate evaluation. Despite the optimistic conclusions in this article, a therapeutic agent for the relief of the buccal-lingual-masticatory movements that develop after prolonged use of phenothiazines and related drugs has not yet been found. — Ed.] ◄

(2) N. Engl. J. Med. 297:524–527, Sept. 8, 1977.

Baclofen, a New Antispastic Drug: Controlled, Multicenter Trial in Patients with Multiple Sclerosis. Baclofen reduces voluntary muscle spasms, probably by hyperpolarizing afferent spinal terminals to reduce monosynaptic extensor and polysynaptic flexor reflex transmission. Clinical trials in several countries have shown baclofen to be an effective, well-tolerated drug in patients with multiple sclerosis. Barry A. Sachais, James N. Logue and Michael S. Carey[3] (Summit, N. J.) conducted a double-blind, multicenter comparison of baclofen and placebo in patients aged 18 and older with spasticity secondary to multiple sclerosis. No muscle relaxant or psychoactive agent was given in the week before the study. Baclofen was given in dosages of 5 mg three times daily for 3 days and then 10 mg three times daily for 4 days to outpatients. Inpatients received 10 mg and then 15 mg three times daily. In the 2d week, outpatients received 15 mg and inpatients received 20 mg three times daily and subsequently higher dosages not to exceed 80 mg daily.

Of 106 patients who completed the study, 54 received baclofen and 52, placebo. Each group had a mean age of 43 years. Most patients were quadriplegic or paraplegic. A dosage of 70–80 mg daily was usually adequate. Depression, euphoria and irritability lessened in both groups. Baclofen-treated patients showed significant decreases in pain and frequency of flexor spasms, resistance to passive joint movement and global severity of disease. Placebo patients showed significant reductions in ankle extension and resistance of passive abduction of the hip. The overall spastic state improved significantly in baclofen-treated patients. Somnolence occurred in 75% of baclofen-treated patients and 36% of placebo patients; it was rarely severe. Excessive weakness occurred in 20% of the former and in 11% of placebo patients. No serious drug-related laboratory abnormalities were observed.

Balcofen is a safe, effective antispasticity agent for patients with multiple sclerosis. Patients often appreciate the relief from spasticity and clonus that is gained and find increased independence in their daily lives. Such patients are

---

(3) Arch. Neurol. 34:422–428, July, 1977.

usually better candidates for nursing care and physical therapy.

▶ [Using patients with spastic syndromes secondary to multiple sclerosis, these investigators have shown that baclofen is an effective drug in relieving symptoms of spasticity such as flexor spasms, pain and stiffness, resistance to passive joint movements and increased muscle stretch reflexes. The side effects were generally mild and transient. — Ed.] ◀

"Disappearing" Spinal Cord Compression: Oncolytic Effect of Glucocorticoids (and Other Chemotherapeutic Agents) on Epidural Metastases. Most workers attribute the salutary effects of corticoids on central nervous system (CNS) tumors to the relief of tumor-related cerebral or spinal cord edema. Failure to appreciate the oncolytic potential of glucocorticoid therapy may lead to inappropriate treatment. Jerome B. Posner, John Howieson and Esteban Cvitkovic[4] report the findings in 4 patients having spinal cord compression due to epidural metastases. Two had prompt relief of symptoms after glucocorticoid therapy alone, with marked shrinkage or disappearance of the metastasis. In 2 patients, glucocorticoids combined with other chemotherapeutic agents led to disappearance of the extradural tumor. One patient had unnecessary surgery because of failure to recognize the oncolytic effects of the chemotherapy, and in a second patient an unnecessary operation was narrowly averted.

The mechanism by which glucocorticoids act on signs and symptoms in patients with brain tumors and other edema-producing neurologic diseases remains unclear. Glucocorticoids are known to have oncolytic effects in a variety of human tumors, particularly lymphomas. One of the present patients had a non-Hodgkin's lymphoma. One patient received cis-platinum as well as glucocorticoid, and 1 received high-dose methotrexate and vinblastine along with steroids. Glucocorticoids should be given to all patients with epidural cord compression by malignancy. Relief of cord edema will lead to clinical improvement in many cases and in a few cases the oncolytic effects of steroids may be of substantial benefit. Definitive treatment should be undertaken as soon as possible after the diagnosis is established. If symptoms resolve rapidly after glucocorticoids are given, myelography should be repeated. If the epidural tumor has regressed,

---

(4) Ann. Neurol. 2:409–413, November, 1977.

definitive therapy should be continued but the patient should henceforth be managed as a glucocorticoid responder.

► [This is an extremely interesting article. It has been shown that for certain patients glucocorticoids and other chemotherapeutic agents may have an oncolytic effect on epidural metastatic neoplasms and make it possible to spare the patients what had been thought to be necessary surgery. — Ed.] ◄

Granulomatous Angiitis of the Brain: Successfully Treated Case. Noninfectious granulomatous angiitis of the nervous system can be a rare cause of a neurologic disorder characterized by focal signs or may present as a presenile dementia. Rodwan K. Rajjoub, James H. Wood and Ayub K. Ommaya[5] (Nat. Inst. of Health) report the first case of granulomatous angiitis of the brain to be diagnosed by surgical biopsy and successfully treated.

Man, 38, had an 18-month history of impaired consciousness, memory loss, confusion, hallucinations, headaches and focal seizures involving the right arm and accompanied by dysphasia. Examination revealed disorientation and dysnomic dysphasia. An opacity was found in the right apical region on chest radiography and a bone scan showed increased activity in this region. A biopsy specimen of a mediastinal node led to a diagnosis of Hodgkin's disease, mixed cell type. A brain scan was normal, but an EEG showed abnormal slow activity in the left anterior and midtemporal regions. Computerized axial tomography showed abnormal areas bilaterally in the frontal and parietal regions (Fig 59). A biopsy specimen of the right frontal lobe showed changes of granulomatous angiitis; viral cultures were negative. Mediastinal irradiation and dexamethasone therapy were followed by significant EEG improvement, and follow-up tomographic studies showed resolution of the abnormalities. Reactivity to purified protein derivative converted to positive. The patient regained his memory, orientation and normal speech. Hodgkin's disease is presently in remission.

Extrapyramidal symptoms, reported in other patients, were not noted in the present patient and no visual disturbances were observed. A clear-cut biopsy diagnosis led to early treatment with steroids and irradiation. Granulomatous angiitis should be considered in the differential diagnosis of a focal disorder associated with presenile dementia and also in suspected space-occupying lesions that may change their

(5) Neurology (Minneap.) 27:588–591, June, 1977.

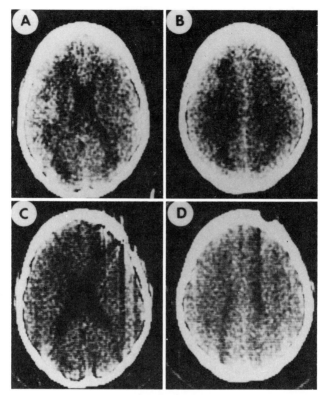

Fig 59.—Computerized axial tomograms without contrast enhancement before and after therapy. **A** and **B**, cerebral edema involving frontal and parietal regions is visualized as diffuse decreased absorption on pretreatment scans. **C** and **D**, note resolution of cerebral edema after dexamethasone and radiation therapy. (Courtesy of Rajjoub, R. K., et al.: Neurology (Minneap.) 27:588–591, June, 1977.)

mass character over time. The disease is potentially reversible.

▶ [This is certainly an extremely important case. It would be interesting to know about the erythrocyte sedimentation rate and changes in it during therapy. One wonders what part the radiation therapy had in the outcome.—Ed.] ◀

NEUROSURGERY

OSCAR SUGAR, M.D.

Introduction

Not all of the information of value to neurosurgeons comes from articles written by "scientists" or "physicians." Paul Sampson, a staff writer for the *Journal of the American Medical Association*, has an interesting article in the Medical News portion of the journal (July 21, 1978, page 195) entitled "Chymopapain: A Case Study in Federal Drug Regulation."

The Food and Drug Administration (FDA) has not yet approved chymopapain for use in human beings. In March, 1974, it was recommended that the drug be given a Phase IV approval, restricting its use to medical specialists trained in its use and requiring reports of results. A double-blind study was started in December, 1974, while a notice was being drafted in the *Federal Register* asking for comment concerning its release. In May, 1975, the officers of the American Association of Neurological Surgeons and of the American Academy of Orthopedic Surgeons were notified of this study and in July, 1975, they were told of the preliminary results that indicated that the drug itself appeared to be no more effective than the medium in which it was delivered, a mixture of cysteine hydrochloride monohydrate, edetate disodium and iothalamate sodium. This material has since been patented by Baxter-Travenol under the name "CEI," and in turn a new double-blind study has been undertaken to compare this material against a saline placebo. Only after these results are known will a determination be made if chymopapain should be tested against a saline placebo. Baxter-Travenol withdrew its new drug application for chymopapain in 1975, after a suggestion from Dr. M. A. Clark of the FDA's Bureau of Drugs that this might be wise pending the outcome of the double-blind studies.

The apparent insistence of the FDA (and consequently, of Baxter-Travenol) on the use of double-blind studies is in conflict with the clinical experience that asserts a benefit to patients, ranging from 60% to 70% from use of the current chymopapain mixture. It also is in conflict with the experience in Canada where the chymopapain mixture is still in use and is conferring benefits on a number of patients, some of whom come from the United States. (To the best of my current knowledge, Discase, Baxter's chymopapain preparation, is being used only in Canada and in Mexico.) Among the users of chymopapain in the United States is Wiltse, a Long Beach, California, orthopedist. His analysis of patients shows that an ideal diskectomy patient has an 85.2% chance of a good or excellent result from injection therapy and only 7.4% of such patients come to surgery in a period averaging 3.5 years after injection. He believes that not only is the drug effective but also that it is safe (because only 2 deaths have occurred in more than 15,000 cases), actually much safer than disk removal by laminectomy (although Sussman, of Howard University, disputes this, saying that chymopapain is the wrong drug, used in the wrong patients — most of whom would get better anyway — and is toxic to nerve tissues). Apfelbach, a Lake Forest, Illinois, orthopedist, believes that clinical experience is adequate without a double-blind study and compares use of chymopapain to that of methyl methacrylate for use in orthopedics, where no double-blind study was possible.

The newspapers are joining in, with most journalists siding with the chymopapain users. The publicity and push for public insistence on availability of the drug have been unfairly compared to those with regard to Laetrile, for which there is no such body of clinical trial. The journalists refer to some statements made by doctors that impute a financial motive for the opposition to use the chemical and attempt to polarize orthopedists (for) against neurosurgeons (against). The facts are otherwise; both orthopedists and neurosurgeons have been prominent in the battle for release of the medicine, and those who have done laminectomies in the past certainly can learn to inject chymopapain instead. It may well turn out to be the last "conservative" or at least nonoperative measure to be used before laminectomy for disk protrusion. It is not a panacea; it sometimes does its work too well and removes all of the disk, allowing collapse of the disk space, with mechanical changes around the nerve root that then require foramenotomy or laminectomy — but so does vigorous disk removal by a direct operative approach. Problems of the low back promise to be with us for some time.

Oscar Sugar, M.D.

Brief Interesting Notes

The scientific detectives have turned again to medical matters in searching in the past. R. T. Steinbeck (*Paleopathological Diagnosis and Interpretation: Bone Diseases in Ancient Human Populations* [Springfield, Ill.: Charles C Thomas, Publisher, 1976]) describes changes in skulls from scalping, as well as from missiles and trephination. Infections that can be reliably diagnosed include syphilis of the skull, osteomyelitis, leprosy and tuberculosis of the spine. Spongy hyperostosis of the skull from thalassemia and other anemias has been recognized. I disagree with the author's statement of rarity of anterior cervical joint changes. Among tumors described are osteomas of the skull, fibrous dysplasia, hemangioma, meningioma, histiocytosis X and multiple myeloma (or carcinoma).

Not quite as ancient are the techniques devised by Golgi, which can be used to demonstrate the dendrites and dendritic (synaptic) spines of pyramidal cells of the human cortex. At the April, 1978, meeting of the Society of Neurological Surgeons in Philadelphia, Dominic Purpura pointed out the relative paucity of the dendritic spines, which are longer and thinner than usual, in some instances of mental retardation. Electron microscopy of tissues from the same child failed to show obvious abnormality. Similar changes are seen with storage diseases, in which strange bulging bodies appear at the region of the origin of the axon.

The influence of isolation rearing (compared to communal rearing) on the dendritic spines of cells of the fish tectum has been described (Science 200:787, 1978). Isolated fish have fewer, but longer and thinner, spines than the more stimulated ones. Perhaps there are some objective reasons for stimulating infants and small children, to their benefit. Someone has said that it was better for a child to be spanked than ignored.

A summary of various definitions and types of nystagmus can be found in Baloh's classification of pathologic nystagmus (Bull. Los Angeles Neurol. Soc. 41:120, 1976). It is based on electro-oculographic recordings but has many clinical observations and points of interest. Thus, he states that lateral deviation of the eyes in eliciting nystagmus should not be beyond 40 degrees, lest so-called physiologic nystagmus be elicited. Fixation of vision inhibits vestibular nystagmus, but gaze paretic, rebound and congenital nystagmus are all prominent with fixation. Frenzel glasses inhibit fixation only in a darkened room. Eye closure is more effective in eliciting vestibular nystagmus and this can be readily recorded with the oculographic technique. Positional change is important in altering central input of otolith input, but altered neck proprioception may also be involved in so-called positional nystagmus. This type is best seen with inhibition of fixation. Paroxysmal positional nystagmus is best induced by rapid change from a sitting to a head-hanging position. There is no completely reliable way of distinguishing peripheral and central origins of vestibular nystagmus, but central vestibular nystagmus is usually associated with other brain stem signs and may not be inhibited by fixation. Isolated vestibular nystagmus completely suppressed by fixation is strongly suggestive of peripheral vestibular disease (especially if there is an associated hearing loss). Stationary positional nystagmus (contrasted with paroxysmal) may occur without known vestibular disease; it may be seen in head lateral but not body lateral positions, suggesting that altered neck proprioceptive input may play a role. Positional nystagmus after intake of alcohol is ascribed to diffusion differences of alcohol into the cupula as compared to the endolymph.

The audiologist with the Otologic Medical Group of Los Angeles, E. W. Johnson, has analyzed the auditory test results in 500 cases of acoustic tumor (Arch. Otolaryngol. 103:152, 1977). Tests included pure-tone air and bone conduction tests, speech tests, adaptation tests including modified tone decay and Bekesy audiometry, short increment sensitivity index (SISI) and alternate binaural loudness balance. The youngest patient was aged 9 years and the oldest, aged 78. Fifteen percent of patients were under age 30 and 2% were over 70. Duration of hearing loss was less than 6 months in 17%, and 40% of patients had had hearing problems for 1–3 years. Ten percent had had hearing loss for over 10 years. The investigation supported the contention that all unilateral sensorineural hearing impairments require thorough investigation. High-frequency pure tone loss was evident in 2 of every 3 patients. Speech discrimination is of considerable importance in the differential diagnosis of retrocochlear versus cochlear involvement. Because findings vary from person to person, it is important to do the entire battery of tests. Johnson suggests that after operation with total hearing loss, the patient have an immediate trial with a contralateral routing of an off-side signal hearing aid (CROS). This is much more apt to be useful if the trial is done soon after operation than if the trial is delayed for weeks or months.

In these days of computerized tomography scanning and sophisticated neuroradiology, one might well ignore the plain x-rays and the pineal calcification. However, cost-conscious committees may well force reconsideration and justification for complicated techniques. Hence, it is worthwhile to learn (Pilling and Hawkins: Br. J. Radiol. 50:796, 1977) that calcification within the pineal gland has its center within 2 mm of the midline of the gland (in 72 of 73 glands). Usually one considers pineal calcification to be normally situated within 2 mm of the midline, and this study reinforces this view.

Progressive enlargement of a diastatic or linear skull fracture is commonly known as "growing skull fracture." A review of 4 cases by Hellbusch, Moiel and Cheek (South. Med. J. 70:555, 1977) indicates the generally unsatisfactory results of operation on such children. The authors believe early operation is indicated; therefore follow-up films should be taken at periodic intervals (3 months, for instance) after linear fracture is first seen. Craniectomy is needed to find the limits of normal dura mater, and grafts are better done with pericranium or fascia lata than with foreign material. A strong dural repair may obviate need for immediate cranioplasty, because young children often re-form their own bone.

At exploration of the optic chiasm in a woman, aged 60, with progressive visual loss, Bosma (Acta Neurochir. (Wien.) 38:305, 1977) found the anterior cerebral artery on the right to pass under (ventral) to the optic nerve. It gave off both interhemispheral anterior cerebral arteries. The right internal carotid artery apparently bifurcated in the cavernous sinus.

There is evidence from experiments in the macaque monkey carried out by Schneider, Kulics and Ducker (J. Neurol. Neurosurg. Psychiatry 40:417, 1977) that limb position information is carried by different mechanisms for distal and proximal portions. Cortical representation of the distal limb volar surface as it moves in space is impaired by lesions of the dorsal funiculus or posterior white column. Proximal limb information may or may not be impaired by similar lesions; this information is initially in dorsal or posterior white columns but shifts to the dorsolateral funiculus as it ascends. Posterior white column damage in the cervical cord impairs only distal, not proximal, information. This fiber sorting may account for a variety of peculiar findings after injuries to the posterior columns in monkeys; as yet, there is little information as to its presence in man.

Orticochea (Br. J. Plast. Surg. 30:223, 1977) has revived the use of a tourniquet around the head to control hemorrhage during operations on the scalp. His apparatus is pneumatic, protects the eyes and is used low on the head and hence it permits access for most scalp operations.

An example of what can be done by an experienced microneurosurgeon is given by Chater, Buncke and Alpert (Surg. Neurol. 7:343, 1977). Two cases are presented in which a full-thickness graft of skin was removed from the right inguinal area, with superficial circumflex iliac artery and vein, and put into place to cover a scalp deficit (due to electric burn), with the artery and vein anastomosed to the superficial temporal vessels in one instance and to the occipital vessels in the other.

Orthopedists are concerned with "amputation neuromas" and have devised a number of techniques to minimize neuroma and scar formation. After studying rabbits, Swanson, Boeve and Lumsden (J. Hand Surg. 2:70, 1977) applied their new silicone capping technique to 18 patients with 38 traumatic neuromas in the upper extremities and 8 patients with 9 neuromas in the lower extremities. Two patients acquired sympathetic dystrophy and were dissatisfied; 1 required reoperation, but the rest were relieved of their complaints. The neuroma was resected until unscarred fasciculi were seen. A silicone cap having a length-diameter ratio of from 5:1 to 10:1 was trimmed. A 5-0 nonabsorbable suture was used to tie the end of the nerve into the cylindrical cap whose distal end was closed but through which the needle could be passed. An absorbable suture was tied over the knot and was then passed through the skin so as to pull the nerve away from area of heavy use or contact. The capping did not prevent phantom pain. Evidence from rabbits is that axons survived for a distance of 5–10 mm from the end of the cap, with fusiform swelling presumably due to "axon damming," that is, blockage of normal flow of axoplasm.

Uninhibited neurogenic bladder is characterized by urinary frequency, urgency, urge incontinence and recurrent urinary tract infections. Anticholinergic drugs and frequent voiding are usually sufficient to give improvement (in 81% of 64 adults with this syndrome). In other patients operation may be needed, and Diokno, Vinson and McGillicuddy (J. Urol. 118:299, 1977) suggest selective sacral rhizotomy, as they have found it to be extremely useful in 6 women and 1 boy aged 12. Cystometrograms were done before and after selective sacral blocks with Xylocaine. If uncontrolled contractions were delayed, the amplitude of uninhibited contractions decreased and the bladder capacity increased, lumbosacral laminectomy was performed, and the nerve roots were stimulated while intravesical pressure was monitored. The root whose stimulation produced the greatest increase of intravesical pressure was selected for transsection. Five patients had right S3 section, 1 had right S2 section, and 1 had right S4 section. All patients had perineal hypoesthesia specifically related to the root severed; it was localized and was not the source of complaint. No patient had stress urinary incontinence and the male patient continued to have nocturnal penile tumescence. Three patients are considered cured and 3 improved; 1 is no better. Criteria for patient selection should include definite diagnosis of uninhibited neurogenic bladder by cystometry. Bladder capacity should be at least 200 ml (after blocking motor impulses). A small contracted bladder contraindicates rhizotomy.

Anatomy and Physiology

Sensory Conduction in Medial Plantar Nerve: Normal Values, Clinical Applications and Comparison with the Sural and Upper Limb Sensory Nerve Action Potentials in Peripheral Neuropathy. Peripheral neuropathies may have a predilection for sensory fibers in the lower extremities, and there is some evidence suggesting that measurement of the sural sensory action potential (SAP) may be more useful than upper limb SAPs in this setting. R. J. Guiloff and R. M. Sherratt[1] (London) developed a method for recording the medial plantar SAP at the ankle with surface electrodes. Sural nerve SAPs are recorded antidromically with the subject lying on a couch, with supramaximal 0.1-ms rectangular stimuli delivered at a point close to the Achilles tendon. Medial plantar SAPs are recorded orthodromically in the same extremity as the sural SAP, with supramaximal stimuli delivered through ring electrodes encircling the hallux.

Studies were done in 69 control subjects aged 13–81 (17 healthy volunteers, 39 patients without evidence of peripheral nerve disease and 13 patients with isolated nerve disease but at least one normal lower extremity) and in 33 patients with clinical criteria for peripheral neuropathy (13) or other disorders involving the nerves to the legs (disk prolapse, trauma, etc.). In control subjects the medial plantar SAP usually consisted of a negative wave, sometimes preceded or followed by a positive wave. It was unmeasurable in only 3 older subjects. Sural SAP was present in all control subjects. Both the sural and medial plantar SAP amplitudes correlated significantly with age and the amplitudes of the two potentials correlated significantly with one another. All 13 patients with peripheral neuropathy had absent medial plantar SAPs. This was the only SAP absent in all 7 patients under age 60 and was the best indicator of involve-

---

(1) J. Neurol. Neurosurg. Psychiatry 40:1168–1181, December, 1977.

ment of peripheral nerves in peripheral neuropathy. Of the 33 patients, 3 with preganglionic L5–S1 root lesions had normal sural and medial plantar SAPs. All 6 patients with drop feet due to lateral popliteal nerve palsy and 2 with L4–L5 disk protrusion had normal medial plantar SAPs. Medial plantar SAPs were absent in 1 patient with a sciatic nerve lesion, 1 with a tarsal tunnel syndrome and 1 with a medial plantar nerve lesion.

Measurement of the medial plantar SAP at the ankle is a more sensitive test for peripheral neuropathy than the sural and median SAPs and the lateral popliteal mixed nerve action potential. It may be useful in patients with drop foot, helping to show or exclude involvement of L4–L5 postganglionic sensory fibers at the nerve root or plexus level.

Pathogenesis of Intracranial Arachnoid Cysts. Setti S. Rengachary, Itaru Watanabe and Charles E. Brackett[2] (Kansas City, Kan.) quote Richard Bright's original description of intracranial arachnoid cyst in 1831 to show that it contained the concept that these cysts are truly intra-arachnoid in location and are formed by splitting or duplication of the arachnoid membrane.

Man, 48, presented with severe depression, insomnia, arterial hypertension, recent weight loss and headaches. He had a history of thoracotomy for caseous granuloma of the lung, removal of a parathyroid adenoma and anemia. A large cystic lesion in the left sylvian fissure area was detected. The patient deteriorated rapidly and died, in ventricular fibrillation, of rupture of a dissecting aortic aneurysm. A 5×5×5-cm cystic lesion in the sylvian fissure was found to represent splitting of the arachnoid membrane, with the pia remaining as a separate intact membrane. The cyst was unquestionably intra-arachnoid. Beneath the cyst the inner layer of the arachnoid and the pia were in direct contact.

Another man, aged 44, with slowly progressive incoordination for 2 years, had a retrovermian avascular mass shown on computerized tomography to be a large midline posterior fossa cyst. This was excised through a posterior fossa craniectomy. The structure of the cyst wall was basically that of normal arachnoid membrane. The light microscopic features were indistinguishable from those of the first patient.

Controversy exists as to the exact histogenesis of the

(2) Surg. Neurol. 9:139–144, February, 1978.

human arachnoid membrane. Most embryologists consider both the arachnoid and pia mater to be derivatives of the primitive mesenchyme surrounding the neural tube. This separates into ectomeninx and endomeninx, the latter differentiating into the pia-arachnoid membrane and the subarachnoid space. An aberration in flow of cerebrospinal fluid in the endomeninx may lead to formation of a blind pocket or potential arachnoid cyst. Splitting and duplication of the arachnoid membrane, as seen in the present cases, show the validity of this hypothesis.

Detection and Localization of Occult Lesions with Brain Stem Auditory Responses. James J. Stockard, Janet E. Stockard and Frank W. Sharbrough[3] (Mayo Clinic and Found.) describe the seven vertex-positive potentials (brain stem auditory responses) which can be recorded from the human scalp within 10 msec of an appropriate acoustic stimulus. Measurement of the relative latencies and amplitudes of the potentials permits the detection of subclinical lesions in patients with suspected multiple sclerosis or neoplasms. The brain stem auditory response is altered in a systematic way by lesions at different levels of the auditory pathway. The electroanatomical correlations schematized in Figure 1 are empirically valid although oversimplified. The first potential is generated in the acoustic nerve, the third in the pons and the fifth in the midbrain. Abnormalities of latency in the tumor group were defined as prolongations in the interwave latencies among waves I, III, IV-V and V by more than the upper limits of the one-tailed 99% confidence limits for the latencies. Abnormalities of amplitude were defined on the basis of wave IV-V only; this is the largest and most reliable of the response components.

Brain stem auditory responses were abnormal in 12 of 15 cases of subtentorial neoplasm, including all 5 cases of acoustic neuroma and all 4 of brain stem glioma. Studies were also done in 30 patients with "definite," 30 with "probable" and 40 with "possible" multiple sclerosis. Response abnormalities were present in 93% of the definite cases, and 60% of these had more definitive latency abnormalities. The respective figures were 77% and 67%, respectively, for probable cases, and 35% of possible cases had response abnor-

(3) Mayo Clin. Proc. 52:761–769, December, 1977.

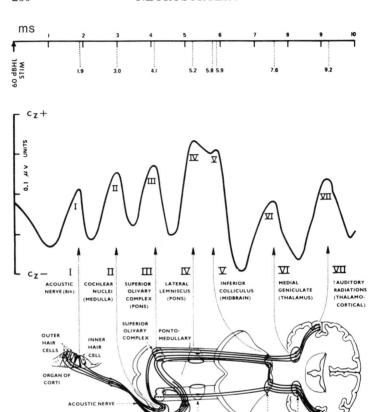

Fig 1.—Diagram of normal latencies for vertex-positive brain stem auditory potentials (waves I through VII) evoked by clicks of 60 dbHL (60 db above normal hearing threshold) at a rate of 10 per second. Lesions at different levels of auditory pathway tend to produce response abnormalities beginning with indicated components, although this does not specify the precise generators of the response; the relative contributions of synaptic and axonal activity to the response are as yet unknown. Intermediate latency (5.8 msec) between those of wave IV and V is mean peak latency of fused wave IV-V when present, C_z+, vertex positivity, represented by an upward pen deflection; C_z-, vertex negativity, represented by a downward pen deflection. (Courtesy of Stockard, J. J., et al.: Mayo Clin. Proc. 52:761–769, December, 1977; courtesy of Ellen Grass, modified with permission.)

malities, half of which involved latency abnormalities, in the absence of clinical evidence of brain stem involvement. In all, 65 of the 100 patients had response abnormalities and in 45 of these there were significant abnormalities in latency, with or without concomitant conduction abnormalities. Over half of 70 patients without clinical evidence of brain stem dysfunction had electrophysiologic evidence of a clinically unsuspected lesion.

The greatest value of scalp recording of brain stem auditory responses lies in complementarity with other diagnostic studies. Used in conjunction with conventional audiometry and long-latency auditory evoked responses, the test allows functional assessment of the auditory pathway from cochlea to cortex. Combination of the test with visual and somatosensory evoked responses should allow the earlier detection of lesions at every level of the central nervous system.

► [Setiey, Revol and Courjon (Lyon Med. 237:847, 1977) use pickup electrodes in the central areas for stimulation results from the median nerve and use electrodes in the rolandic-vertex area when the external popliteal (common peroneal) nerve is stimulated. They use brief (0.5 msec) shocks separated by a fixed interval of 1,300 msec delivered to the wrist or at the head of the fibula. Stimulation should produce a feeble muscular contraction but not be painful. Three series of 150 stimulations are averaged. The first peak corresponds to arrival at the cortex of the impulse from the thalamus. The second peak is caused by electric changes in the parietal area due to the lemniscal activity. Some believe there is a late phase of this response modified by attention and level of alertness. If the parietal cortex is removed, the total evoked potential disappears.

In recent lesions of the parietal lobe (verified by scans, angiography or operation), the evoked response disappears or is reduced or the third spike disappears, although the EEG remains normal. The evoked potentials are normal during migraine episodes and in hysterical anesthesia. In sensory epilepsy, suppression of response speaks for a lesion such as a tumor. In 2 of 3 paraplegics, the evoked response was absent and there was no recovery; in a third, there were subnormal evoked responses and there was a good sensory-motor recovery, indicating the value of this test in acute spinal lesions.

Electric potentials of the spinal cord can be evoked by stimulating the tibial nerve and recording from electrodes placed percutaneously into the epidural space. Shimoji, Matsuki and Shimizu (J. Neurosurg. 46:304, 1977) were unable to elicit these from skin stimulation alone, whereas both techniques of stimulation were capable of evoking somatosensory potentials from the scalp. The cord potentials are quite similar to those evoked directly from the spinal cord dorsum in rabbits. The immediate application of this information is not yet at hand. – Ed.] ◄

Neurosurgical Intensive Care is discussed by M. Lou

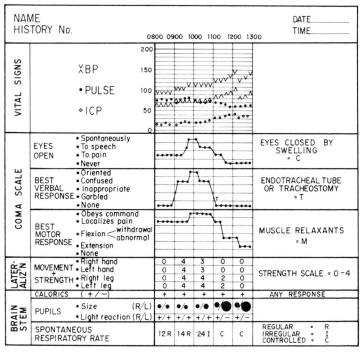

Fig 2. – Example of neurologic status record, showing course of patient admitted to neurologic intensive care unit after head injury. Initial examination revealed comatose patient lacking spontaneous movements but responding to pain. After 1 hour, patient emerged from coma, only to experience exacerbation with concurrent intracranial pressure (*ICP*) elevation and clinical evidence of impending transtentorial herniation. Trachea was intubated and patient hyperventilated before surgical evacuation of large hematoma. (Courtesy of Marsh, M. L., et al.: Anesthesiology 47:149–163, August, 1977.)

Marsh, Lawrence F. Marshall and Harvey M. Shapiro[4] (Univ. of California, San Diego). The enhanced monitoring capabilities and physician input associated with a neurologic intensive care facility do much to aid recruitment of nursing personnel. Accurate continuing assessment and recording of neurologic status is the first priority. The Glasgow coma score has been incorporated in the neurologic status recording form (Fig 2). A combination of computed tomographic (CT) scanning and continuous intracranial pressure

(4) Anesthesiology 47:149–163, August, 1977.

recording is important in neurosurgical monitoring. Interest in electrophysiologic monitoring techniques has increased. Occasionally intracranial pressure monitoring is initiated in the emergency room, but in most cases a CT scan is done as soon as possible in head injury cases. Stroke, brain tumor and metabolic encephalopathies are other reasons for monitoring. In comatose patients blood should be taken for a toxicology screen and glucose determination. Intracranial pressure reduction in a nonsurgical setting may involve osmotherapy, controlled hyperventilation and high-dose steroid therapy. Adequate cerebral perfusion presupposes a stable cardiovascular system, and patients with arrhythmias and hypotension must be treated vigorously.

Barbiturates have been shown to reduce ischemic brain damage in monkeys after stroke and cerebral circulatory arrest. Barbiturates and hypothermia have been used to reduce persistently elevated intracranial pressure in critically ill head-injured patients, with good results. Pentobarbital alone has effectively reduced intracranial pressure in most comatose head-injured patients with significant midline shifts and intracranial hypertension after hyperventilation, steroids and mannitol. The mechanism of action of barbiturates on ischemic cerebral tissue is not understood, and more studies are needed before large-scale clinical trials are begun. Barbiturates can rapidly reduce intracranial pressure and control the pressure for prolonged periods in certain patients, in both the operating room and the intensive care unit. Here a special ischemic brain protective effect need not be cited as a reason to use barbiturates.

Treatment of Intracranial Hypertension: Analysis of 105 Consecutive, Continuous Recordings of Intracranial Pressure. H. E. James, Th. W. Langfitt, V. S. Kumar and S. Y. Ghostine[5] (Univ. of Pennsylvania) analyzed 105 continuous intracranial pressure (ICP) recordings obtained in a 3-year period from 95 patients with the use of an intraventricular cannula. The 60 male and 35 female patients were aged 1–73. The most common clinical diagnoses were intracranial tumor, head injury and vascular disease. Hydrocephalus was present in 25 patients. The indications for recording ICP were evidence of a severe brain

(5)   Acta Neurochir. (Wien) 36:189–200, 1977.

insult, cerebral swelling of unknown cause or due to systemic disease, and clinical evidence of intracranial hypertension after craniotomy. Seventy patients were stuporous or comatose at the time of study. A Scott cannula was inserted through a bur hole or twist drill hole made 2 cm from the midline, usually into the right frontal horn of the lateral ventricle.

The ICP exceeded 20 mm Hg at least once in 86 patients, with the exclusion of transient changes due to patient movement or suction. The plateau waves of Lundberg were noted in 19 recordings, and B waves were observed in 19 recordings. Forty patients had drainage of cerebrospinal fluid through the ventricular cannula on 46 occasions; ICP fell immediately in all instances. Hypertonic mannitol led to a reduction in ICP in 67 of 73 instances in the 44 patients treated, with a mean reduction of 52%. Hyperventilation was effective in 34 of 50 trials, which led to a mean reduction in ICP of 46.6%. Hypothermia was tried 40 times in 40 patients and was effective in 17 trials. Moderate hypothermia of 27 – 31 C was not more effective than mild hypothermia of 32 – 36 C. Twenty autopsies showed no significant hematoma along the track of the cannula. Six patients had clinical signs of infection, and infection appeared to contribute to 3 deaths, but 4 infections occurred in one of the four hospitals participating in the study. Two of 29 patients studied for 5 days or longer had clinical infections. Risk of intracranial contamination seemed to increase with length of recording time.

Hypertonic mannitol reduced the ICP in nearly all patients in this trial, but the time course of the reduction was quite variable. Hyperventilation was less effective, and the data on hypothermia are more difficult to interpret. The advantages of continuous monitoring of ICP responses to treatment in very ill patients outweigh the risks of intracranial infection in these patients.

Effect of Routine Bedside Procedures on Intracranial Pressure. M. N. Shalit (Petah Tikva, Israel) and F. Umansky[6] (Tel Aviv Univ.) observed the effects of common bedside management procedures on intracranial pressure (ICP) in 21 comatose patients with brain edema and in-

(6) Isr. J. Med. Sci. 13:881–886, September, 1977.

creased ICP of various causes. Nine patients had an acute subdural hematoma, 5 had brain edema after head injury and 7 had infiltrating gliomas of the brain. All had had operations. An intraventricular cannula was used to record ICP in 6 patients, a subdural transducer in 6 and a small subdural cannula in 9. In 3 patients the ICP was recorded simultaneously from the ventricle and subdural space for 3 – 4 days.

Coughing after tracheal suction was accompanied by an increase in ICP, sometimes to very high levels and sometimes for a prolonged period. Where the trachea was blocked by secretions, suction had a favorable effect on the ICP. In most patients tested, all changes in body position were accompanied by considerable changes in ICP, without significant changes in arterial pressure or blood gases. Rotation and flexion-extension of the head usually considerably increased the ICP rapidly, especially in patients with relatively high initial pressures. Increases in jugular venous pressure were also observed. The ICP often increased gradually when both jugular veins were compressed in the neck, but less than on movements of the head. Elevation of the head of the bed often was followed by a 10- to 30-mm Hg fall in ICP.

Common patient management procedures may markedly affect the ICP in patients with brain edema and increased ICP. Often proper patient positioning may be more effective in reducing ICP than mannitol administration. Sideward rotation of the head at craniotomy should be avoided unless the whole body is rotated in the same direction. Venous outflow obstruction is not the chief cause of increased ICP with a change in positioning. The cumulative effect of ICP increases occurring during routine patient management may be a major factor in determining the outcome of the illness.

▶ [The admonitions from Shalit and Umansky may prevent serious problems during craniotomy (when the brain seems to expand as soon as the dura mater is opened, despite use of mannitol, when the position of the head and neck is poor). Certainly we must teach our nurses to turn the patient "logwise" not only when there is a spine operation but also with head problems, and an examiner of the patient's eyes should not just turn the head but have the patient flat when the patient is at risk for raised intracranial pressure. The benefits of the head-up position can be seriously compromised if, in this position, the tongue or other soft tissue obstructs the airway. The authors believe the problems with raising pressure from turning the head are more likely due to interference with cerebrospinal fluid flow near the foramen magnum (temporary incarceration) than with venous outflow. – Ed.] ◄

Mannitol Dose Requirements in Brain-Injured Patients. Osmotic diuretics have a major role in reducing intracranial hypertension in neurosurgical patients, but little documentation of dose requirements is available. Current dose schedules suggest 0.5 – 1.5 gm/kg, but are based on urea doses and on studies in many patients with little or no intracranial hypertension. Lawrence F. Marshall, Randall W. Smith, L. Andrew Rauscher and Harvey M. Shapiro[7] (San Diego, Calif.) attempted to determine the minimum effective dose of mannitol in 8 patients with acute closed head injuries complicated by an intracranial pressure exceeding 30 mm Hg. The patients did not respond to verbal stimuli when admitted, and they had ventriculostomies placed. The mean intracranial pressure was 44.1 mm Hg, despite controlled ventilation and high-dose dexamethasone therapy. The doses of mannitol, given at 8-hour or greater intervals, were 0.25, 0.5 and 1 gm/kg. The indications for mannitol included a cerebral perfusion pressure below 50 mm Hg.

There were no significant differences in intracranial pressures, volume-pressure responses or the times required to achieve the maximum fall in intracranial pressure. A significantly increased osmotic gradient was noted in patients given 0.5 and 1 gm mannitol per kg. Three patients given 1 gm/kg had a rise in intracranial pressure with a rise in systemic arterial pressure of less than 10 mg Hg; the increases were transient and not clinically significant. Two patients required cerebrospinal fluid (CSF) venting between doses, but the volume pressure response at the time of the next mannitol administration was not significantly different.

Doses of mannitol much lower than those previously recommended for controlling intracranial hypertension are effective in reducing intracranial pressure. Smaller doses permit more frequent administration if chronic mannitol therapy is necessary. Severe dehydration can be avoided in most cases when a low-dose regimen is used. A dose of 1 gm/kg did not result in significantly greater pressure reductions than a smaller dose in any of the present patients.

(7)   J. Neurosurg. 48:169–172, February, 1978.

▶ [Noteworthy is the rate of administration (5 gm= 20 cc/minute) and the lack of apparent benefit from high doses of dexamethasone (20 mg every 6 hours). Gobiet (Neurochirurgia (Stuttg.) 20:35, 1977) monitored intracranial pressure with extradural transducers in 100 cases of severe head injury and compared the effects of various osmotic diuretics and saluretics; only mannitol (20% solution, 1 gm/kg given in 15 minutes) and sorbitol (40% solution, 1 gm/kg given in 15 minutes) were beneficial compared to 5% glycerin, 20% glucose and 20% human albumin. Glycerin in 20% solution did drop pressure in 16 of 22 cases with the first dose, but only in 6 of 20 cases with a second dose. Frusemide, 250 mg, failed to drop the pressure in 12 of 32 cases, but maximum effect was reached in 48 minutes and lasted slightly over 2 hours. Dexamethasone "in usual doses" did not appear to affect the outcome, but there was distinct benefit in morbidity and mortality with the use of "very high doses." Initial adult dose was 48 mg, and 8 mg every 2 hours thereafter on day 1 and 4 mg every 2 hours on days 2 and 4 (increased to 8 mg on day 3). Children over age 10 received 24 mg, and 4 mg every 2 hours thereafter. Children under age 10 received 20 mg initially and 4 mg every 3 hours thereafter. The increased dosage on day 3 was made because of findings of a delayed rise in intracranial pressure. Gobiet considers a free airway, hyperventilation, balanced infusion therapy, high caloric nutrition and high doses of dexamethasone to be prophylactic, while therapy is with hypertonic solutions for intracranial pressure over 50 mm Hg or for cerebral perfusion pressure under 50 mm Hg.

Rottenberg, Hurwitz and Posner (Neurology (Minneap.) 27:600–608, 1977) used patients with implanted ventricular catheters and Ommaya reservoirs to study effect of oral glycerol on intraventricular pressure. The patients had meningeal carcinomatosis or acute leukemia. The investigators determined that a single 1 gm/kg-dose of oral glycerol is adequate to lower acutely raised intracranial pressure, but its effect is short-lived. If doses are spaced at 6 hours, the pressure will return to baseline between doses. At 4-hour intervals, the patient may be unable to metabolize the glycerol, and eventual deterioration from reverse osmotic gradient may occur. They suggest it is safer to let the pressure return to baseline by the 6-hour interval technique, especially with the addition of corticosteroids.

A simple method of continuous measurement of cerebrospinal fluid pressure is described by Hartmann and Alberti (Acta Neurochir. (Wien) 36: 201, 1977). It has been applied in cases of subarachnoid pressure, ischemic infarcts, supratentorial space-occupying lesions and communicating hydrocephalus. The puncture was made with the head lower than the feet in those patients with raised intracranial pressure, and less than 2 drops of fluid was lost during the procedure, so no fear of herniation was realized.

Gaab and Pflughaupt (ibid. 37:17, 1977) believe that 10% glycerin (glycerol) solution in doses of up to 1 gm/kg body weight and with rates of up to 5 ml/minute is an effective material to dehydrate brain tissue, without rebound. Obvious diuresis occurs only with infusion rates of over 2.5 ml/minute. Hemolysis, which followed use of 20–30% solution, did not occur with the more dilute solution. In 3 cases, increased blood sugar concentration after severe head trauma returned to normal levels.—Ed.]

Continuous Lumbar Drainage of Cerebrospinal Fluid in Neurosurgical Patients. External cerebrospinal fluid (CSF) drainage by the lumbar route seems adequate when the CSF pressure or volume needs to be reduced for a limited period. Gideon Findler, Abraham Sahar and Aaron J. Beller[8] (Hadassah Hebrew Univ.) have used this method before and after a variety of neurosurgical operations and at times as a substitute for surgery. Fifty patients had continuous lumbar CSF drainage in 1971–76 for such conditions as CSF fistula, benign increased intracranial pressure and intrathecal medication. A polyethylene catheter was placed in the L3–L4 interspace and directed cephalad in the subarachnoid space. The amount of CSF drained was gradually increased over 2–3 days. The collecting system was changed daily.

Drainage prevented fluid collection in 17 of 20 patients with CSF accumulation or leakage at a cranial operative site. The average period of drainage was 10 days, and an average of 370 ml of fluid was removed daily. Two patients had leaks at the lumbar puncture site after 5–7 days. All but 3 patients received prophylactic antibiotics and no patient had signs of infection. Cerebrospinal fluid rhinorrhea ceased in 8 of 14 patients after an average of 8 days of lumbar CSF drainage. An average of 350 ml was drained daily. All these patients received prophylactic antibiotics. Drainage of CSF was effective in 3 of 5 patients with postoperative rhinorrhea. None of 3 patients having drainage begun just before surgery had rhinorrhea. Drainage was effective in 2 patients with fistulas after meningocele repair and in 2 having intradural tumors removed.

Few complications occurred in this series. Both deaths were related to preceding infection. The simplicity of this method, its possible use as a substitute for an operation, and the paucity of complications favor its wider use.

(8)   Surg. Neurol. 8:455–457, December, 1977.

Diagnosis

▶ Although computerized tomographic (CT) scanning is more costly than isotope brain scanning, it is more accurate by about 25%; CT scanning is therefore cost beneficial. Substituting CT scanning for radioactive scanning has the further benefit that rarely will an isotope scan be requested after CT scanning, whereas a radioactive scan may well be followed by a CT scan in order to check accuracy or to get more information. The relative costs of a CT scan ($130 per patient) and isotope scan ($51 per patient) become wider if an extra charge is made for contrast studies in the CT scan. Evens and Jost (Semin. Nucl. Med. 7:129, 1977) list advantages of CT scan as greater sensitivity and accuracy, improvement in differential diagnosis, usefulness in patients with atrophy and ventricular abnormalities and granting of important information in patients with trauma, hemorrhage and postoperative complications. Radioactive scans are cheaper, the equipment is more versatile, scanning is readily available and no contrast material is required and hence there is essentially no morbidity. The authors do not mention that one advantage of isotope scanning is that it permits study of cerebral blood flow with the same injection, giving a type of information not available from CT scan. (I do not know where the data base for this study came from; the price ranges for scans in the Chicago area are far different!)

In these cost-conscious days, anything that legitimately reduces costs should be noted. Delays in scanning, repetition of scans and hospitalizations can be due to restlessness of the patient, especially a child. A satisfactory sedation for children suggested by Anderson and Osborn (Radiology 124:739, 1977) is a mixture of meperidine (Demerol), 25 mg/ml; chlorpromazine (Thorazine), 6.25 mg/ml; and promethazine (Phenergan), 6.25 mg/ml. A volume of 0.55 ml was used for children weighing 15 lb (6.8 kg); 1.1 ml was used for those weighing 30 lb (13.6 kg), and a 1.8-ml cocktail was used for those weighing 50 lb (22.8 kg). The children were given no food or liquids for several hours, and the medication was given intramuscularly. Sedation was usually satisfactory within 20–30 minutes. Agitation produced by inflating the water bag around the head usually disappeared within a few minutes.

Titanium clips 0.2 mm thick are nontoxic, easy to handle, apparently reliable and cheaper than silver clips. Although they are visible on plain x-ray film, they do not cause disturbance in CT images. An article by von Holst et al. (Acta Neurochir. (Wien) 38:101, 1977) emphasizes the disturbance produced by movement in the presence of metal clips of ordinary types (silver, tantalum). Aluminium clips also can be used for this purpose, but their manufacture is more difficult than those made of 99.9% titanium. The titanium clips can be obtained from Stille-Werner AB, of Stockholm.

Computerized tomographic scan findings, while not specific, may alert the radiologist to the possibility of venous angioma of the brain. Only 16 cases have been previously reported, according to Michels, Bentson and Winter (J. Comput. Assist. Tomogr. 1:149, 1977), who add 6 cases, studied with CT scans and angiography. Typically there are irregularly sized venules without dilated adjacent arteries; there is usually an umbrella or Medusa-like pattern radiating toward the draining vein. Edema and mass effect were not found in these cases, which help differentiate them from hematoma in the CT scan. Some were seen as focal densities and others were manifested only by a draining vein in contrast studies. — Ed. ◄

Computed Tomography of Intraspinal and Paraspinal Neoplasms. Hiroshi Nakagawa, Yun Peng Huang, Leonard I. Malis and Bernard S. Wolf[9] (City Univ. of New York) studied 36 cases of spinal neoplasm in 1975–77 with the use of a body scanner with a 256×256 matrix. Slices 8 mm thick were used in all but the very early cases, in which 13-mm collimation was used. Most adult patients received 300 ml of 30% meglumine diatrizoate; some children received none. There were 19 intraspinal and 17 paraspinal tumors in the series. Eleven patients with intraspinal tumors had positive, 4 had equivocal and 4 had negative computed tomography (CT) scans. Three of 4 meningiomas that were positive had dense calcification. All 3 lipomas were easily diagnosed. Five of 9 intradural extramedullary tumors showed positive CT images but only 1 of 4 intramedullary tumors was positive. Three of 4 extradural intraspinal neoplasms were positive. All scans of paraspinal tumors were diagnostic. Of the 17, 11 extended into the spinal canal and 13 involved bony structures. All 5 metastatic carcinomas, the 3 chordomas and the multiple myeloma involved the vertebrae.

Computed tomography is extremely sensitive in detecting fine intraspinal calcifications but may not be diagnostic of neurofibroma unless it is highly enhanced or causes bony changes. Computed tomography is diagnostic of lipoma because of its low attenuation coefficients. Intramedullary tumors are not usually detected by present scanners unless water-soluble contrast material is used. Bone destruction by chordoma is visualized on CT scans. Osteolytic and osteoblastic vertebral lesions from spinal metastases can be demonstrated by CT scanning (Fig 3).

The limitations of present CT scanners are related to their inability to demonstrate the normal anatomy of the intra-

(9) J. Comput. Assist. Tomogr. 1:377–390, October, 1977.

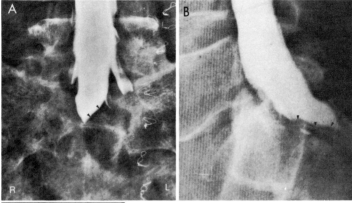

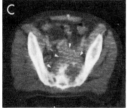

Fig 3. — Metastatic carcinoma of the sacrum in a man, aged 59, with a history of rectal carcinoma, who was referred because of low back pain and bladder dysfunction. **A,** lumbrosacral myelogram in anteroposterior view shows slight indentation *(arrowheads)* of the Pantopaque column at S1 level. **B,** myelogram in lateral projection again discloses slight anterior defect *(arrowheads)*. The posterior border of the vertebral body of the upper sacrum is not clearly seen. **C,** CT scan at this level outlines a large soft-tissue mass *(arrowheads)* with marked destruction of the sacrum. (Courtesy of Nakagawa, H., et al.: J. Comput. Assist. Tomogr. 1:377–390, October, 1977.)

spinal space. This problem may be solved by the development of higher-resolution devices. The use of water-soluble contrast medium is an important adjunct to CT of the spine.

▶ [Studies with CT scanning are being expanded in all sorts of disorders of the spinal canal, including dysrhaphia. James and Oliff (J. Comput. Assist. Tomogr. 1:391, 1977) describe 8 patients in whom sufficient information was obtained with this technique to obviate the use of invasive diagnostic studies, desirable especially in children and those with low conus medullaris. The scanner permitted direct linear measurement of objects with error of only $\pm$ 1.5% with appropriate matrix and software. Lesions found included spina bifida occulta with filum tethered to skin dimple, lipomeningocele and syringocele, lipomeningocele, sacral agenesis and syringomyelia with spina bifida. Operation confirmed diagnosis in 6 cases. Scans with the patient supine were found to be misleading because cerebrospinal fluid was compressed out of the masses; sedation was as necessary as with head scanning (phenobarbital, intramuscularly, for infants under age 1 year; general anesthesia with intubation for children in the prone position; and ketamine, intramuscularly, for patients in the supine or lateral decubitus positions). Hounsefield units were used to determine the nature of the soft tissue mass found within the canal.

Apparently the study on computer-assisted myelography by Coin, Chan, Keranen and Pennink (ibid., p. 398) was done before meglumine iocarmate was removed from the American market. The authors carried out conventional radiographic lumbar myelography with this water-soluble material (or, in a few cases, with metrizamide (Amipaque)). Lumbar studies with the body scanner were done with the patient's head and shoulders elevated. Thoracic and cervical CT studies were done 6 hours after lumbar instillation of iocarmate. In a few cases, tomography was done after diskography with these materials. The comparative photographs of myelograms versus CT scans are quite instructive. – Ed.] ◄

Tentorium in Axial Section. – *I. Normal CT appearance and nonneoplastic pathology* are described by Thomas P. Naidich, Norman E. Leeds, Irvin I. Kricheff, Rochelle M. Pudlowski, James B. Naidich and Robert D. Zimmerman.[1] Familiarity with the normal computerized tomography (CT) appearance and anatomical relationships of the tentorium provides a basis for understanding the CT manifestations of many nonneoplastic disease processes. The tentorium was visualized in 99% of 100 contrast-enhanced CT scans of good quality and was seen well in two thirds of cases. The torcular was well demonstrated in 30% of enhanced scans. The transverse sinuses were well shown bilaterally in 30% of scans and unilaterally in 10%. A section in the plane of the incisura will show the full contour of the tentorial margin. Any section exiting above the torcular will show converging V-shaped tentorial bands. Below the plane through the torcular the tentorial leaves diverge laterally toward their lateral calvarial attachments. A section passing directly through the torcular shows an M-shaped tentorial image (Fig 4).

A number of pathologic states such as calcification may make the tentorium more evident on CT scanning without contrast enhancement. Dilatation of the juxtatentorial cisterns from cerebral or cerebellar atrophy creates pools of cerebrospinal fluid that outline the surfaces of the tentorium. Severe ventricular dilatation delineates the position of the tentorium on CT without contrast enhancement. Conditions that enlarge tentorial channels and cause tentorial hypervascularity occasionally cause recognizable changes in the tentorial bands on CT scans both with and without contrast enhancement. Unusually wide, dense, "blushlike" tentorial bands on contrast-enhanced scans may be a sign of

(1) Radiology 123:631–638, June, 1977.

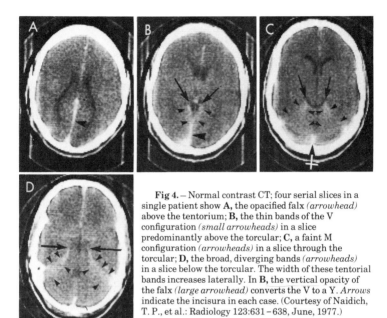

Fig 4. – Normal contrast CT; four serial slices in a single patient show **A,** the opacified falx *(arrowhead)* above the tentorium; **B,** the thin bands of the V configuration *(small arrowheads)* in a slice predominantly above the torcular; **C,** a faint M configuration *(arrowheads)* in a slice through the torcular; **D,** the broad, diverging bands *(arrowheads)* in a slice below the torcular. The width of these tentorial bands increases laterally. In **B,** the vertical opacity of the falx *(large arrowhead)* converts the V to a Y. *Arrows* indicate the incisura in each case. (Courtesy of Naidich, T. P., et al.: Radiology 123:631–638, June, 1977.)

tentorial hypervascularity. Arteriovenous malformations and venous sinus thrombosis may produce unusual prominence of the tentorial bands on contrast-enhanced CT scans.

II. Lesion localization is reviewed by Naidich, Leeds, Kricheff, Pudlowski, Naidich and Zimmerman.[2] The opacified tentorium provides an important landmark for localizing intracranial pathology on axial section, contrast-enhanced computerized tomography (CT) scans. Medial posterior temporal lesions lie anterolateral to the opacified lateral edge of the tentorium and may show flattening of their posteromedial contour. Lateral cerebellar lesions may show flattening of their anterolateral border. Occipital masses may show concavity of their medial aspects, and flattening of their medial borders to conform to the falx cerebri is sometimes noted. The lateral margins of posteromedial cerebellar lesions may be flattened, with the medial margins round. The

(2)   Radiology 123:639–648, June, 1977.

exact relationship of a mass to the incisura is clearly shown on contrast CT study. Larger incisural masses distort or obliterate the cisterns and may have flattened posterolateral margins.

Masses of the superior vermis, brain stem and aqueduct may be distinguished by their relationships to the tentorium and quadrigeminal cistern. Flattening of the tentorial border of an extra-axial posterior fossa mass indicates confluence with the roof of the posterior fossa and shows that the mass is growing up toward the incisura. Most tentorial meningiomas arise from the undersurface of the tentorium. Infratentorial tentorial meningiomas that grow up through the incisura often assume a "comma" configuration. At present it is extremely difficult to identify infratentorial meningiomas that have invaded the tentorium to grow into the supratentorial compartment. Large, long-standing purely infratentorial meningiomas may bulge the tentorium far upward and may even cause a supratentorial mass effect, with amputation or obliteration of the ipsilateral temporal horn, occipital horn or atrium.

▶ [Osborn (Radiology 123:93, 1977) has also described the anatomy and CT scan of the tentorium and has illustrated transtentorial herniation secondary to supratentorial mass effect. Further material on this topic is to be found in an article by Osborn, "The Medial Tentorium and Incisura: Normal and Pathologic Anatomy" (Neuroradiology 13:109, 1977). – Ed.]

Computer Tomography of Cerebellopontine Angle Lesions. Jens Thomsen, Carsten Gyldensted and Jack Lester[3] (Copenhagen) performed computerized tomography (CT) in 53 consecutive patients seen in 1974 – 76 with a working diagnosis of cerebellopontine angle tumor. The 160×160-matrix scanner obtaining 13-mm sections was used. Metrizoate sodium (Isopaque) was used for tumor enhancement. Seventeen patients had abnormal tumor signs at CT examination. A tumor was found at exploration in 15 of 16 patients. Reduced acoustic function was present in 16 tumor patients, reduced caloric function in 16 and 7th nerve involvement in 10. Seven patients had 5th nerve involvement, 5 had cerebellar symptoms, 2 had brain stem symptoms and 4 had choked disks. The cerebrospinal fluid protein level was elevated in all 14 patients evaluated. Tomography of the internal auditory meatus was negative in 8 patients; 2

(3) Arch. Otolaryngol. 103:65 – 69, February, 1977.

patients may have had false negative CT studies. Three of 36 petrous tomographic studies gave abnormal results.

A CT examination should be included in the workup for cerebellopontine angle tumor, preceding invasive procedures like pneumoencephalography and iophendylate cisternography. It can be used safely in patients with increased intracranial pressure. It is, however, not an alternative to cisternography because it does not demonstrate intrameatal or small tumors. The smallest tumor demonstrated by CT in the present series extended 7 mm into the angle. Further diagnostic procedures are not necessary in cases with clearly positive CT scans with tumor enhancement. Cisternography is indicated in cases with normal CT scans. In normal cases with increased intracranial pressure and normal CT scans, vertebral angiography can be performed to elucidate the diagnosis.

▶ [Bergeron, Cohen and Pinto (Arch. Otolaryngol. 103:314, 1977) take exception to the concept that CT scanning makes routine roentgenography and tomography superfluous for diagnosis of acoustic tumors. Computerized tomographic scanning is insensitive and unreliable for delineating size and configuration of the internal auditory canals and, with current technology, will not reliably show neuromas less than 1.5 cm in diameter. Uncommonly, CT scanning may also be falsely negative in the presence of relatively large lesions. The situation may change with further advances in CT scanning, especially with the advent of metrizamide cisternography.

Davis et al. (Radiology 124:81, 1977) have evaluated preoperative CT scans and operative findings in 49 consecutive patients with verified acoustic neuroma. The incidence of false negative scans was 20%; 10 false negative scans were with lesions of less than 2 cm at operation, but 3 of these were intracanalicular tumors. Currently, the sequence of study may well be plain films followed by contrast enhancement CT scanning. If the CT scan is positive, and plain films or polytomograms show erosion of the internal auditory meatus, nothing more need be done. If the scan is positive and no erosion is seen, angiography is advocated to determine if a meningioma is present or to exclude unusual vascular lesions, tortuous vertebrobasilar vessels and similar disorders. With tumors less than 2 cm in diameter, the scan will often be normal and should then be followed by polytomography and positive contrast study (Pantopaque or metrizamide). Computer reconstruction and coronal scanning may make possible detection of small lesions and of residual tumor.

Limitations of CT scanning in acoustic neuromas are also described by Hoffman and Cox (Arch. Otolaryngol. 103:594, 1977). They report two cases in which small acoustic tumors were not detected by CT scanning. One case involved a man, aged 58, with tomographic evidence of erosion, a negative CT scan and a Pantopaque study indicating a 1-cm lesion which was found and removed at operation. The other involved a boy, aged 17, with bilaterally enlarged canals with neurofibromatosis and also with an astrocytoma of the right cerebellum (which was detected by CT scanning and was removed); the acoustic neuromas were not removed in view of the minimal hearing loss.

Computerized tomography signs of acoustic neuroma given in order of frequency by Wortzman, et al. (J. Otolaryngol. (Suppl. 3) 6:63, 1977) are: a mass of increased density after contrast enhancement, obliterated 4th ventricle, displaced 4th ventricle, widened angle of the cistern, a mass of normal or increased density without enhancement, adjacent cerebellar edema, and a defect in metrizamide-filled cistern (when this study is available). The authors recommend the following scheme for study of a patient with retrocochlear hearing loss and vestibular dysfunction: temporal bone evaluation with plain films and polytome tomography, then CT scanning. If the result is negative, posterior fossa myelography is done with surgery if myelography is positive and follow-up if it is negative. If the CT scan is positive they advise angiography. A positive result is followed by surgery and a negative one, by pneumography or myelography. Operation follows if the result of myelography is positive, and if it is negative, the CT scan is said to be falsely positive. — Ed.] ◄

Serial Computed Tomography of Primary Brain Tumors Following Surgery, Irradiation and Chemotherapy.

James E. Marks and Mokhtar Gado[4] (Washington Univ.) studied the lesions in 55 patients having primary brain tumors by computed tomographic (CT) scanning before, during and after treatment. Patients had a mean of 3.7 CT studies performed, with a mean interval between the first and last studies of 10.1 months. Postirradiation follow-up ranged from 1 to 29 months. There were 18 glioblastomas, 18 low-grade astrocytomas, 14 unbiopsied tumors and 5 optic nerve gliomas in the series. All but 3 of the glioblastomas and astrocytomas were in the cerebral hemispheres. All these patients were treated surgically and also received 5,000 – 6,000 rad in 5 – 6 weeks to the entire brain or to generous local fields. All patients with optic nerve gliomas and unbiopsied tumors were irradiated. Chemotherapy was given to 17 patients.

Pretreatment scans showed reduced density in most glioblastomas and astrocytomas and normal density in most unbiopsied tumors and optic nerve gliomas. All the glioblastomas and 40% of the astrocytomas were enhanced by contrast medium injection, as were almost all unbiopsied tumors and 75% of optic nerve gliomas. Lesion size decreased after treatment in 62% of patients, stabilized in 29% and increased in 9%. The CT findings correlated with the clinical course in 93% of cases; 73% of tumors persisted, 20% disap-

(4)   Radiology 125:119–125, October, 1977.

peared and 7% recurred during follow-up. Hydrocephalus was noted on the last scan in 24% of patients. Persistent or reduced tumor density compatible with "brain softening" with or without contrast medium enhancement or a mass effect occurred in 73% of cases in this series.

The general lack of morphological-pathologic correlation makes pathophysiologic interpretation of CT scans somewhat conjectural. Nevertheless, the presence of contrast enhancement in all glioblastomas but only 40% of low-grade astrocytomas suggests that the latter tumor may have a worse prognosis if contrast enhancement is present. Indeed, it may be that contrast enhancement may be more accurate in prognosis than pathologic studies, with their sampling errors. Serial CT scans are not routinely justified, but in the presence of clinical deterioration are useful in confirming progression, recurrence, radiation injury or the development of hydrocephalus. They should be used on a research basis until the chronology of the morphologic events after the treatment of primary brain tumors is thoroughly understood.

Diagnosis of Isodense Subdural Hematomas by Computed Tomography. An "isodense" subdural hematoma is found at the intermediate stage of development of a hematoma, 30–90 days after the initial insult. Marco A. Amendola and Bernard J. Ostrum[5] (Albert Einstein Med. Center, Philadelphia) evaluated delayed CT scanning after contrast medium injection for demonstrating these hematomas. A total of 2,500 patients were studied in a 10-month period with use of a CT scanner with a 256×256 matrix. Four pairs of slices 13 mm thick were obtained in a plane angled 20 degrees to the canthomeatal line. Nine patients with unilateral effacement of sulci were restudied after the infusion of 100 ml Renografin 60; 7 of these also had delayed studies 4–6 hours after contrast medium injection. The 9 patients were aged 47–85. Only 3 had a history of trauma. Brain scans were reported as compatible with subdural hematoma in 3 patients, as completely negative in 4 and as compatible with infarct or tumor in 1. Subdural hematoma was proved at angiography and surgery in all cases.

All 9 patients showed effacement of cortical sulci over the

(5) Am. J. Roentgenol. 129:693–697, October, 1977.

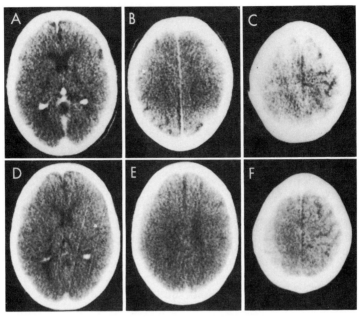

Fig 5.—No mass effect with enhancement. **A**–**C**, scans 5 minutes after contrast, showing no mass effect or other abnormality at ventricular level; unilaterally effaced sulci raised possibility of isodense subdural hematoma (**C**). **D**–**F**, delayed scans 6 hours later, showing enhanced subdural hematoma (**E** and **F**). (Courtesy of Amendola, M. A., and Ostrum, B. J.: Am. J. Roentgenol. 129:693–697, October, 1977.)

convexity. In 8 the effacement was ipsilateral and in 1, effacement was bilateral but a hematoma was present on only one side. Seven patients showed a mass effect on the precontrast scan with no change in density of the brain parenchyma. No hematoma was visualized immediately after contrast enhancement, but 3 of 7 patients having delayed scans exhibited the hematoma 4–6 hours after contrast medium injection.

The effacement sign is most often seen in subdural hematomas over the convexity of the cerebral hemisphere near the frontal and parietal lobes. The sign results from obliteration of the normal cerebrospinal fluid paths between the cerebral gyri by the isodense subdural collection. The findings in 1 patient are shown in Figure 5. A mass effect in the precontrast CT scan or unilateral effacement of cortical sulci over the convexity should lead to a suspicion of an isodense subdural hematoma. Delayed postcontrast scans show a hematoma in at least 40% of cases. The rest can only be demonstrated by cerebral angiography.

► ["Hare's ears sign" is the term applied by Marcu and Becker (Neuroradiology 14:81, 1977) to sharply pointed small anterior ventricular horns seen in CT scans of patients with bilateral chronic isodense subdural hematomas. They report 3 cases. This sign is found only when the two hematomas are in the parietal areas predominantly.

With the use of the 160×160 matrix, CT scanning of subdural hematomas becomes much more effective according to Scotti, Terbrugge, Melacon and Bélanger (J. Neurosurg. 47:311, 1977). Subdural hematomas were found to be more dense than surrounding brain in 100% of acute hematomas, of the same density in 70% of subacute hematomas and less dense than surrounding brain in 76% of those with chronic subdural hematomas.

Sequential CT scanning in 40 patients with intracerebral hematomas shows a decreasing density by an average of 0.7 EMI units per day. The mass effect (ventricular shift, for instance) does not decrease in proportion to this decrease in density of the hematoma. Residua include decreased parenchymatous density, focal atrophy and ventricular enlargement, according to Dolinskas, Bilaniuk, Zimmerman and Kuhl (Am. J. Roentgenol. 129:681, 1977).

Tomodensitometric measurements were made in 5,000 cases with CT scans by Collard, Dupont and San (J. Radiol. Electrol. Med. Nucl. 58:405, 1977). Diffuse hemorrhages with densities of 25–35 EMI units generally resorb quickly and leave little long-term residue. Collections of 35–45 EMI units are more slowly resorbed, but sometimes may be accompanied by spontaneous improvement. Persistence of values over 35 EMI units a week after hemorrhage has a bad prognosis and may support the decision to operate. The authors believe that tomodensitometric illustration of a capsulolenticular hemorrhage in a hypertensive patient contraindicates angiography; blood in the subarachnoid space supports angiography. Even when there is certainty of aneurysm rupture, CT evaluation may indicate whether angiography should be carotid or vertebral. At times, hemorrhage may be isodense and the lesion may pass unseen. Density measurements may be important in decisions as to when the patient may return to work and use of anticoagulants and those cases which may be medicolegal. – Ed.] ◄

Electron Density and Atomic Number Determination by Computed Tomography are reported by I. Isherwood, B. R. Pullan, R. A. Rutherford and F. A. Strang[6] (Univ. of Manchester). The feasibility of computed tomography (CT) scans obtained with two different beam energies permit calculation of attenuation coefficients in such a way as to allow extraction of electron densities and effective atomic num-

(6) Br. J. Radiol. 50:613–619, September, 1977.

bers for the measurements. Variations of as little as 1 part in 400 in effective atomic number could be detected with beams of 40 and 80 kev. It may be that such determinations may permit better detection of disease, more accurate differentiation of disease processes and study of biologic pathways.

Twelve patients with colloid cysts who had bilateral ventriculocisternostomy 1–23 years previously were studied. Nine patients and the colloid cyst of 1 patient who died before treatment could be instituted were subjected to double-energy CT scanning. Movement between successive scans made calculations impracticable in 2 other patients. The mean age at operation was 40.4; 8 patients were men. The estimated duration of symptoms indicated a possible tumor age up to 27 years. The definitive diagnostic procedure in most cases was Myodil ventriculography. Size did not appear to have any relation to estimated tumor age. Electron density of the colloid cysts, expressed as a function of attenuation value at 140 kev, showed a consistent relationship. Effective atomic number showed no such relationship. Chemical analysis gave no evidence of material of high

Fig 6. – Computed tomography scan of colloid cyst before (**A**) and after (**B**) ventricular drainage. (Courtesy of Isherwood, I., et al.: Br. J. Radiol. 50:613–619, September, 1977.)

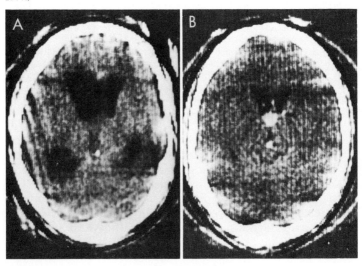

atomic number within an excised colloid cyst. One cyst was not detected at initial CT study, almost certainly because the initial sections were not low enough to include the tumor (Fig 6). Sections must include the suprasellar structures.

The high attenuation values of colloid cysts seem to be due to increased electron density, not to any increase in elements of high atomic number. The cysts do not appear to change in size or content over long periods. The long-term survival of patients treated solely by bilateral Torkildsen's ventriculocisternostomies suggests that this simple approach to the problem is a safe and effective one.

▶ [Colloid cysts of the 3d ventricle appear as rounded areas of normal or increased density located at the foramen of Monro, with increased attenuation after intravenous infusion of contrast materials. Four cases were found in 4,000 consecutive CT scans by Osborn and Wing (Radiology 124: 257, 1977). They found variable degrees of ventricular enlargement, lack of visualization of the anterior end of the 3d ventricle, and separation of the posteromedial portions of the frontal horns. Thin sections (8-mm overlapping sections) through the foramen of Monro are useful when there is no obvious obstructive hydrocephalus, for a 13-mm section may show the lesion only extremely faintly. Conversely, 13-mm slices may show an apparent cyst that turns out to be normal vasculature on 8-mm overlapping sections; choroid plexus, fornix and confluence of septal and thalamostriate veins may contribute to the confusion. – Ed.] ◀

Metrizamide Computed Tomography Cisternography: Pediatric Applications. Intrathecal enhancement of computed tomography (CT) scanning with use of water-soluble metrizamide can obviate many of the limitations of routine CT scanning. Burton P. Drayer, Arthur E. Rosenbaum, Donald B. Reigel, William O. Bank and Ziad L. Deeb[7] (Univ. of Pittsburgh) performed metrizamide CT cisternography on 22 children aged 1 month to 18 years. No premedication was usually necessary for children aged 12 and over. Intrathecal instillation of metrizamide was monitored by brief fluoroscopic screening. After instillation the patient was turned supine, tilted to a 60-degree Trendelenberg position for about 1 minute and returned slowly to a 15-degree Trendelenberg position for scanning with a 160×160 matrix. All patients had CT scanning before and after intravenous enhancement before the intrathecally enhanced scan.

(7) Radiology 124:349–357, August, 1977.

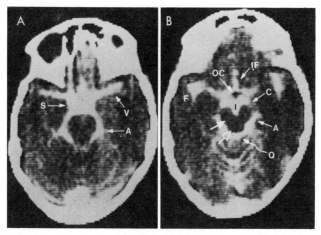

Fig 7.—Normal basal subarachnoid cisterns on metrizamide CT cisternography. **A,** pons-midbrain junction surrounded by metrizamide in ambient cistern *(A)*. Suprasellar cistern *(S)* filled with metrizamide communicates laterally with the sylvian cistern (of the middle cerebral artery, *V*). **B,** midbrain delineated by metrizamide in the interpeduncular *(I)*, crural *(C)*, ambient *(A)* and quadrigeminal *(Q)* cisterns. The tegmentum *(closed arrow)* of the midbrain is wide and the tectum *(open arrow)* is narrow. The suprasellar cistern is a broad polygon with a central transverse linear filling defect produced by the optic chiasm *(OC)*. The sylvian fissure *(F)* and interhemispheric fissure *(IF)* are also visualized. (Courtesy of Drayer, B. P., et al.: Radiology 124:349–357, August, 1977.)

Precise visualization of the basal subarachnoid spaces was obtained in each child (Fig 7). Distinct "blushing" of the superficial brain substance was noted in all normal subjects on the cranial CT 6-hour postinjection scan. The basal subarachnoid cisterns and ventricular system were free of contrast material at 24 hours. Accurate brain stem tumor delineation was obtained in all 3 children with brain stem masses. Filling defects were seen in patients with suprasellar space-occupying lesions. The cisternographic study was helpful in demonstrating posterior fossa extra-axial cysts. Abnormal cisternographic findings were obtained in 2 of 7 children with hydrocephalus. Encephalomalacia was demonstrated in a patient with CT findings suggestive of porencephaly. No child under age 6 had adverse reactions, and reactions in older children were not severe and were transient. Electroencephlograms showed epileptiform activity in 1 of 4 children, but no clinical seizure occurred and this child had had intracranial surgery.

Intrathecal contrast enhancement with cranial CT scanning provides a new approach to the study of basal mass lesions and to the physiologic study of cerebrospinal fluid flow patterns. Newer CT scanners and nonionic contrast agents should make possible better and even safer applications of this technique.

▶ [The authors considered 5 of the hydrocephalic children to have normal flow patterns, with no ventricular stasis beyond 12 hours and with normal evolution of typical cerebral blush in the parasagittal and convexity regions. The reactions to metrizamide in the children aged 6 or older included headache (3), nausea (3), vomiting (2) and apprehension with crying and olfactory phenomena (1). The reactions have been delayed 3–6 hours in onset, with the lag corresponding to the appearance of the cerebral blush. These results should be compared with those in the following article, in which cisternography was done with ¹¹¹In-DPTA. —Ed.] ◀

Computed Cranial Tomography and Radionuclide Cisternography in Hydrocephalus. John C. Harbert, David C. McCullough and Dieter Schellinger[8] (Georgetown Univ.) discuss the relations between computerized cranial tomography (CCT) and radionuclide cisternography in the evaluation of adult and pediatric hydrocephalus. The screening test of choice for adults with presenile dementia is CCT. It can strongly suggest normal-pressure hydrocephalus, but is does not indicate the degree of cerebrospinal fluid (CSF) obstruction present in hydrocephalus. The results of CCT and cisternography correlate reasonably well, but significant discrepancies may occur. Firm criteria for installing shunts in patients with normal-pressure hydrocephalus do not exist. A decision to install a shunt in a patient with a borderline case who has CCT evidence of moderate ventricular dilatation and few dilated sulci may be supported by cisternographic evidence of ventricular reflux and delayed clearance. Cisternography is useful in estimating CSF shunt patency.

Scanning by CCT has now largely supplanted cisternography as a screening procedure for macrocephaly in children. Obstructive noncommunicating hydrocephalus may be strongly suspected and basal and cerebellar tumors readily detected. Brain stem and posterior fossa abnormalities are often evident. Among patients without high CSF pressure who do not require immediate shunting, cisternography is

(8) Semin. Nucl. Med. 7:197–200, April, 1977.

useful in identifying those who may compensate without shunting. Patients with normal or delayed radionuclide clearance may be watched, but ventricular activity persisting at 24 hours is generally an indication for shunting, unless the child is exceptionally alert without evidence of psychomotor retardation. Convexity or cisternal block does not affect the decision to shunt; delayed ventricular clearance is the chief cisternographic indication.

► [It now becomes important to find out if there are significant advantages to CCT scanning with metrizamide compared to nuclide (indium) cisternography. The obvious immediate concern is one of safety and reactions; unfortunately these are not mentioned in the article by Harbert et al., and I am curious as to how the CCT scan changes when indium is in the subarachnoid spaces or ventricles.

In some cases of hydrocephalus studied with CCT scanning, there is decreased density around the ventricles, often associated with acute hypertensive hydrocephalus. The decrease has a gradient, being greatest nearest the ventricles, and the hypodensity usually disappears after the ventricles are reduced in size by shunting. It is thought by Pasquini et al. (J. Comput. Assist. Tomogr. 1:442, 1977) to be due to transit of cerebrospinal fluid from the ventricles to the white matter. The disappearance is taken as evidence of conservation of resilience of the intracranial structures. In study of 10 patients with normotensive hydrocephalus, the authors found the hypodensity to be less frequent than in hypertensive hydrocephalus, and there was little correlation between clinical status or recovery and disappearance of the hypodensity in these patients.—Ed.]

Confirmation of Brain Death at Bedside by Isotope Angiography. Laboratory documentation of brain death is often desirable, especially when the underlying disease is obscure and when there are legal and transplant considerations. Angiography demonstrates brain death, but radionuclide angiography is a less invasive technique for documenting the absence of cerebral blood flow. The method has been criticized because of the risk of transporting an apneic, potentially salvageable patient to the nuclear medicine department. Julius M. Goodman and Larry L. Heck[9] (Indiana Univ.) describe the use of a mobile gamma camera for diagnosis of brain death at the bedside. An anterior scan is obtained with 20 mCi ^{99m}Tc-labeled human albumin in a volume of less than 0.3 ml, with a 10-ml saline flush. Serial images are recorded every 3 seconds for 1 minute. Posterior and lateral static views are then obtained to assess filling of the sagittal sinus better.

(9)   J.A.M.A. 238:966–968, Aug. 29, 1977.

Typically in brain death the radionuclide bolus stops at the base of the skull and the intracranial circulation is not visualized. The picture is striking when a tourniquet is used to occlude the scalp circulation. The superior sagittal sinus is never seen on the dynamic or static studies. No condition producing similar scan findings has been encountered in a 6-year experience with over 25,000 brain scans. The results are usually clear-cut. An EEG is no longer considered to be necessary to confirm brain death. Brain death is not diagnosed if there is even the slightest suggestion of intracranial circulation, but if no flow is seen and the sagittal sinus is not demonstrated, the radionuclide scan need not be repeated. Life support has been continued in patients with severe drug intoxication in whom intracranial circulation has been demonstrated, sometimes with recovery.

The mobile gamma camera has been used at the bedside to diagnose the last 14 of 90 cases of brain death verified by radionuclide angiography. Portability has not detracted from the accuracy of the examination, and the method is less risky to the potentially salvageable patient. A single technologist can perform the examination.

Clinically Silent Brain Metastases: Can Radionuclide Scintigraphy Detect Them? The utility of brain scintigraphy in screening asymptomatic cancer patients for silent brain metastases is controversial. Frank Vieras and Charles M. Boyd[1] (Univ. of Arkansas) evaluated the results of brain scintigraphy in 136 patients with proved primary malignancies seen in 1973 – 75. The patients, male veterans, were asymptomatic for brain metastases and had normal neurologic findings at scintigraphy. Images were recorded after injection of 15 – 20 mCi pertechnetate, which followed an oral dose of potassium perchlorate. Dynamic studies were performed in 99 patients. A gamma camera with parallel-hole collimator was used.

Lung carcinoma was present in 52% of patients in this series. Two patients (1.5%) had abnormal static studies. One had two proved dural metastases and multiple microscopic foci of cerebral involvement by lung adenocarcinoma and the other had findings of skull metastases from prostatic

---

(1) Clin. Nucl. Med. 2:131–133, April, 1977.

carcinoma, which were also shown on bone scanning. Thirteen patients without established metastases had equivocal scan findings, due to physiologic variation or technical artifacts. Only 1 of 99 cerebral flow studies was reported as abnormal, in a patient with a history of cerebrovascular disease.

Dynamic brain scintigraphy did not show occult metastases in this series. Although a screening technique for detecting silent intracranial metastases would be extremely helpful, the present findings suggest that radionuclide brain imaging provides little added information in this group of patients.

► [Actually, this study does not answer the question in the title; what it does show is that the great majority of patients with cancer do not have isotopically detectable metastases in the brain. This is also true in autopsy series. The same conclusion may be drawn from the report by Wittes and Yeh (J.A.M.A. 238:506, 1977), who studied liver scans in 21 patients with oat cell cancer of the lung and found only 1 positive scan; only 1 of 35 patients with brain scan was found to have evidence of pickup. The authors conclude that liver and brain scans with isotopes are not useful in screening a patient with no clinical evidence of spread of oat cell carcinoma, even though the disease is prone to produce early and widespread metastases. — Ed.] ◄

Complications of Cerebral Angiography. Hans Olivecrona[2] (Stockholm) investigated the complications occurring in 5,531 consecutive cerebral angiographies done in 1970 – 74 on 3,730 patients, 54.4% of them male. Light sedation and local anesthesia were used in 78.3% of patients. A total of 3,978 artery punctures were performed. Most studies were done by the percutaneous femoral route. Carotid arteries were used in 37.8% of patients. Angiography of more than one vessel was done at the same sitting in 34.1% of patients. Isopaque cerebral contrast medium was used, usually in a dose of 8 ml per injection with use of a pressure injector. The catheter was flushed every minute with heparinized saline. The ECG was always recorded during cerebral angiography.

Complications occurred in 26.3% of patients. Of 1,220 complications, 861 were local, 191 general and 168 neurologic. The most frequent general symptoms were nausea and vomiting. A sensitivity reaction with urticaria was seen in 1.6% of patients. Hematoma was the most common local

(2) Neuroradiology 14:175–181, 1977.

complication. Perivascular contrast medium injection occurred only with carotid puncture in the neck. Vascular spasm related to the catheter tip was noted in 0.4% of all angiographies. Signs of intracranial embolism occurred in 0.4% of carotid angiographies. Fourteen patients had cerebral complications with resulting paresis; 12 had carotid and 2, vertebral angiography. Four patients had permanent neurologic sequelae with hemiparesis. Left carotid angiography was responsible for half the neurologic complications. Agitation was noted in 65 patients and increased somnolence in 44 patients. Six patients were comatose during angiography but none of them died. Seizures were seen in 6 patients with intracranial tumors. The duration of examination was not related to the occurrence of complications. No definite association of serious neurologic complications with less experienced investigators was apparent.

The overall rate of neurologic complications in this series was 4.6% and of paresis with or without aphasia, 0.4%. It is reasonable to assume that the risk of serious neurologic complications increases with increasing difficulty in selective catheterization of a vessel. Less experienced examiners may be more apt to occasion a greater number of local complications than more experienced ones.

▶ [This investigation was done in a unique manner, with an angiographic journal kept for each patient before, during and after the angiogram and the recording of all the incidents which might be called complications as well as notes on the position of the catheter tip, duration of the procedure, quantity of contrast medium and similar data. Hematoma was the most common local complication (18.9%) but did not require surgical intervention or, in the neck, tracheostomy. Even mild headache, slight nausea and occasional allergic skin reaction not causing patient distress were included. However, overall neurologic complications of 4.6% included agitation, drowsiness, confusion, vertigo, seizures, paresis, stupor and coma. Two patients acquired signs of anterior spinal syndrome with cervical myelopathy after catheter vertebral angiography. Left vertebral catheter angiography was the safest, and right vertebral angiography was the most dangerous. Somewhat fewer complications are encountered with right than with left carotid angiography, in accordance with the concept that the risk becomes greater with the increasing difficulty of catheterization of the various arteries. It is of interest that the 14 cerebral complications occurred in patients aged 20–59, and only 1 involved atherosclerosis!

Pinto et al. (Radiology 124:157, 1977) point out that computerized tomographic scanning may not always differentiate intra-axial from extra-axial lesions, especially when anteriorly placed. They advocate (during angiography) a base view which permits demonstration of posterior arcuate displacement of the anterior inferior cerebellar artery (AICA). Medial displacement of either the prepontine segment of the AICA or of the circum-mesencephalic portion of the superior cerebellar artery indicates brain stem involvement. Marked displacement of the superior cerebellar artery with little movement of the AICA indicates a high cerebellopontine angle mass (meningioma of incisura, trigeminal neurinoma), whereas marked displacement of the AICA with little movement of the superior cerebellar artery indicates a low cerebellopontine angle tumor, as with acoustic tumor.

By the time this YEAR BOOK appears, metrizamide should have been approved for use in myelography in the United States. Its use for cerebral angiography may be delayed but should be approved also, especially when it is realized that it is at least as safe as the current choice, the ionic material meglumine metrizoate (Isopaque Cerebral). A comparative study with double-blind technique was reported by Skalpe, Lundervold and Tjørstad (Neuroradiology 14:15, 1977), in 40 patients, aged 15–60 years, who were informed of the test. One patient who had a migraine syndrome had transient hemiplegia and dysarthria after meglumine angiography, but otherwise there were no statistical changes in blood pressure, EEG and circulation time. There was a statistically significant decrease in deterioration of EEG and bradycardia using metrizamide. In a report from the same clinic concerning meglumine angiography, transient hemiparesis lasting minutes to several days was found in about 1% of 554 patients. In the double-blind series, all angiograms were done via the femoral route, with 10 ml in the carotid artery and 8 ml in the vertebral artery. Total doses were not given, but the sequence generally used was that of left vertebral, right common carotid and left common carotid arteries. – Ed.] ◄

Ventriculography with Nonionic Water-Soluble Contrast Medium Amipaque (Metrizamide): Comparative Experimental and Clinical Studies. Shigeharu Suzuki, Kenjiro Ito and Takashi Iwabuchi[3] (Hirosaki Univ.) carried out animal and clinical studies of metrizamide for use in ventriculography. Metrizamide has been identified as extremely safe in toxicity studies. Twenty adult mongrel dogs received 1.5–5-ml doses of metrizamide by tube into the right lateral ventricle or by cisternal puncture. The ventriculograms were about as sharp as those obtained with 60% Conray. No marked EEG abnormalities were observed. Cerebrospinal fluid cell counts increased an average of 35/cu mm after cisternal injections of metrizamide. There were no signs of localized myoclonus or general convulsions after the injections. No abnormalities were seen in the ventricular wall or choroid plexus a month after contrast was injected into the ventricle.

Thirteen patients aged 6–74 years had 17 ventriculo-

(3) J. Neurosurg. 47:79–85, July, 1977.

graphic studies with 4–15 ml metrizamide. The contrast material was injected through a ventricular cannula or percutaneously in patients who were having shunt procedures. All the ventriculograms and a cisternogram were of adequate diagnostic quality. One patient had a mild headache after the examination. No abnormal EEG changes were found in the 3 patients so studied, and no significant cerebrospinal fluid changes were seen in 6 cases. None of the 3 deaths were related to the use of metrizamide.

Long-term observations after metrizamide administration are necessary, but the present findings indicate this agent is a superior contrast medium with respect to safety.

► [An excellent recounting of the development of metrizamide by its proponent, Per Amundsen of Oslo, is to be found (Wis. Med. J. 76:63, 1977). He is frank to admit that it is not a completely inert contrast medium, but points out that with proper technique (not permitting the material to reach the cerebral hemispheres undiluted), the serious reactions (seizures) should be avoided. – Ed.] ◄

Myelography with Metrizamide is discussed by F. L. M. Peeters[4] (Univ. of Amsterdam). Metrizamide is the first water-soluble contrast medium suitable for myelography of the cervical and thoracic as well as the lumbar region. Unlike other water-soluble mediums, it is nonionic. Headache can last 3 days after lumbar myelography with metrizamide. More serious side effects have not been reported. About 40% of patients have headache after cervical and thoracic myelography with metrizamide, which appears to compare favorably with other water-soluble mediums with respect to the risk of arachnitis. Water-soluble positive-contrast mediums are superior to gas, a negative-contrast medium, though gas is preferable for visualizing large spaces. Water-soluble mediums give better contrast and may penetrate channels which obstruct gas.

High cervical introduction of metrizamide is preferred for cervical myelography. Either cisterna magna puncture or puncture at C2–C3 may be carried out, with the head elevated so that the clivus is slightly higher than the cervical canal. If cervical puncture is contraindicated, contrast medium can be introduced into the lumbar subarachnoid space and guided cervically by cautious tilting. Lumbar puncture is preferable for thoracic myelography and the patient is

---

(4)   Radiol. Clin. (Basel) 46:203–213, 1977.

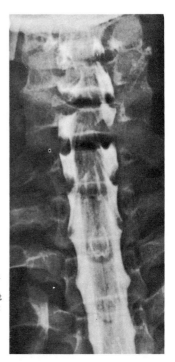

Fig 8. — Cervical myelogram of a woman with neurofibromatosis. All radices show neurinomas, both left and right. Full stop at level C2–C3. (Courtesy of Peeters, F. L. M.: Radiol. Clin. (Basel) 46:203–213, 1977.)

placed in the supine position. The prone position is preferable for examining the lumbar region. Patients examined with 10 ml metrizamide with an iodine concentration of 290 mg/ml also receive oral diazepam for up to 3 days after examination.

The findings in a patient with neurofibromatosis are shown in Figure 8. Both the quality of myelograms and the limited morbidity make metrizamide the current contrast medium of choice for nearly all myelographic studies.

▶ [The benefits of metrizamide outweigh its risks, according to Sackett et al. (Radiology 123:779, 1977). Intrathecal injections were made in 215 patients. Moderate to severe reactions occurred in 32% of those with cervical and 43% with lumbar studies, chiefly 6–8 hours after injection, when the contrast material was apt to be over the cerebral hemispheres. Headache responded well to mild narcotics. Nausea and vomiting were usually associated with headache, but required no specific medication. Three patients had seizures, all with higher than usual amounts of metrizamide in the upper canal. Two patients had significant hypotension

(1 with adrenal insufficiency that had not been provided for). Other symptoms included back and leg pain, neck and shoulder pain, fever, tinnitus and mental status change. The overall group of adverse reactions was similar to those with lumbar instillation alone of meglumine iocarmate (Dimer-X, Dimeray). Cervical injections of metrizamide are best done with fluoroscopic monitoring.

Metrizamide is the material of choice for enhancement of computerized tomography scanning when a chiasmatic lesion is suspected and conventional scan is negative, according to Drayer et al. (ibid., p. 339). Lumbar injection of 5–6 ml of material containing 190 mg iodine/ml was followed by head-down tilting with the patient prone or more often supine. With this low dose and immediate intracranial placement, most side effects have been mild, and no seizures have occurred in 10 cases.

Arachnoiditis does follow use of meglumine iocarmate (Dimer-X) and metrizamide (Amipaque) in monkeys, according to Haughton et al. (ibid., p. 681). Reduced volumes and concentrations of water-soluble materials probably result in less risk of arachnoiditis. The authors point out the value of a primate model for these studies, for only these animals (in contrast to carnivores) have a cauda equina with surrounding large quantities of cerebrospinal fluid. – Ed.] ◄

Postoperative Myelogram: Radiographic Evaluation of Arachnoiditis and Dural-Arachnoidal Tears is discussed by Robert M. Quencer, Michael Tenner and Lewis Rothman[5] (Downstate Med. Center, New York). Myelography of the postoperative spinal patient is usually done because of recurrent or worsening symptoms, and noninfectious meningeal inflammation is often encountered. Both water-soluble and water-insoluble myelographic contrast materials may cause meningeal irritation and arachnoiditis. The amount of Pantopaque remaining after myelography is not important compared to the sensitivity of the patient to the material. Metrizamide appears to be far superior to other water-soluble agents in this respect. Myelography per se can cause arachnoiditis. The changes of adhesive arachnoiditis can range from mild to severe. The mildest changes are root-sleeve blunting and small, irregular lateral defects. The end-stage is a completely obliterated subarachnoid space. A rootless, smoothly narrowed Pantopaque column may be observed, as may a smooth solitary extradural mass. Arachnoiditis may remain static or progress to a more severe form.

Loculated cysts may develop within the dura as a result of adhesive arachnoiditis, and secondary distortion or com-

(5) Radiology 123:667–679, June, 1977.

pression of the cord, spinal nerve roots or spinal vessels may result. An intramedullary cavity or syrinx may also be encountered. Interruption of the dura or arachnoid, or both, at surgery can lead to the formation of extradural cysts that are demonstrable at myelography. The severity of the symptoms are not related to the size of the cyst. A cerebrospinal fluid fistula may form if the tear is large or the cerebrospinal fluid can easily dissect through surrounding soft-tissue planes.

▶ [The most useful sign of recurrent disk prolapse (after initial lumbar disk surgery) is anterior indentation of the iophendylate column opposite a disk space, according to Moseley (Clin. Radiol. 28:267, 1977). Inflammatory changes were indicated by loculation of the subarachnoid space, matting or marked swelling of the nerve roots, irregularity of the theca, and the absence of the posterior bulge at the level of the operation. Waisting of the contrast column, nonfilling of nerve root sheaths, complete myelographic block and posterior indentations were confirmatory evidence of the presence of disease, but not helpful in determining its nature. — Ed.] ◀

Myelographic Features of Mucopolysaccharidoses: New Sign. Dural thickening secondary to abnormal collagenous deposition is an uncommon cause of myelopathy in the mucopolysaccharidoses. Robert D. Sostrin, Anton N. Hasso, Donald I. Peterson and Joseph R. Thompson[6] (Loma Linda Univ.) recently saw 2 patients with progressive myelopathy secondary to dural thickening in the cervical region. One had the Maroteaux-Lamy syndrome (MPS-VI), whereas 1 had a variant of the Hurler-Schie compound (MPS-I H/S).

Man, 22, had had progressive weakness of all extremities for 4 years but was well oriented with good intellectual function. Generalized weakness was noted throughout the extremities, and pain sensation was reduced in the distal lower extremities. Vibratory sense was markedly reduced in the feet and the gait was somewhat staggering and wide based. Reflexes were normal to slightly hyperactive throughout. Sustained bilateral ankle clonus was noted. Coarse facies and short stature were apparent, as was an apical systolic murmur. Absence of α-L-iduronidase confirmed the diagnosis of Hurler-Schie compound. Spinal x-rays showed moderate platyspondyly in the upper thoracic region and oar-shaped ribs. A Pantopaque myelogram showed marked concentric impingement on the subarachnoid space in the cervical region (Fig 9). Attempted intubation at planned cord decompression failed because of abnor-

(6) Radiology 125:421–424, November, 1977.

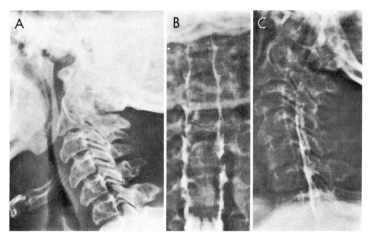

Fig 9.—**A,** lateral cervical spine. The vertebral structures are dysplastic but the spinal canal is not narrowed. **B** and **C,** oil contrast myelograms, posteroanterior and lateral prone views, respectively. The cord is compressed in the sagittal plane with marked separation of the spinal structures from the lateral and ventral surfaces of the bony canal. (Courtesy of Sostrin, R. D., et al.: Radiology 125:421–424, November, 1977.)

mal airway anatomy, and the patient died after a respiratory arrest. Autopsy showed marked dural thickening in the cervical region with cord compression.

The other patient had similar myelographic findings. Opening of the dura was followed by improved neurologic findings in this case. Both these patients had features of an upper motor neuron disorder with spastic gait abnormalities. The clinical manifestations were progressive in nature. Myelograms showed near-complete obliteration of the contrast-filled subarachnoid space and compression of the spinal cord. The dura was thickened in both cases.

Signs of progressive cord compression in patients with mucopolysaccharidosis should be evaluated myelographically and not directly ascribed to acquired narrowing of the bony canal. Laminectomy and dural splitting may relieve the myelopathic symptoms in patients with constriction of the subarachnoid space.

Techniques

▶ Volume 4 of *Advances and Technical Standards in Neurosurgery* (New York: Springer-Verlag New York, Inc., 1977), edited by H. Krayenbuhl, has continued the excellent series on technical details in neurosurgery. These begin with the chapter by N. A. Lassen and D. H. Ingvar, "Clinical Relevance of Cerebral Blood Flow Measurements." These studies have been done with ^{133}Xe injections into the exposed internal carotid artery during carotid endarterectomies and carotid ligations for aneurysms. In the former, the flow studies give objective evidence for or against the need for an arterial bypass or shunt. In focal cortical epilepsy, the regional blood flow was measured by a multidetector scintillation counter, reading 254 regions simultaneously with a maximal counting rate 100 times greater than the conventional gamma counter. The focus of abnormal (increased) blood flow was easily found in 9 patients studied interictally, while the EEG was distinctly focally abnormal in 2 and completely normal in 2. During a seizure, there was marked increase in focus, which promptly became smaller when the seizure was stopped with diazepam. In patients with severe brain damage the severity can be assessed by measuring reduction of blood flow and oxygen consumption (syndromes with coma, akinetic mutism and dementia). Sensory stimuli changes the blood flow by varying amounts in these patients. The predictive value of such tests is unknown and comparisons have not yet been made with evoked potentials.

W. G. Taylor and J. S. P. Lumley (ibid., p. 15) contend that surgery should be the treatment of choice for patients with transient ischemic attacks (TIA) and proved extracranial stenotic lesions. The operative mortality should be about 1% and severe neurologic sequelae less than 4%. Surgery should generally be avoided in the developing stroke. Completed stroke cases will not be improved by operation. To justify operations on an asymptomatic patient, the mortality should be less than 1% and the complication rate no more than 2%. These authors believe shunts should always be used. Operations should not be done during an acute stroke nor within 2 weeks of an acute episode.

"Intrathecal Injection of a Neurolytic Solution for the Relief of Intractable Pain" (ibid., p. 43), by J. Rétif, discusses the relative merits and difficulties with use of alcohol and phenol solutions. Neither is advocated for pain associated with benign lesions. Phenol is used in 5% solution or 7.5% solution in glycerin; Rétif prefers this hyperbaric solution to alcohol because it is more easily manipulated than alcohol. Complications are uncommon if fractional injections are made over 20–30 minutes. Chemical rhizotomy appears better than percutaneous cordotomy for bilateral pelvic and lower extremity pain syndromes. It is less useful in upper extremity pain where failures rise to 60–75% of cases.

The "technical standards" in this volume include L. Symon's "Olfactory Groove and Suprasellar Meningiomas" (ibid., p. 67), "Microsurgical Approach to Acoustic Neurinomas," by M. G. Yaşargil, R. D. Smith and J. C. Gasser (ibid., p. 93), and "Balloon Arterial Catheter Techniques in the Treatment of Arterial Intracranial Diseases" (ibid., p. 131), by G. Debrun, P. Lacour and J. P. Caron.

Tumors of the olfactory groove and suprasellar region account for about 10% of all meningiomas. Brief descriptions of the symptoms, signs and diagnostic techniques are illustrated. Discussions of anesthesia, position and bone-flap placement are followed by techniques of excision, including "uncapping" of olfactory groove tumors by frontal lobe resection. The importance of control of blood supply and care to avoid damage to optic apparatus and carotid arteries is stressed for each tumor locus. Brief tabulation of results in 40 cases is given (2.5% operative mortality = I case). Details of closure are given, including use of tissue glue to cover sinus defects.

The extraordinary results of operations on acoustic neurinomas by the Zurich neurosurgeons are detailed by Yaşargil et al. The detailed step-by-step procedures are well described and illustrated. The importance of position, anesthesia, microscopy and knowledge of the anatomy are stressed.

Debrun and co-workers make their own latex balloons and attach them to the intra-arterial catheters on the day of their use in arterial disease. Release of the balloon is sometimes difficult and there are numerous pitfalls. The balloons are kept distended with a quick-setting plastic after proper placement. Treatment of carotid-cavernous fistula, vertebrovertebral fistula and intracavernous aneurysm of the internal carotid artery is illustrated. The authors' account of the catheter construction is in marked contrast to the secrecy that appears to envelope technical details of similar procedures carried out by Serbinenko.

It is to be hoped that a cumulative index will be available when a sufficient number (10?) of these volumes have appeared. — Ed. ◄

Operative Techniques for Management of Lesions Involving Dural Venous Sinuses.

John P. Kapp, Isaac Gielchinsky and Steven L. Deardourff[7] describe a surgical approach to the management of dural venous sinus lesions developed at an evacuation hospital in Vietnam and report the results obtained in 16 patients who had penetrating craniocerebral injuries with involvement of the dural sinuses. A series of 79 consecutive cases seen in Vietnam in 1968–70 was reviewed. An intravenous tube was placed in a large vein (usually saphenous) initially, and if grafting was a possibility, a vein segment was obtained at that time. Bleeding was controlled by inflating balloons within the sinus lumen. An internal shunt was used to prevent venous stasis if it was necessary to occlude a critical sinus

(7) Surg. Neurol. 7:339–342, June, 1977.

temporarily. Nonessential sinuses were ligated if this was technically easier than primary repair. Essential sinuses were repaired primarily if possible or with a vein graft if there was extensive tissue loss after débridement.

In the Vietnam series, there was 1 death among 22 cases involving the anterior sagittal sinus, 15 deaths among 35 cases involving the posterior sagittal sinus and 5 deaths among 21 cases involving the transverse sinus. In the present series, no deaths occurred among 5 cases in which the anterior sagittal sinus was ligated and none among 8 in which the posterior sagittal sinus was repaired. One of 3 patients undergoing repair of the transverse sinus died.

Often repair of a simple laceration is quicker and easier than ligation of a sinus, but the transverse sinuses should be repaired. Primary repair is indicated if it can be done without narrowing the lumen by more than half. Otherwise, reversed saphenous vein segments are used as grafts, as shown in Figures 10 and 11. This approach permits lesions of the dural venous sinuses to be managed in a relatively bloodless field. Repair can be achieved while blood loss is reduced, and

Fig 10 (left). – Shunt in place with balloons inflated within lumen of sinus. Saphenous vein graft has been sutured to wall of sinus on right side.

Fig 11 (right). – Interrupted sutures have been placed between wall of sinus on left side and vein graft, to be tied when shunt is removed.

(Courtesy of Kapp, J. P., et al.: Surg. Neurol. 7:339 – 342, June, 1977.)

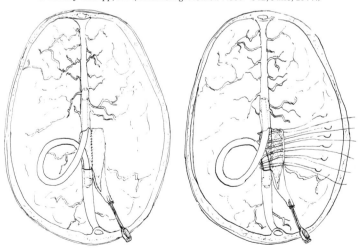

the problem of brain swelling secondary to venous stasis during repair is eliminated. The greatest benefit from sinus reconstruction is in patients with injury of the posterior sagittal sinus.

► [Repair or replacement of most of the superior longitudinal sinus may be necessary if a meningioma involving the sinus is to be removed well enough to prevent recurrence. – Ed.] ◄

Subgaleal Shunt for Temporary Ventricle Decompression and Subdural Drainage has been evaluated by George E. Perret and Carl J. Graf[8] (Univ. of Iowa). The usual methods of temporarily reducing intraventricular pressure are designed to be closed systems, but the risk of infection and its complications is always present. In ventriculo-subgaleal shunting, trephine openings are made in the posterior parietal area and a cannula introduced into the ventricle to estimate brain thickness. A shunt tube is then passed into the ventricle, a pocket is made in the subgaleal space and the distal end of the ventricular tube is placed in the space. The procedure can conveniently be done at the time of air ventriculography. The subgaleal space has remained functional with apparent fluid-absorbing surfaces for 3 weeks and longer. In subdural-subgaleal shunting a trephine opening is made over the hematoma, usually in the parietal region, and shunt tubing is placed in the subdural space before its distal end is led to the subgaleal space.

The ventriculosubgaleal shunt technique was useful in 2 tumor patients. The subdural-subgaleal shunt has been used in 26 patients to drain recurrent subdural hematomas after initial surgical evacuation of fluid hematomas or symptomatic hygromas. Usually the shunt was as effective as the more complicated subdural-peritoneal shunt.

The ventriculosubgaleal shunt immediately decompresses the ventricular system after ventriculography, especially in the presence of a tumor obstructing the 3d or 4th ventricle. Other indications for the shunt are decompression before definitive surgery, decompression during radiotherapy for brain tumors and the control of increased intracranial pressure and hydrocephalus secondary to subarachnoid hemorrhage. Small lateral ventricles contraindicate the procedure. Complications are few. The ventriculosubgaleal

(8)   J. Neurosurg. 47:590–595, October, 1977

shunt requires little postoperative care. The subdural-sub-galeal shunt avoids the risk of subdural infection from repeated subdural puncture, is simpler to perform than the subdural-peritoneal shunt and is as effective in draining the subdural space.

► [Such shunts have been used in 173 cases since 1967, according to the authors. There were 55 supratentorial and 87 infratentorial tumors and 57 nonneoplastic cases. These included 27 cases of hydrocephalus, and these would be the ones of great interest in determining how long the subgaleal shunts work. Historical accounts of development of treatment of hydrocephalus usually speak disparagingly of subgaleal shunts because they do not work indefinitely, but Perret and Graf have now shown how effective they can be for temporary ventricular decompression. They also emphasize the need to create a blood-free subgaleal pocket 10 cm in diameter to harbor the fluid, in contrast to the ancient procedure of just putting a catheter tip under the galea. Those who have seen children with accumulation of subgaleal fluid after skull fractures are familiar with the innocuous nature of these masses — and the suddenness with which they may disappear, as well as the rarity with which they have to be tapped. However, for instances of tumor in which a long-term or intermittent need for ventricular decompression can be foreseen, a preliminary ventriculo-peritoneal shunt may still be the best way of dealing with the problem. — Ed.] ◄

Cisternoatrial, Ventriculocisternal and Other Cisternal Shunts Simplified: Percutaneous Technique. Robert F. Spetzler, Philip R. Weinstein, Norman Chater and Charles B. Wilson[9] (Univ. of California, San Francisco) use lateral C1–C2 puncture to introduce a catheter into the cisterna magna for treating communicating hydrocephalus and aqueductal stenosis, to drain noncommunicating tumor cysts and to administer intrathecal antibiotics.

A spring-reinforced Silastic catheter with a radiopaque marker in the end of a multiperforated tip has been designed to fit through a no. 16 Touhy needle, which is inserted through a 1-cm skin incision into the subarachnoid space between the C1 and C2 laminae. The catheter is passed into the cisterna magna, and the needle is withdrawn over the shunt tubing. The catheter can then be connected to a reservoir inserted through a mastoid incision. In communicating hydrocephalus a needle is inserted into the internal jugular vein, and through this a catheter is placed into the atrium. In aqueductal stenosis a catheter is passed into the ventricle through a needle placed through a posterior

(9) J. Neurosurg. 47:299–302, August, 1977.

parietal twist drill opening. It then is connected via a reservoir to the cisternal catheter. The catheter may be placed directly into a cyst that is to be shunted. A cisterna magna catheter can be used in coccidioidomycosis when lumbar puncture is precluded by secondary arachnoiditis.

The percutaneous approach to the cisterna magna is simple and safe and requires minimal operative intervention. No operative complications have resulted. Variations of cisternal shunts have been used in 11 patients. The lateral percutaneous route to the subarachnoid space has been used well over 200 times in the past 4 years without any complications. Vertebral artery puncture remains a potential hazard, as does puncture of the spinal cord. Cord puncture can be avoided by verifying proper needle position radiographically. The percutaneous route to the jugular vein is safe and reliable.

▶ [Diversion of cerebrospinal fluid into the lymphatic system has been carried out in adults by Kempe and Blaylock (J. Neurosurg. 47:86, 1977). Experiences with a supraclavicular approach to sympathectomy led to the use of this "vascular" channel that has its own valvular system. Thus none of the mechanical problems of ordinary ventriculoatrial shunts are encountered, nor does blood come in contact with the single silicone tube that goes from ventricle to thoracic duct. Ten of the 16 patients have done well with this system.

A much older shunting system, using the ureter, is no longer employed. Its complications had included meningitis, scoliosis, cauda equina syndromes and arachnoiditis. Fischer, Welch and Shillito (ibid., p. 96) report 3 instances of syringomyelia long after such lumboureteral shunts. The exact cause is unclear, although crowding of neural tissues into the foramen magnum due to lowered lumbar spinal pressure may be implicated. The authors emphasize the indolent nature of the disorder and advise search for early symptoms in patients who have had such ureteral shunts. — Ed.] ◀

Mechanical and Physiologic Effects of Dentatotomy. Controversy exists as to whether patients with spondylotic myelopathy should be operated on. Some clinical observations suggest tethering of the spinal cord by the dentate ligaments in this condition. Joseph F. Cusick, James J. Ackmann and Sanford J. Larson[1] examined in 14 dogs the role of the dentate ligaments in the pathogenesis of myelopathy secondary to diseases that alter the normal biomechanics of the spinal canal. The effects of elevation of the cord posteriorly on somatosensory evoked potentials

---

(1) J. Neurosurg. 46:767–775, June, 1977.

and tension requirements were compared before and after dentate ligament section in acute studies.

At levels of posterior displacement usually within the confines of the canine spinal canal, the dentate ligaments were found to be the most significant element increasing tension requirements and evoked potential changes. Findings in the dog studies confirmed other observations that the degree of cord deficit is proportional to the number of cord segments involved. In human cadavers, for a given increment of posterior displacement, tension was greater before the dentate ligaments were cut. With moderate degrees of cord elevation, tension decreased markedly after dentate section. Tension in the elevated cord was increased when the spine was flexed and reduced with extension, both before and after dentate ligament section.

These observations show a restrictive influence of the intact dentate ligaments on posterior spinal cord elevation. Cord blood flow studies were not done, but it does not appear likely that the rapid recovery seen would be due to a reversal of cord ischemia. If a laminectomy is done for spondylotic myelopathy, division of the dentate ligaments appears justifiable, especially if gas myelography shows persistent adherence of the spinal cord to the floor of the spinal canal. A single illustrative case report is presented.

▶ [At times, the influence of multiple spondylotic bars is such that when the dentate ligaments are cut the entire cord migrates within the dural sheath; therefore, when the latter is to be sutured, there appears not to be enough room. In such instances, a dural graft may give adequate room for the spinal cord and cerebrospinal fluid, but then there is the risk of cerebrospinal fluid leak. — Ed.] ◀

Terminal Ventriculostomy for Syringomyelia. W. James Gardner, Herbert S. Bell, Pete N. Poolos, Donald F. Dohn and Marta Steinberg[2] (Cleveland Clinic Found.) reviewed records of 12 patients who underwent terminal (lumbar) ventriculostomy in 1973–75 for syringomyelia. Average patient age was 22 years, and the average interval from onset of symptoms to ventriculostomy was 17 years. The tip of the conus was at or below the level of L2 in 11 cases. Nine patients were scoliotic, and 7 had basilar impression. Seven had had a previous craniovertebral decompression, after which 5 improved and 1 became worse.

(2)   J. Neurosurg. 46:609–617, May, 1977.

Pneumoencephalography remains by far the most reliable radiographic procedure for demonstrating syringomyelia. Placement of the film cassette on the shoulder in contact with the flexed head eliminates the need for tomography. The head is flexed forward and the patient tilted until the cervical spine is straight. Air (30 cc) is injected by lumbar puncture under thiopental analgesia without intubation. In half the cases, fluid did not escape from the divided terminal ventricle at operation, presumably because of the recommended head-down position at operation.

All but 2 patients have improved on follow-up for up to 30 months after surgery. Anhidrosis and muscle fasciculations cleared immediately, and other signs and symptoms improved in all cases. The only postoperative complication, a hematomyelia, contributed to a poor result.

Terminal ventriculostomy deserves further trial as a substitute for craniovertebral decompression in the management of syringomyelia. All syringomyelia is symptomatic hydromeylia; noncommunicating syringomyelia does not occur. Intradural arachnoid diverticula, filling from above, constitute the subarachnoidal counterpart of the syrinx. The erect posture may aggravate the symptoms of syringomyelia, perhaps by increasing the downward thrust of the ventricular pressure wave.

Safety of Minidose Heparin Administration for Neurosurgical Patients. Deep vein thrombosis and pulmonary embolism continue to cause postoperative morbidity and mortality. Hugh G. Barnett, John R. Clifford and Raeburn C. Llewellyn[3] (New Orleans) evaluated the safety of minidose heparin therapy in 150 adult patients who were having elective neurosurgical procedures. No patient had a history of bleeding disorders, deep vein thrombosis or pulmonary embolism. Heparin was given subcutaneously with preoperative medication and every 12 hours postoperatively while patients were confined to bed. All patients were treated for at least 3 days postoperatively. The most common surgical procedures were craniotomy for tumor, anterior cervical fusion and lumbar disk surgery.

No complications related to heparin administration were observed. There was no excessive bleeding or difficulty with

(3) J. Neurosurg. 47:27–30, July, 1977.

hemostasis. Four wound seromas required aspiration post-operatively. There were 2 wound hematomas. One patient had a nonfatal pulmonary embolus. Seven patients died; autopsies were performed in 6. Four autopsies showed no evidence of deep vein thrombosis or pulmonary emboli. One patient, who died of myocardial infarction, had many small pulmonary emboli. The other autopsied patient had a massive, fatal pulmonary embolus, which occurred 15 days after removal of a meningioma; heparin therapy had been stopped 5 days postoperatively. The 1 death in a nonautopsied patient was due to pneumonia.

Administration of minidose heparin perioperatively to neurosurgical patients, especially high-risk patients, may well reduce the incidence of deep vein thrombosis and pulmonary embolism. The treatment is simple, safe and inexpensive and does not place the patient at any increased risk.

► [The authors wisely point out that their study was done primarily to determine the safety of the program of heparin therapy they used. "The purpose of this study was not to test the effectiveness of minidose heparin in preventing deep venous thrombosis or pulmonary emboli, and we do not believe any valid conclusions in this regard can be drawn." I was brought up, neurosurgically, in an era that favored the use of aspirin for pain and temperature control — and the incidence of pulmonary embolism was extremely small. Gastric bleeding *did* occur, and I would certainly rather give up aspirin than steroids which also produce this complication. Perhaps a double-blind study could be done with aspirin plus antacid, steroid plus antacid, and minidose heparin in lumbar disk surgery or other non-life-threatening neurosurgical procedures, with the use of clinical response and perhaps nuclide imaging to determine the frequency of deep vein thrombosis. Obviously, the duration of bed rest and early ambulation would also have to be considered. — Ed.] ◄

► ↓ Or perhaps a more mechanical means of preventing complications should be undertaken, as in the following article. — Ed. ◄

Prevention of Deep Vein Thrombosis in Neurosurgical Patients: Controlled, Randomized Trial of External Pneumatic Compression Boots. John J. Skillman, Richard E. C. Collins, Nicholas P. Coe, Betty S. Goldstein, Ruth M. Shapiro. Nicholas T. Zervas, Michael A. Bettmann and Edwin W. Salzman[4] (Harvard Med. School) evaluated effectiveness of external pneumatic compression of the calves in the prevention of deep vein thrombosis (DVT) in 95 patients having neurosurgical procedures. Study patients

(4) Surgery 83:354–358, March, 1978.

wore inflatable boots from induction of anesthesia to the end of the period of bed rest. The boots produce an inflation cycle of 10 seconds of rapid inflation to 35 – 40 mm Hg, followed by slower deflation and recycling once per minute. Development of deep vein thrombosis was monitored by the ^{125}I-fibrinogen technique.

The study and control patients were comparable in age and duration of anesthesia. Twice as many craniotomies were done for tumor in the control group. Seven of 20 control patients having craniotomy had deep vein thrombosis compared with 1 of 11 patients in the study group. About three fourths of all patients received drugs known to interfere with platelet function before or after surgery. The rate of deep vein thrombosis was 25% in the control group and 8.5% in the study group. The positive benefit from compression was greater if the 2 patients with positive scans and no phlebograms done were excluded from statistical analysis. The incidence of false positive scans was 24%. No patient had symptomatic pulmonary embolization in the hospital, but 1 control patient who died had autopsy evidence of embolism although death was considered due to pneumonia. Another control patient had pulmonary embolization after discharge.

These results strongly suggest that intermittent calf compression by inflatable plastic boots is an effective means of preventing deep vein thrombosis in patients having neurosurgery, in whom anticoagulants are contraindicated because of the risk of hemorrhage. The effect of compression was especially apparent in patients having craniotomy for tumor. Similar results have been obtained in patients having open urologic operations, a group in whom the use of anticoagulants is also of concern.

Use of Microfibrillar Collagen as Topical Hemostatic Agent in Brain Tissue. John D. Rybock and Don M. Long[5] (Johns Hopkins Hosp.) assessed the long-term effects of applying microfibrillar collagen (MFC), a water-insoluble partial acid salt of collagen prepared from purified bovine corium and processed into microcrystals of submicron size, to neural tissue of dogs. The product is a dry, fluffy substance that is self-adherent; it is also available in a nonwoven sheet form. After bilateral craniotomies were made

(5) J. Neurosurg. 46:501–505, April, 1977.

in 12 mongrel dogs, hemostasis was attempted with MFC alone on one side and with gelatin foam alone on the other. The animals were killed after 2, 4 and 6 months.

When gelatin foam was used, bone wax was always necessary to control diploic hemorrhage and bipolar coagulation to control bleeding from pial vessels. Except for an occasional large pial vessel, MFC alone provided effective hemostasis. The material adhered tightly as soon as it was applied to a wound, and hemostasis was usually immediate and complete. No hematoma, increased intracranial pressure, cysts or abscesses were observed. Marked glial proliferation was seen at lesion margins in 2-month specimens, and islands of fibrous material were present on the MFC-treated side. An even better-defined superficial collagen layer was present at 4 months, with persistent moderate chronic cell infiltration. A well-defined collagen layer with few fibroblasts replicated the dura at 6 months. Few chronic inflammatory cells remained at this time. The gliotic margin of the lesion was unremarkable.

Although MFC is a "foreign" protein, the potential for antibody induction appears small. Microfibrillar collagen appears to be as good as or better than gelatin foam by most criteria. It is absorbable, does not provoke a major tissue reaction and is not significantly neurotoxic. Controlled studies in patients are needed to reach a final conclusion, but MFC appears definitely to improve the control of surface bleeding.

▶ [In human beings, gelatin foam may be used with considerable success to stop bleeding from bone. Several exhibits at meetings of the American Association of Neurological Surgeons have demonstrated the problems with use of gelatin foam in hemostasis and the importance of prompt application of a cotton patty and suction. Microfibrillar collagen has some advantages in this regard. We have not found any difference in perineural scarring in dogs when microfibrillar collagen was compared with gelatin foam sponge. I have suggested to the Avicon Company that cost is a great hindrance to use of the collagen preparation and have proposed smaller packets to avoid the waste which may occur when the usual container is used. — Ed.] ◀

Technique of the Transbuccal Approach. M. Jomin and N. Bouasakao[6] emphasize the need for certain preoperative precautions to avoid postoperative problems. Prevention of sepsis in the mouth and pharynx includes repair

---

(6) Neurochirurgie 23:259–264, 1977.

of dental cavities, systematic bacteriologic investigation and a program of local-regional disinfection instituted 5 days before surgery. Buccal morphology varies from patient to patient and may interfere with the normal course of surgery. One may have to repair an ogival palate, remove bare-necked teeth and evaluate the maximal aperture of temporomaxillary articulations.

TECHNIQUE. — With the patient in the dorsal decubitus position and the head and neck hyperextended by a block, maximum opening of the mouth is obtained with Guillaume or ORL tonsil retractors. The tongue is placed behind the lower dental arch. Opening of the velum and palate is necessary to achieve transvelopalatine entry and to reach the clivus and cerebrospinal junction. A median incision is made in the velum and palatine mucosa after local anesthesia with Xylocaine and epinephrine. According to the specific anatomy that is present, the palate and palatine apophysis are then resected from the superior maxilla, opening the choanae and cavum. Opening of the posterior pharyngeal wall is an indispensable step in reaching the clivus. A vertical incision is most convenient. After lateral scaling of the fibromucosa and musculoligamentous plane, the osseous plane is bared with a Cloward self-retaining blade retractor. Osseous formations are then opened with long and fine punches and pneumatic or electric drills. The clival resection is some 2.5 cm long and 1.5 cm wide; spinal resection is as required. The rigid dura adheres quite firmly to the clivus. Its incision allows good access to the lesion and an airtight, fine closure. Closure of the dura is achieved with separate stitches. Reinforcement with musculoaponeurotic material may be used to avoid escape of cerebrospinal fluid. The posterior pharyngeal wall is closed in two layers, on the fibromuscular level with synthetic catgut and on the mucosal level with silk sutures. Repair of the velum must be meticulous to avoid postoperative functional difficulties. A nasopharyngeal tube, placed after the end of operation, allows postoperative alimentation.

A major postoperative risk is the escape of cerebrospinal fluid within a septic situation. The risk of meningitis is limited by diminishing as much as possible such escape and assuring antiseptic local conditions.

Although seemingly complex, this approach is technically simple and rapid and requires a minimum of instruments. Two less favorable aspects are the necessity for a tracheotomy of several days' duration and the risk of infection, since the immediate airtight meningeal closure is only relative.

▶ [The illustrations in the original article, too numerous to include here, are extremely useful. The operation is done with general anesthesia administered via a low tracheostomy. — Ed.] ◀

Cerebrospinal Rhinorrhea: Extracranial Surgical Repair. Although intracranial repair of cerebrospinal fluid leaks has become routine, extracranial repair has become more attractive because of reduced morbidity. Such procedures have been done in 14 patients since 1970 by Thomas C. Calcaterra, John I. Moseley and Robert W. Rand[7] (Univ of California, Los Angeles).

Acute leaks due to head trauma or cranial surgery were managed conservatively when possible. Bed rest in a sitting position was used for 2 weeks. Lumbar punctures were done twice daily or continuous cerebrospinal fluid drainage instituted along with prophylactic antibiotics. Immediate repair was done when operative intervention was otherwise indicated or when there was intracranial air. When meningitis was a complication, this was cleared by antibiotic therapy before operation. Precise localization of the dural defect was considered essential before operation.

TECHNIQUE. — Nasal cavities are sprayed with a 4% solution of cocaine. Cottonoid pledgets are then placed in the various recesses (Fig 12). At least 10 ml cerebrospinal fluid is removed, mixed with fluorescein or indigo carmine and slowly reinjected. After 30 min-

Fig 12. — Placement of cottonoid pledgets. **A,** sagittal view of the nasal cavity showing anatomical location of pledgets. **B,** coronal view of nasal cavity showing the same pledgets. (Courtesy of Calcaterra, T. C., et al.: West. J. Med. 127:279–283, October, 1977.)

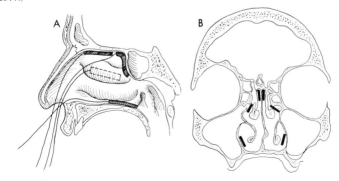

(7) West. J. Med. 127:279–283, October, 1977.

utes of recumbency, the cottonoids are removed to identify the site of the leak. Similar testing with intrathecal dye is also used for intraoperative localization of the leak. An extracranial approach to the frontal sinus leak is made with an osteoplastic frontal bone flap through a coronal or eyebrow incision. Bone adjacent to the tear is removed with a drill bur, and the dura mater is closed directly or with a graft of frontalis fascia. Leaks from the cribriform plate and ethmoid roof are approached by complete ethmoidectomy via a curved naso-orbital incision. Tissue adhesives may be placed (with the use of the operating microscope) to seal mucoperiosteal flaps to cover the leak. Sphenoid sinus leaks may be approached through the ethmoidal sinuses or via the nasal septum. The sphenoidal mucosa is removed and the sinus packed with thigh muscle fragments buttressed by septal bone. For the leaks through the ear, the middle ear may be packed through the eustachian tube or a dural graft to cover the leak may be used via a mastoidectomy.

The extracranial operations successfully and permanently sealed the leaks in these 14 patients. Intracranial repair earlier via craniotomy had failed in 6 of them. The authors believe that extracranial repair should be the first line of attack if the cerebrospinal fluid leak is not due to brain tumor.

▶ [Metrizamide has been useful in demonstrating cerebrospinal fluid rhinorrhea. Drayer et al. (Am. J. Roentgenol. 129:149, 1977) put 6 ml 190 mg iodine/ml metrizamide into the lumbar sac of a woman aged 56 and put her in a prone head-down position at − 60 degrees for 1 minute, then returned her to − 10 degrees while she was being transferred to a computerized tomography scanner. The contrast material layered in the left nasal passage and was seen to occupy the left sphenoid sinus, thus demarcating the site of leakage. Incidentally, the patient was treated by packing of the left sphenoid sinus with recurrent drainage only 2 months later. Arseni (Seara Med. Neurocirurg. 6:129, 1977) finds that posttraumatic cerebrospinal rhinorrhea is due to a tear from a fragment of ethmoid or orbital roof. Fistula of the petrous bone is due to dehiscence of the lips of the dural wound adhering to the petrous bone edges. In the latter case, the dura is detached 2 – 3 cm around the fissure through a temporal flap, without suturing the dura. In rhinorrhea, he removes the bone sliver extradurally, separates the dura for 2 – 3 cm on each side, then opens the dura to detach adhesions, but does not suture the basal dura. Of 161 patients with rhinorrhea, 121 (75%) healed spontaneously and the others were operated on and recovered. Of 190 patients with otorrhea, 95% recovered spontaneously and only 9 (5%) needed operation, and they had good results. − Ed.] ◀

Replacement Laminotomy. Extensive laminectomy results in a loss of the protective and supportive functions of the bony arches and connecting ligaments of the spine, often deterring the surgeon from treating benign lesions fully or leading him to compromise exposure. Dwight Parkinson[8] (Univ. of Manitoba) was unaware of Raimondi's answer to this problem, but when faced with such a situation devised a very similar solution.

The procedure was facilitated by great widening of the spinal canal from a congenital intraspinal extradural cyst. A set of two opposed drill holes was placed as far laterally as possible on each side of each lamina and, with the use of an aneurysm needle, a wire was threaded through the ligament beneath the lamina and used to pull a Gigli saw back through (Fig 13). Care should be taken to leave as much ligament intact as possible. A cut was made between each set of holes on either side, the procedure repeated at each arch and the string of arches removed with the connecting ligaments intact. After cyst removal the string of arches was wired back in place and the upper- and lower-most liga-

Fig 13. – **A,** drill holes are placed in each lamina laterally. **B,** an aneurysm needle is introduced through the ligament beneath the lamina and back out through the ligament above. It is usually necessary to initiate the openings with a small curet. Saw cuts are placed on either side between the corresponding drill holes; then the entire string of connected arches is removed. **C,** at the termination, the connected string of arches is wired back into place. (Courtesy of Parkinson, D.: Surg. Neurol. 8:277–279, October, 1977.)

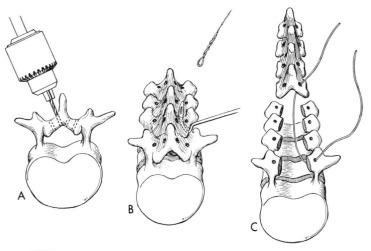

(8) Surg. Neurol. 8:277–279, October, 1977.

ments were sutured to the margins of the ligaments on the adjacent intact arches. The patient walked the next day with no restrictions in activity and he recovered uneventfully. Radiographs taken 9 months later showed the arches to be well united and well mineralized. The interpedicular spaces had narrowed an average of 4 mm, indicating the restitution of normal architecture.

This procedure can be done on a normal neural arch, even in children, as shown by Raimondi, who used a power drill and sutured rather than wired the arches back in place. Recently, Parkinson used it again in an adult with an arteriovenous malformation and a normal spinal canal.

Choice of Transplant in Cranial Defects: Analysis of 73 Cases is presented by N. Hardt and J. Ammann[9] (Lucerne). Spontaneous closure is not expected in these posttraumatic (primary) or postoperative (secondary) osseous defects, making plastic reconstruction necessary. In such a procedure the principal differences of the various calvarial regions must be considered, including the latent risk of infection in frontobasal areas and the generally aseptic conditions in other regions. Autologous transplants or alloplastic implants have been used. The correct choices of material and technique are decisive for primary healing, which in the case of autoplasty, occurs within the first 72 hours under optimal conditions by connection to the capillary circulation. The advantage of autoplasty lies in its mechanical stability and vital healing, which insures against inflammatory complications and is easily amenable to renewed plastic coverage in case of repeated injury of the suprastructure.

In the authors' experience, reimplantation of the autologous bone flap, freezer preserved, gave excellent results; no disturbances of healing were noted, given good wound edge contact. The use of pelvic bone was suggested by Converse mainly for reconstruction of large frontal defects with the risk of latent infection. The material was taken from the inner aspect of the ilium because its concave shape was, by reversal, easily adaptable to the convex cranial contour. The use of rib was particularly indicated in extensive defects in children and young adults, with a combination of rib transplant and costal cartilage considered especially favorable.

(9) Chirurg 48:32–36, January, 1977.

Peer's use of costal cartilage had the advantage of rapid connective tissue fixation without significant resorptive loss.

Among alloplastic materials, methyl methacrylate and silicone polymer are presently preferred, due to their good biocompatibility. Although they give the best cosmetic results, they carry a considerable risk of secondary loosening with infection. The complication rate is 10-30% according to several authors. The reactive formation of a connective tissue capsule, followed by atrophy in the peripheral regions of the defect causes the secondary loosening, which in turn further stimulates the exudative and proliferative reactions of the base.

In the present series 73 plastic procedures were carried out during 1965-75. Sixty-nine defects were treated by autoplasty and 4 by alloplastic methods. The rate of disturbance-free healing was 95-100% in the alloplastic cases. Although functional results were always satisfactory, within 1-2 years a loss of contour was noted in 50% after use of large pelvic chips and in about 40% after plastic revision using rib material. Cosmetic results were best in autoplastic revisions, although in 2 of 4 patients so treated, the material had to be removed due to secondary loosening and infection.

Autotransplants are generally preferred, with the choice of material dictated by the criteria of defect size and localization and patient age. Pelvic material is most advantageous in moderate or pulsating defects in the adult; in children pelvic chips may be removed only in limited measure, sparing the iliac crest, to avoid disturbances of growth. In case of small, nonpulsating defects within the frontal sphere, cartilage chips in the form of diced cartilage are preferred. Alloplastic techniques are justified in some limited cases but are frequently used only for temporary management of large defects in the temporoparietal sphere, to be replaced by autoplastic transplant if complications arise. Given careful choice of surgical technique and transplant material, the autoplastic calvarian revision may yield cosmetic results equal to those of alloplastic methods.

▶ [Subczynski (J. Trauma 17:467, 1977) reminds the reader that methyl methacrylate is a strong antibacterial agent during polymerization and is fairly resistant to infection. Such infection as does occur usually results when the plate is ill-adjusted and movable. He describes a series of 25 patients with compound comminuted depressed skull fractures with one-stage débridement and plastic repair. The 23 male and 2 female patients were aged 4–63 years. Antibiotics were used on admission, with operation usually done within 24 hours (or 48 hours at the outside). Débridement was followed by saline wash, and if foreign materials were present, bacitracin solution was also used. The plate was put in place while the material was still doughy, and it was washed with ice-cold saline during polymerization. This permitted perfect fit, and sutures were not used for fixation. Extensive plates were perforated to allow drainage of fluid. Periosteum and galea were closed with catgut, and skin was closed with nylon. In the 1 patient who developed infection, bilateral frontal and ethmoidal sinus involvement was present. The flap was removed after meningitis developed; further mucosal débridement was done, the sinuses were covered with periosteum and fascia lata, and later plastic repair was done without incident. In 2 other patients with sinus involvement, viable periosteum was used to separate off the sinuses from the epidural space, and plating was done without infection.

Tysvaer and Hovind (ibid., p. 231) prefer to have stainless steel mesh cut and put in place before the acrylic is added. Two of 24 plates had to be removed because of infection and 1 more because of aseptic exudate, presumably allergic response to the plastic. None of these plates were put in at the time of primary skull operation. – Ed.] ◄

First Attempts with Laser Beams in Treatment of Neurosurgical Diseases are reported by F. Heppner and P. W. Ascher[1] (Univ. of Graz).

The two major requirements of a laser device applicable for use on the nervous system are that the depth effect of the beam be shallow and that it may be guided and dosed with utmost precision. There must be the assurance that the separation, coagulation and vaporizing effects are strictly limited to the intended region, leaving cold the immediately adjacent areas of the organ in question. The beam must be visible and easy to handle, without endangering attending personnel.

The Sharplan 791 type CO_2 laser, especially adapted to meet these requirements, was used in the treatment of 9 gliomas, 10 meningiomas, 6 patients with metastases, 1 vascular malformation, 3 intracerebral interventions, 1 hippocampectomy, 2 neurinomas, 2 intramedullary tumors of the spinal cord, 1 thoracic commissurotomy, 1 thoracic prolapse of an intravertebral disk, 1 vertebral metastasis and 3 stump neurinomas.

The CO_2 laser penetrates about 10 times less deep into the tissue than the Nd-YAG laser, namely 0.2 mm, and contains

(1) Zentralbl. Neurochir. 38:77–86, 1977.

as medium a gas mixture of 4.5% CO_2, 13.5% N_2 and helium. This gas mixture is pumped under a working pressure of 25–35 mm Hg through a plasma tube that contains an anode at the center and one cathode at each end; high voltage of 12 kv ionizes the gas.

The admitted beam is differentiated from the usual infrared rays by the following parameters: high intensity (maximal 5 watt continuously); monochromatism (narrow spectral band breadth at 10.6 μ); coherence (spatially and temporally the waves are in the same phase); collimation (parallel bundling with 2.2 mrad, divergence angle). Distancing of the instrument and enlargement of the focus cause diminution of energy output and the beam no longer cuts but coagulates.

After appropriate testing the Sharplan 791 was first used for removal of a brain tumor. The epidermis, periosteum, dura and cortex were incised with the laser beam; the sharply delineated lesion was circumcised and prepared, with the remaining cavity carefully vaporized in order to destroy any remaining microscopic glioblastomous cellular units. The healing process was unremarkable. The cutting effect was mainly used for incision of soft tissue, though in some cases also for the formation of bony cover.

Observations to date suggest that in terms of precision, preservation of tissue and hemostatic effect, the expectations of the CO_2 laser have been justified. It is appropriate for use in nervous regions previously inaccessible, such as the brain stem, and under the surgical microscope. Topographic precision and the possibility of energetic dosing make this equipment a valuable supplement to presently available surgical instruments.

Is Rib Resection Necessary for Relief of Thoracic Outlet Syndrome? The recent trend has, in general, been toward resecting the 1st rib more or less empirically to relieve thoracic outlet syndrome. J. Manly Stallworth, Gerald J. Quinn and Albert F. Aiken[2] (Med. Univ. of South Carolina) found rib resections necessary in only 9 of 103 patients having 146 operative procedures for thoracic outlet syndrome in 1966–75, to achieve a success rate of 92.5%. Four of the 9 patients had accessory cervical ribs removed and 1

(2) Ann. Surg. 185:581–589, May, 1977.

had removal of the clavicle. Conservative measures were tried before surgery; cervical traction was sometimes prescribed as a therapeutic trial. More recently the transaxillary approach has been used. Division of tendons, muscles or anomalous bands was carried out in 135 instances. In 107 patients the pectoralis minor, scalene anterior or subclavian muscle was markedly thickened and tendinous. In no case was a structure divided or resected unless it was compressing the neurovascular bundle.

No intrapleural complications have occurred. Two patients had a hematoma and 1 had temporary diaphragmatic paralysis after scalenotomy. No residual neurologic or vascular deficit was present in 135 patients 6 months postoperatively; 8 patients were unimproved. One patient had already had bilateral 1st rib resection and one remained unimproved after resection of a cervical rib.

Each patient with thoracic outlet syndrome must be individually evaluated and managed accordingly. Routine resection of the 1st rib should be avoided.

► [The complications of resection of the 1st rib have, at times, been disastrous. Certainly partial brachial plexus palsy or long-lasting causalgia are enough to warrant caution in approach to the thoracic outlet syndrome. It certainly seems more logical to assume a soft tissue disorder (hypertrophied muscle, tendinous muscle) than a bony compression by a structure (the 1st rib) usually considered a normal part of the body. The authors point out the accuracy of electric testing in the carpal tunnel syndrome — and the lack of value of electromyogram and nerve conduction measurements in the thoracic outlet syndrome. Arterial flow evaluations with the portable recording oscillograph have been relatively simple and accurate in determining involvement of the neurovascular bundle by the various maneuvers designed to show compromise at the outlet. — Ed.] ◄

Intracranial Biopsy Assisted by Computerized Tomography. The computerized tomogram (CT) provides an excellent template when combined with external landmarks for accurate placement of a needle or probe within a lesion of interest. Joseph C. Maroon, William O. Bank, Burton P. Drayer and Arthur E. Rosenbaum[3] (Pittsburgh) describe a CT biopsy and aspiration technique and the preliminary results obtained. Computerized tomography scans are made until a mass is visualized and aligned with tape markers on a cap worn by the subject, and the site for a twist-drill hole is selected. A hole is then made and the dura incised; a flexible

(3) J. Neurosurg. 46:740–744, June, 1977.

opaque Formocath 6 F catheter, tapered to fit around a metal stylet, is inserted about one fourth of the calculated distance to the mass. The stylet is then removed and additional scans are made before advancing the needle to the calculated depth. Another scan is made to determine the precise location of the needle tip before biopsy or cyst drainage.

Three patients had CT-assisted brain-tumor biopsy or needle aspiration, or both. All 3 were scanned initially at 15 degrees to the orbitomeatal baseline with an EMI instrument having a 160 × 160 matrix. The findings in a patient with a cyst are shown in Figure 14. A second patient responded to aspiration of fluid and debris from a glioblastoma multiforme. A third had biopsy confirmation of a glioblastoma multiforme. Preoperative hemiparesis was worsened by needle aspiration of the highly vascular neoplasm in this case.

This technique of CT-assisted biopsy appears to have its greatest application in patients with suspected malignant tumors, either inaccessible to removal by standard approaches or when bulk removal would likely be of little benefit or result in neurologic deterioration. Both biopsy and percutaneous evacuation are feasible with this technique.

Fig 14. – Computerized tomography scans. **A,** preprocedural scan demonstrates the cystic mass in the right thalamus without evidence of enhancement. The thin extracalvarial markers (frontal) were used to determine the point of entry. **B,** after calculation of the desired trajectory and depth, the needle is inserted halfway to the lesion and the scan repeated to confirm optimal positioning. **C,** further advancement of the needle pierces the capsule of the cyst at the calculated depth, with slight reduction in size after initial aspiration. (Courtesy of Maroon, J. C., et al.: J. Neurosurg. 46:740–744, June, 1977.)

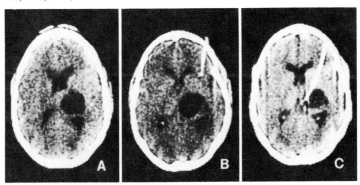

Multiple needle thrusts can be avoided and immediate confirmation of successful evacuation of cyst-abscesses should be possible. Completely automated CT stereotactic systems being developed will produce numerous orthogonal displays, have a much reduced scan time and be capable of three-dimensional reconstructions.

Trauma

Prognostic and Therapeutic Importance of Changes in CSF during Acute Stage of Brain Injury. H. D. Seitz and K. Ocker[4] (Medical School of Hannover) examined the effects of gaseous and biochemical changes in cerebrospinal fluid on cerebral blood flow and metabolism in the acute stage of brain injury. Femoral artery, jugular vein and cerebrospinal fluid samples were taken simultaneously within 12–24 hours after injury and then at 1- to 2-day intervals. Cerebrospinal fluid was taken by suboccipital puncture of the cisterna magna. Cerebral blood flow was measured by the xenon clearance method, with the use of an autofluoroscope. Studies were done in 27 patients who had had a short period of unconsciousness and no neurologic defect (stage 1), 33 with unconsciousness for over 72 hours and slight neurologic signs as well as a pathologic EEG (stage 2) and 40 in coma with severe neurologic and vegetative changes, a highly abnormal EEG and an intracranial pressure over 30 mm Hg (stage 3).

The blood Po_2 and cerebrospinal fluid Po_2 were reduced in all stages, but increased to normal in survivors. Similar changes in Pco_2 were observed. A tendency to respiratory alkalosis resulted from the fall in Pco_2. Metabolic acidosis developed in time in cases with a poor prognosis. A primary metabolic acidosis was always found in the cerebrospinal fluid, in accord with the severity of damage. The acidosis normalized in more favorable cases, but increased to death in the prognostically poor cases. An unfavorable prognosis was related to a fall in O_2 tension, a greatly reduced bicarbonate level, an elevated lactate level and a decline in pH in the cerebrospinal fluid.

Thirty-five stage 3 patients were treated with intrathecal 8.4% bicarbonate. Distinct clinical improvement resulted in 60% of the cases, but no significant effect was noted in 8

(4) Acta Neurochir. (Wien) 38:211–231, 1977.

cases. Mean blood flow was reduced, and gray matter flow
was decreased to about half of normal. Cerebral cortical perfusion was reduced by 30% in these cases. After bicarbonate
administration, the blood flow increased in all patients but
1, and metabolic rates in the damaged hemisphere were
improved. Blood flow improved in both gray and white matter.

Arterial hypoxia and hypoxemia are associated with
brain injury. Treatment of the cerebrospinal fluid acidosis
by the intrathecal injection of buffer substances can improve
cerebral blood flow and metabolism in cases of severe brain
injury. In many cases the rehabilitation of patients is improved and mortality reduced.

**Outcome from Severe Head Injury with Early Diag-
nosis and Intensive Management.** Donald P. Becker, J.
Douglas Miller, John D. Ward, Richard P. Greenberg, Harold F. Young and Romas Sakalas[5] (Med. College of Virginia)
reviewed data on 160 patients, seen in 1972 – 76 with severe
head injury, who have died or been followed for at least 3
months. All were seen within 12 hours of injury, and most
within 4 hours. No patient was able to obey simple commands on admission. Cases of coma due to alcohol, drug
overdosage or epilepsy were excluded, as were patients with
gunshot wounds of the head and those who, on admission,
were apneic and had bilaterally fixed, dilated pupils and no
motor response to painful stimuli. Mannitol was given before surgical decompression. All patients were initially arti-
ficially ventilated. Increased intracranial pressure of over
40 mm Hg was treated.

Intracranial mass lesions were treated by surgical decompression in 39% of the cases. Most patients in the series were
male and young; average age was 27 years. Nearly half the
patients were decorticate or decerebrate at best, or gave no
motor response to pain at all. Although 36% of the patients
made a good recovery, 24% were moderately disabled, 8%
were left severely disabled and 2% were vegetative. The
mortality was 30%. Patients with mass lesions had a mortality of 40%, compared with 23% for those with diffuse
brain injury; fewer good recoveries occurred in the former
group. A significant midline brain shift was associated with

(5)   J. Neurosurg. 47:491 – 502, October, 1977.

a higher mortality, as was increasing age. Abnormal motor response and the oculocephalic response were related to a poor outcome, and bilateral absence of pupillary light responses was similarly related. Of 29 patients with abnormal motor responses, impaired or absent oculocephalic responses and bilaterally absent pupillary light reactions, 76% died.

Mortality in this series compares favorably with that reported from other centers. Vigorous surgical and medical management apparently permits some patients who would have died to recover well, without increasing the proportion of severely disabled patients. A generous craniotomy and artificial ventilation are important aspects of management. Any upset in cardiopulmonary function, fluid and electrolyte balance, or body temperature must be promptly corrected.

▶ [Becker's group used a frontal twist drill to measure ventricular pressure in the emergency room. Air was injected in the frontal horn for radiographs to see if there was a shift of 5 mm or more; such shifts led to exploration and decompression. Large decompressions have been used by others and appear to save lives but not necessarily improve them. Computerized tomography (CT) scans may not always be readily available, and, in such instances, angiography or ventriculography may be useful. It was not always necessary to give muscle relaxants for artificial ventilation, and arterial Pco_2 was maintained at 25–35 mm Hg. However, Bruce (Philadelphia meeting of the Society of Neurological Surgeons, 1978) described the custom at the University of Pennsylvania to treat children by paralyzing them and keeping the Pco_2 to 25 mm Hg (torr). Ventricles are shown by CT scan to be so small that I doubt that it is always possible to monitor children with swollen brains by ventricular catheter. Bruce contends there is some risk in early use of mannitol in the first 24 hours due to the subsequent temporary increase in blood volume and intracranial pressure before the osmotic effect is manifest. The dose of dexamethasone used by Becker et al. in intensive care management was 10 mg immediately and 4 mg every 6 hours for at least 3 days and that of phenytoin, 100 mg three times daily. The current tendency is to use much larger doses of steroids, but one should be aware of the interactions between steroids and phenytoin—and indeed, with other materials. Thus, Rose et al. (J.A.M.A. 237:2630, 1977) report a case in which a woman receiving phenytoin for seizures associated with a vascular malformation was also given chloramphenicol for septic shock. On three separate occasions, she became stuporous and confused when the antibiotic was given, and on each occasion the phenytoin level in the serum was found to be markedly elevated. Others have reported a drop in steroid efficiency when phenytoin is given.

Rose, Valtonen and Jennett (Br. Med. J. 2:615, 1977) analyzed with regard to the avoidable factors contributing to death, the outcome of 116 patients who died of head injury or its complications, since each of these patients was known to have talked after the injury. An avoidable factor was identified for 74%; for 54%, the avoidable factor was considered to have contributed to death directly. Regrettably, the most common avoidable factor was delay in treatment of an intracranial hematoma. Others included poorly controlled epilepsy, meningitis, hypotension and hypoxia. —Ed.] ◄

Value of Computerized Tomography in Management of 1,000 Consecutive Head Injuries. Barry N. French and Arthur B. Dublin[6] (Univ. of California, Davis) reviewed information on 1,000 consecutive head-injured patients seen in 14 months in 1975 and 1976, 316 of whom had computerized tomography (CT). A standard EMI head unit with a 160×160 matrix was used to obtain a four-level unenhanced scan. A total of 474 studies were carried out, 20 with contrast enhancement. Indications for CT scanning early in the series were liberal. About a fourth of patients were alert and neurologically normal at the time of study, whereas 14% were deeply comatose or showed brain stem posturing. About half the patients were scanned within 24 hours of injury. About 35 patients underwent angiography at some time during their illnesses. About a fourth of the patients were intubated before the CT scan.

Scans were abnormal in 51% of patients, and in 38% of these more than one abnormality was demonstrated. Six patients had a normal first scan and developed abnormality on repeat scanning. In most cases the abnormality demonstrated did not require surgery and did not alter management. An epidural hematoma was demonstrated in 6 patients and 87 subdural hematomas were shown in 69 patients. Thirty-nine patients had a diagnosis of intracerebral hematoma, and 22 of them had other CT scan abnormalities. Contusion and edema were observed in 54 patients, and about half had other abnormalities. Contused areas had a "mottled" or "salt-and-pepper" appearance on the CT scan. Only 25 patients had significant ventricular enlargement; in 5 this was the only abnormality on the initial scan. Nine patients had intraventricular hemorrhage, all with other lesions also. Delayed scans showed lucent extracerebral collections representing subdural hygromas in 10 patients. Eighteen of 40 patients with "brain stem contusion" had surgically significant abnormalities. Seven had abnormalities on repeat CT scanning.

(6) Surg. Neurol. 7:171–183, April, 1977.

The yield of abnormalities in this series was high. No significant abnormalities were missed by CT scanning in 9 autopsy cases. Cost effectiveness for use of the CT scan in head trauma cannot be calculated.

▶ [The authors state that they now manage head injuries with CT scans rather than with angiography except for instances of isodense bilateral hematomas, posttraumatic cerebral vasospasm, fistulas and possible aneurysms. Repetitive CT scanning is certainly to be preferred to repetitive angiograms.

One criticism: the title of the article gives the impression that CT scans were used to manage 1,000 cases of head injury. In fact, the scans were done only in 316 cases, so that, to be exact, one would have to say that the CT scans had no value in 684 cases — because no scans were done! — Ed.]

Post-Head Trauma Syndrome in an Adolescent Treated with Lithium Carbonate: Case Report. Alternatives are being sought to phenothiazine therapy for controlling manifestations of the posttraumatic syndrome. Cal K. Cohn, James R. Wright III and Richard A. DeVaul[7] (Univ. of Texas Med. School, Houston) describe a boy with closed head trauma and agitated hypomanic behavior who responded to lithium carbonate after he failed to respond to several other treatments.

Boy, 12, sustained multiple injuries including injury to the right frontal area in an automobile accident and was admitted in coma. A dense left hemiparesis was present. An EEG showed bilateral slowing with more delta activity in the right posterior quadrant and attenuation over the left frontocentral area. Angiography showed an area of contusion in the right frontoparietal area. The patient was extremely agitated, coprolalic and echolalic after the procedure and required restraint and sedation with phenothiazines. After 7 days he was discharged with mild hemiparesis, but he returned after another 7 days because agitation, verbal abuse, insomnia and pressured speech had ensued, and he attempted to stab himself. An extremely mild hemiparesis was present. Mental examination showed decreased concentration, grandiosity and flight of ideas. The patient was mildly depressed and acknowledged suicidal ideation. A repeat EEG was normal. Lithium carbonate was given in a dosage of 300 mg twice daily. Agitation and emotional lability decreased and attention span increased. The patient rapidly resumed his premorbid level of function after discharge. Lithium was stopped after 6 months, and on follow-up 4 months later there was no recurrence of symptoms.

Illness manifested by manic or hypomanic behavior may

---

(7) Dis. Nerv. Syst. 38:630–631, August, 1977.

respond to lithium carbonate. Manic-depressive disease or recurrent depressions need not be present. Target symptoms of mania or hypomania may in themselves warrant a trial of lithium.

▶ [One wonders if the same medication might be used during the acute episode of unruliness that so often follows head injuries and that makes nursing care so difficult. — Ed.] ◀

Decerebrate Rigidity in Acute Head Injury. Albino Bricolo, Sergio Turazzi, Alberto Alexandre and Nicola Rizzuto[8] (Verona, Italy) studied the motor patterns of 800 patients with severe head injuries seen consecutively in 1973–75. Most injuries were due to traffic accidents. All patients were unconscious for 24 hours or longer, immediately or very shortly after injury, and had evidence of anatomical or functional impairment of the central nervous system (CNS). Nearly all patients had electromyography. Decerebrate rigidity developed in 317 (39.6%) patients in the acute stage. The clinical picture was quite varied and often unstable.

Full decerebrate rigidity was observed in 109 patients, unilateral rigidity in 37 and decorticate rigidity in 21. Twenty patients exhibited extensor rigidity on one side and a decorticate attitude on the other. Only 5 patients showed mixed decerebrate rigidity. Alternating decerebrate rigidity was observed in 125 patients. Magnus and de Kleijn reflexes were evoked by head turning in a small number of patients. Tetraplegia was sometimes observed when no cervical cord lesions were present. Breakdown of function of the autonomic system was almost invariable. Deep coma was present in 282 (89%) of patients with decerebrate rigidity, and about half the patients had dysfunction of brain stem ocular motility. Angiography showed expanding intracranial lesions in 233 patients, with a mortality of 75.9%, compared with 60.7% for patients without such lesions.

A total of 146 patients with angiographic indications were treated surgically. Patients having operations had a mortality of 76%, compared with 75.8% for patients not having operations with abnormal angiograms. Patients without extensor motor abnormalities who had operations had a mortality of 37.5%, compared to 43.7% for nonsurgical pa-

(8) J. Neurosurg. 47:680–698, November, 1977.

tients. Mortality in the decerebrate group was constant and nearly independent of age. Signs of brain stem involvement were often associated with postural abnormalities in the groups with the highest mortality. Anoxic neocortical damage was found in all 31 autopsied patients. Of 17 patients with full decerebrate rigidity, 14 had gross brain stem lesions due to increased intracranial pressure. Five of 6 patients with alternating decerebrate rigidity had either hemorrhagic lesions or foci of softening in the mesencephalon and upper pons or both. Similar changes were found in the brain stem in 2 of 3 patients with combined decerebrate rigidity.

The phenomena of decerebrate rigidity are important unfavorable signs indicating severe, diffuse brain damage and a serious clinical state with increased metabolic demands. The localizing value of extensor motor abnormalities in patients with severe head injuries is not proved, but a stable, complete extensor posture, combined with deep coma and brain stem ocular signs, indicates severe midbrain dysfunction. However, structural brain stem damage is not always conclusively indicated. Good recovery was achieved in 16% of decerebrate patients, whereas 12.1% survived in prolonged coma or with severe disabilities.

Five Years' Experience with Penetrating Craniocerebral Gunshot Wounds. Patrick L. Lillard[9] (Univ. of Mississippi) reviewed experience with 83 cases of penetrating craniocerebral gunshot wounds in civilians seen in 1971–75 among 147 patients admitted in this period with gunshot wounds to the head. Yearly rates have been quite consistent. About 80% of patients were male and nearly 75% were black. The average patient age was 29.6. There were 15 suicide attempts in the series. The overall mortality was 43.4%. Only 18 of 36 patients who died were autopsied. Suicide attempts carried the highest mortality in the series. The course and extent of the missile tract was an extremely significant mortality factor. Other than those with posterior fossa wounds, patients with single lobe injuries did much better than those in whom the missle crossed either the midsagittal or midcoronal plane. Age and retained missile fragments did not significantly affect mortality. The average

(9)   Surg. Neurol. 9:79–83, February, 1978.

interval to definitive therapy was 2.8 hours in fatal cases and 5.9 hours in survivors, excluding 1 patient who was seen at 72 hours and died 10 days later. Missile fragments were retained in 57 patients. Multiple missile injuries that included other areas of the body did not alter mortality.

Forty-seven survivors have been followed, 16 for over 1 year and 7 of these for over 4 years. Only 19 survivors are judged capable of work and only 3 are known to be working. Fifteen survivors have required follow-up admissions or been admitted to facilities for chronic care or rehabilitation. Only 4 patients had cerebral angiography before surgery. Antibiotics and steroids were given to all patients considered viable when admitted. Twenty patients were placed on anticonvulsant therapy initially. Six survivors had post-traumatic seizures. Surgery was done in 64 patients, with a surgical mortality of 32.8%. Surgery itself did not appear to contribute to mortality. Intracranial pressure monitoring was performed for at least 72 hours postoperatively in 12 patients in the last year of the study.

The overall mortality of 43.4% indicates that a more vigorous approach is needed in monitoring and controlling pressure effects in more severely injured patients with penetrating craniocerebral gunshot wounds.

Delayed Facial Palsy after Head Injury. There is much disagreement about the precise place of surgical exploration of the injured facial nerve. K. Puvanendran, M. Vitharana and P. K. Wong[1] (Singapore) conducted a prospective study of this complication of head injury in a series of 6,304 cases of head injury seen in 1974–75. All cases of bleeding ear after closed head injury were followed from the time of injury. Thirty-nine patients had bleeding ears and 16 of them had delayed facial palsy. Three others had facial palsy immediately after injury. Three of the 16 patients with delayed palsy had bilateral facial palsies. The chance of a patient with bleeding ear developing delayed facial palsy after head injury was 49%.

The 12 male and 4 female patients with delayed facial palsy were aged 9–58. Eleven were involved in traffic accidents. The palsy was complete in 14 cases, partial in 3 and subclinical in 2. No patient reported pain in the appropriate

(1) J. Neurol. Neurosurg. Psychiatry 40:342–350, April, 1977.

ear apart from that at the site of impact. In 9 patients the site of impact was around the ear. In 10 patients the lesion was at the geniculate ganglion, whereas in 7 it was distal to the chorda tympani branch.

The delay in onset of facial palsy ranged from 2 to 21 days; in most cases it was 2–7 days. Eight patients had a definite petrous bone fracture on the side of the facial palsy. Conduction block occurred in 3 patients with clinical palsy and 2 with subclinical palsy. The other 14 patients showed denervation, which in 6 was complete. In cases of conduction block, clinical recovery began by about day 5 and was complete by a mean of 36 days. The mean time for onset of recovery was 13 days in patients with partial denervation and 35 days in patients with complete denervation. None of the latter patients has shown complete recovery from facial weakness to date. Patients with partial denervation recovered full voluntary movement, but were not without sequelae of abnormal reinnervation. No patient with a conduction block had a contracture or abnormal movement. All patients but 1 with denervation had some form of abnormal movement. Ten patients had perceptive or mixed deafness; 7 had abnormal vestibular function on the side of the facial palsy. One patient had a contralateral 6th nerve palsy. None had olfactory nerve involvement. One patient had an associated subdural hematoma that was evacuated.

Facial nerve decompression in the facial canal should be considered at the earliest indication of denervation. Because the lesion often extends up to the geniculate ganglion, the entire facial nerve in the temporal bone should be decompressed, which would involve a combined translabyrinthine and middle fossa approach. If the geniculate ganglion is intact, a mastoid approach is adequate.

► [I am not sure that I know how important it is to look with minute care (e.g., tomography) for skull fracture in a case of facial nerve palsy after head injury. The outcome does not depend on absence or presence of fracture, and I do not know that the presence of fracture makes a difference in the only therapy offered—surgical decompression.—Ed.] ◄

Acute Fractures of the Odontoid Process: Analysis of 45 Cases. Michael L. J. Apuzzo, James S. Heiden, Martin H. Weiss, Truman T. Ackerson, J. Paul Harvey and Theodore Kurze[2] (Univ. of Southern California) treated 45 pa-

(2) J. Neurosurg. 48:85–91, January, 1978.

tients for acute fractures of the odontoid process in 1969–74. Of the 35 men and 10 women in the series, 21 were over age 40. Fractures resulted from auto accidents in 25 patients and from falls in 11. Detectable myelopathy was evident in 8 patients. Except for an elderly tetraplegic woman who died of pulmonary complications, all patients had full neurologic recovery within 4 weeks of injury. Tomography was performed in 73% of cases before treatment and in 77% after treatment. All fractures were treated within 72 hours of admission. All displaced fractures were reduced by skeletal traction (10–12 lbs). Undisplaced fractures were managed by cervical halter or skeletal traction.

External immobilization was maintained for at least 14 weeks in 41 patients. Minerva plaster jackets were used in 22 patients. Thirteen of 40 evaluable patients did not show fusion, but 2 of these had evidence of fibrous union and no instability on flexion-extension or cineradiographic studies. Thirteen patients had posterior wiring and fusion, 3 initially and 10 after failure of fusion by external immobilization. In 1 patient the occiput was included in the fusion process because of a fracture of the posterior ring of the atlas. Patients were kept in modified Thomas braces for 3–4 months after operative fusion. Ten of the 13 fractures were initially displaced and 7 involved the body of the axis. No significant operative complications occurred and no adverse effects of the fusion procedure were noted on follow-up for 6–18 months. Complete stability was obtained at the atlantoaxial level in all patients despite persistent nonunion of the dens in 9.

All undisplaced odontoid fractures should be immobilized externally. All those displaced more than 4 mm should be considered for primary operative treatment. Displaced fractures in patients over age 40 are probably best managed by initial surgery. In experienced hands, posterior wiring and fusion of C1–3 carries low mortality and morbidity. Iliac donor sites have been used.

Effect of Mannitol in a Patient with Spinal Cord Injury: Case Report. Hyperosmolar solutions may help reduce intracranial pressure in head-injured patients, and urea has been shown to benefit the walking ability of animals with cord injury. B. Magnaes[3] (Rikshosp., Oslo) reports relief

(3) Acta Neurochir. (Wien) 39:59–61, 1977.

from spinal cord compression after mannitol therapy in a patient with a spinal injury.

Girl, 16, reported chest pain after a motorcycle accident, and x-rays showed a compression fracture at T6–T7 without dislocation. Several hours later she was found to be paraplegic, with sensory loss from the costal margin downward. The Queckenstedt test showed a complete block. A volume of 500 ml of 20% mannitol was given intravenously in 20 minutes, and Queckenstedt testing showed a normal response after 20 and 60 minutes. Mannitol was given in a dosage of 250 ml every 4 hours, with 4 mg dexamethasone every 6 hours. The Queckenstedt response was normal on day 3, and the patient had regained some sensation in the legs. Motor activity began to return in the 2d week, and 10 months after injury the patient was able to walk with crutches.

This effect was most likely due to mannitol, because the patient was thought to have a stable fracture, and body position was unchanged during initial pressure recording. The change from a complete block to a normal square wave response on Queckenstedt testing indicated at least some relief from mechanical spinal cord compression.

▶ [Fracture of the spine in ankylosing spondylitis is uncommon. A case is reported by Leslie (Injury 9:53, 1977). He points out that all fractures of such spines are unstable, and there is a high incidence of spinal cord damage in these instances. Management is difficult. Leslie's case is the second one reported with operative treatment (suggested if conservative therapy fails or if there is early neurologic involvement). Spinous process fixation was thwarted by fractures of these parts, so plates were wired onto the laminae of the 2 vertebrae above and the 2 below the fracture.

Most patients with kyphoscoliosis do not have severe neurologic complications; acquired kyphosis is more apt to be accompanied by paraplegia than scoliosis. Sudden paraplegia after trauma in a patient with kyphoscoliosis is reported by Cho and Myers (Arch. Phys. Med. Rehab. 58: 229, 1977). This patient fortunately improved after conservative therapy in bed (without steroids). In general, these authors believe that the treatment should be the same as with injury to hitherto normal spines — namely, that advocated by Guttmann. — Ed.] ◀

Infections

► An important and helpful manual, *Manual on Control of Infection in Surgical Patients* (Philadelphia: J. B. Lippincott Co., 1976), was put out by the American College of Surgeons.

Spinal epidural abscess should be considered, say Schlossberg and Shulman (South. Med. J. 70:669, 1977), in any patient who has fever, leukocytosis, back pain and recent infection or back trauma. Immediate spinal puncture with manometry is indicated, followed by myelography and, if the diagnosis is established, prompt operation. Increased white blood cells and protein in the cerebrospinal fluid is usual. In comparison with transverse myelopathy, spinal abscess can be distinguished by the presence of pain and the slower development of paraplegia. Vertebral osteomyelitis favors the presence of an abscess, as does a recent pyogenic infection elsewhere in the body, or a positive blood culture. In their series of 6 patients, the only patient who made a full recovery was the one who had only minimal defect before laminectomy. Antibiotic therapy should, of course, be given along with operative treatment. Most epidural abscesses occur in the midthoracic or upper lumbar spine (where the epidural space is normally largest); the size and shape of this space also account for the preponderance of posterior abscess compared to anterior placement. — Ed. ◄

Hospital-Acquired Bacterial Meningitis in Neurosurgical Patients is an infrequent but devastating postoperative complication. Frederick J. Buckwold, Roger Hand and Robert R. Hansebout[4] (McGill Univ.) noted that gram-negative organisms frequently caused nosocomial meningitis in their neurosurgical unit and carried out a retrospective survey of all neurosurgical patients seen in the past 15 years with hospital-acquired bacterial meningitis. Of the 10,634 neurosurgical operations done in this period, about half were craniotomies and about a third were laminectomies. Figures on the placement of ventricular drainage tubes were not included in the study.

The overall rate of postoperative infection was 0.65%. Twenty-three patients had hospital-acquired meningitis, 18 of them after craniotomy (0.34%) and 1 after laminectomy (0.03%). Only 0.55% of 1,100 patients admitted with skull

---

(4) J. Neurosurg. 46:494–500, April, 1977.

fracture or cerebrospinal fluid leakage acquired meningitis in the hospital. Five of the 6 had craniotomy for lesions other than cerebrospinal fluid leakage per se. None of 46 patients who had craniotomy for repair of persistent cerebrospinal fluid leakage acquired meningitis. The 23 patients with hospital-acquired meningitis had a mean age of 41.6 years; 12 of them died. The most common associated factor was craniotomy; 5 patients had multiple craniotomies. No single factor appreciably affected mortality. Over 60% of the patients acquired meningitis more than a week after the last neurosurgical procedure. The etiologic agent was *Staphylococcus epidermidis* in 4 cases and a gram-negative bacillus in the rest. *Klebsiella-Enterobacter-Serratia* organisms were implicated in 14 cases. The mortality from gram-negative infection was 57.9%. About half the deaths occurred within the 1st week of treatment. One of 8 other patients admitted with bacterial meningitis after head trauma or neurosurgery in an earlier admission died.

Over 80% of the cases in this series were caused by gram-negative enteric bacilli. Intrathecal gentamicin was not shown to be more effective than systemic therapy. Direct intraventricular administration of gentamicin may be more effective treatment for gram-negative meningitis.

► ["Wash your gloves!" is the message from Dunkley and Lewis (Br. Med. J. 2:1391, 1977). They report a meningeal reaction to surgical glove powder in cerebrospinal fluid. Pyrexia, malaise and neck stiffness developed in a man, aged 53, who had removal of subependymoma from the 4th ventricle 3 days earlier. Lumbar puncture revealed yellow fluid with 150 white blood cells per cu mm. Particles with Maltese-cross birefringence typical of starch granules were found in the fluid. Betamethasone treatment and repeated cerebrospinal fluid removal (30 ml) was followed by improvement. — Ed.] ◄

Factors Affecting the Incidence of Wound Infection in Neurosurgery. L. A. Quadery, A. V. Medlery and J. Miles[5] (Liverpool, England) carried out a prospective survey of wound infection in 357 consecutive patients having neurosurgical procedures in a 10-month period in 1973; emergency operations and cases already known to be infected were excluded. Some surgeons used crystalline penicillin, 1 megaunit 6-hourly, and sulfadiazine, 1 gm 6-hourly for 1 week, prophylactically. The suture materials used included

---

(5) Acta Neurochir. (Wien) 39:133–141, 1977.

wax-coated braided black silk, silicone-coated braided black silk and silicone-treated braided polyester. Steroids were used on clinical grounds, usually as dexamethasone in a dose of 4 mg every 6 hours.

Seventeen patients (4.9%) had postoperative wound infection. Infection occurred in 1 of 43 steroid-treated patients. Organisms were isolated in 5 of 17 patients. The infection rate was 20% in 5 elective craniotomies for complications of trauma. Rates of about 5% were found in other elective craniotomies, elective laminectomy and elective bur hole placement. Elective disk surgery carried an infection rate of 3%. Comparable infection rates were found with the different types of suture material used. Patients not given antibiotics had an infection rate of 2.3%, compared with 7.4% for those given local antibiotics alone and 11.8% for those given systemic antibiotics. When both topical and systemic antibiotics were used, the rate of infection was 3.3%. Only 1 of 40 patients who were reexplored had wound infection. The performance time of surgery did not affect the rate of sepsis. No patient died of postoperative wound infection or its sequelae.

The overall rate of infection in this neurosurgical series was 4.8%. Steroids were not implicated in wound infections, and systemic antibiotics were not associated with a reduction in wound infection. Antibiotics are expensive, carry a risk of "immunologic hypersensitivity" to both patients and staff and through indiscriminate use can encourage the emergence of resistant strains of "hospital organisms." Prophylactic antibiotics appear to confer no protection against wound infection in elective neurosurgery.

▶ [The reasons for the marked disparity in infection rates at the Liverpool and Montreal hospitals are not immediately apparent. In the latter hospitals, the operating rooms are not shared with other surgical services, and ultraviolet light is used over the instrument trays in the operating room. All the patients in the Montreal series were treated with an antibacterial agent at the time of operation (sulfonamide before 1970 and ampicillin thereafter). Buckwold et al. believe many cases of postoperative meningitis arise from nosocomial infections from catheters. – Ed.] ◀

Hydatid Cysts of the Brain: Diagnostic and Therapeutic Problems in 100 Cases in Algeria are reviewed by M. Abada, I. Galli, A. Bousallah and G. Lehmann.[6] Hyda-

(6) Neurochirurgie 23:195–204, 1977.

tidosis is an endemic parasitosis occurring in sheep-raising areas such as the Mediterranean, South America, New Zealand and Australia. The hexacanthous embryo eliminated by the carnivore (dog) is absorbed by the herbivore, which it infests via the portal route, and settles in the tissue where it undergoes cystic involution, enclosing scolices which may infect yet another carnivore. Human beings, particularly children, may take the place of the herbivore in this cycle, developing a hepatic (60%), pulmonary (30%) or cerebral cyst (1.4%).

Among the 100 evaluable cases considered, the hydatidosis was exclusively cerebral in all but 3. It was largely a pediatric disease. All cysts observed were supratentorial, involving both hemispheres with equal frequency. They were generally less than 2 cm from the brain surface. Three lesions were juxtaventricular. Eighty-two cysts were solitary. Most were retrorolandic. In the 18 patients with multiple cysts, the vesicles were always grouped in one region.

Eighty cases were characterized by progressive intracranial hypertension, which had evolved over an average of 9 months before hospitalization, although actual onset undoubtedly dated back much further. In 11 cases cerebral trauma caused decompensation of a previously unrecognized hydatid cyst; an epileptic seizure, most frequently generalized, was the first symptom of the disease in 9 cases. Intracranial hypertension was manifested by clear symptoms (optic stasis or atrophy) in 94 patients, although general health was good. Thirty-four patients were blind on admission. Among the signs of deficit, those signaling a supratentorial expansive process (motor disturbances, hemiparesis in adults) were of greatest diagnostic value. An EEG, done in 65 cases, did not pinpoint a silent zone hemmed by delta waves, though it was useful in terms of localization in 42 cases. Standard skull films almost always furnished indirect "historical" signs of a cerebral hydatid cyst, particularly cranial asymmetry, with bulging of the involved side. Larger cysts posed few diagnostic problems on carotid angiography. An avascular mass was seen, surrounded by a circle of displaced vessels and showing no structural anomalies save elongation. Smaller cysts, displacing fewer vessels, were more difficult to diagnose. The presence of a peculiar border, seen in some 10% of cases, at times allowed diagnosis. Multiple cysts grouped in one region gave the image of a large single cyst. Ventriculography is clearly contraindicated because of the resultant dissemination of scolices. Nevertheless, it was carried out in some cases as an emergency measure for decompression.

Surgical treatment of single cysts consists of en bloc excision after corticectomy. The field is protected by formol-impregnated compresses or compresses soaked in hypertonic solutions. The authors used the technique of Arana Iniguez and San Julian in 77 patients. It consists of injection of serum between the cyst and the cerebrum to "deliver" the "water bomb." In cases of multiple cysts, ablation of vesicles is carried out as required, the residual cavity is rinsed with formol, serum with hypertonic saline or glucose and rinsed again with isotonic serum, which is left in place to prevent collapse of the hemisphere. The postoperative period was marked in 50% of cases by immediate or delayed hyperthermia of some 5 days' duration.

Of the 90 patients who could be traced, 73 survived and 26 of these were considered to be cured.

Intracranial Tuberculomas. The occurrence of intracranial tuberculomas has declined in recent years, but in Turkey a certain percentage of intracranial tumors are still tuberculomas. H. Gökalp, E. Özkal and B. Tümer[7] (Ankara Univ.) reviewed the findings in 8 patients seen in 1967–75 with a histologic diagnosis of intracranial tuberculoma. The 8 were among 1,015 patients with histologically verified intracranial tumors seen during this period.

Brain tuberculomas mainly develop from a primary tuberculous focus elsewhere; the focus need not necessarily be clinically active. Tuberculomas are generally seen in the first 3 decades of life; the present patients had a mean age of 23 years. Tuberculomas can occur anywhere in the brain; 5 of the present patients had hemispheric lesions, with 2 in the optochiasmatic region. One patient had 2 lesions in the cerebellum. The signs and symptoms are those of an intracranial space-occupying lesion. Severe headache is always present, and most patients acquire severe papilledema. Visual disturbances occur early; they were the initial complaints in 4 patients. Seizures were an early feature in 3 pa-

(7)   Clin. Neurol. Neurosurg. 79:228–236, 1977.

tients with hemispheric lesions. Motor weakness was an early symptom in 6 cases. The duration of symptoms is generally 3–12 months.

The clinical diagnosis of tuberculoma is difficult. The finding of tuberculous disease elsewhere in the body or a history of contact is important in making a correct diagnosis. Brain scanning is useful. If the angiogram shows hydrocephalus, indicating a posterior fossa lesion, contrast ventriculography should be carried out. The diagnosis can only be confirmed histologically. Streptomycin therapy has reduced the mortality substantially. One of the present patients died in status epilepticus, and another died of postoperative coliform infection.

Congenital Disorders

Subtotal Neonatal Calvariectomy for Severe Craniosynostosis. Synostosis of multiple cranial sutures, especially the coronal and sagittal sutures, may produce visual and central nervous system (CNS) problems or severe craniofacial deformities, or both. Early surgical decompression can often ameliorate or prevent these sequelae, but the success of past surgery has been variable. James W. Hanson, Martin P. Sayers, Lawrence M. Knopp, Constance Macdonald and David W. Smith[8] used early, more radical calvariectomy as an alternative procedure.

Female infant, born at term and weighing 2.8 kg, had a severe cranoifacial deformity secondary to synostosis of sagittal, coronal and lambdoidal sutures. The brain had grown through the open metopic suture and anterior fontanel. Hypotonia, lethargy, exotropia and poor feeding were evident by age 10 days. At age 13 days the calvarium was excised to the supraorbital margins, to near the foramen magnum and to the region of the squamosal sutures. The entire extent of the coronal sutures was excised. Lateral venous sinuses were absent. The skin was closed directly over the intact dura. Abnormal neurologic signs disappeared except for mild hypotonia. Bone islands were seen within 2 weeks and a new calvarium was well developed by age 4 months, with coronal and sagittal sutures and "fontanels" in the usual sites. No protective headgear was used. Subsequent head circumference measurements have followed the 50th percentile up to age 2 years. Cosmetic results have been excellent. Mild frontal prominence appears to be a normal family characteristic. Maxillofacial growth has been somewhat greater than average for age (Fig 15). Development has been normal except for mild hypotonia and slightly delayed gross motor skills.

The improved facial appearance of this child is particularly pleasing. Early partial calvariectomy for coronal synostosis should permit more normal forward growth of the cranial base and limit secondary deformities. A more complete expansion of dura over a wide area is possible than with linear

---

(8)   J. Pediatr. 91:257–260, August, 1977.

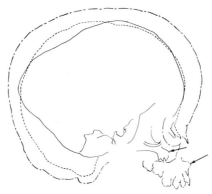

Fig 15.—Cephalometric tracings aligned at the sella and anterior cranial base preoperatively at age 3 days *(solid line)* and postoperatively at age 4 months *(dotted line)* and at age 18 months *(outer interrupted line)*. The arrows point to the anterior point of the maxilla at age 3 days and again at age 18 months. Note the extent of forward growth of the face as well as the remodeling of the calvarium. (Courtesy of Hanson, J. W., et al.: J. Pediatr. 91:257–260, August, 1977.)

craniotomy methods. Staged procedures are usually not necessary. Morbidity has been low with this approach and the need for reoperation has been lessened.

▶ [From the meeting of the Société de Neuro-Chirurgie de Langue Française at Nice in May, 1977, comes an excellent French monograph (Neurochirurgie 23 (Suppl. 2:1, 1977) dealing with craniofacial dysmorphism: premature synostoses, including cranio-synostoses and facial synostoses, by Montaut and Stricker of Nancy, France, with the collaboration of 10 others. There are chapters on history, mythology, phylogenesis, morphogenesis and development, anatomopathologic studies of craniosynostosis, surgical anatomy, signs and symptoms, craniometry, radiology, scanning, clinical course, diagnosis, etiology, pathogenesis, surgical treatment, results, indications and conclusions. This monograph should be translated into English to make its full impact on American neurosurgery. — Ed.] ◀

Parieto-Occipital Overlap in Normal and Hydrocephalic Infants. J. C. Bouzige, J. L. Ferran, E. Castan-Tarbouriech and Ph. Castan[9] (Montpellier, France) state that such overlap is fairly common in the newborn. It is the result of cranial molding by overlap of the bones of the vault, compressing the sutures. In the normal infant, reexpansion of these bones, particularly in the region of the lambdoid suture, generally takes place within 3 days after birth.

_____

(9)   J. Radiol. Electrol. Med. Nucl. 58:111–114, February, 1977.

However, there may be pathologic consequences even in the normal infant, and particularly in the hydrocephalic newborn, due to compression of the superior longitudinal sinus and the resultant effect on the cerebral circulation. Deep cerebral infarctions may ensue, due to shunting of the blood supply. The overlapping may vary in intensity and is clearest on profile films. Usually the parietal bone overlaps the occipital bone, although the reverse may occur. The phenomenon is well demonstrated on sinusographic examination performed with the newborn in the dorsal decubitus position and with older infants in the lateral decubitus position. The superior longitudinal sinus appears to be flattened or interrupted. Chronic compression at the level of the superior longitudinal sinus in the dorsal decubitus position may be responsible for a rerouting of venous blood toward deeper systems and thus causes stasis by obstruction and venous hypertension, with exclusion of peripheral venous dynamics.

Practically, such overlapping should be avoided as much as possible, particularly during resuscitation of a newborn in respiratory distress. The "true" lateral decubitus position, without rotation of the head, is considered to be ideal for the infant.

Aqueduct Stenosis: Case Review and Discussion. James J. McMillan and Bernard Williams[1] review 27 cases of hydrocephalus associated with aqueduct stenosis seen at Midland Centre for Neurosurgery and Neurology, Smethwick, England, during 1964–74 and discuss 9 other cases in which hydrocephalus occurred and the aqueduct stenosed and some additional feature was present—either a meningocele or encephalocele or incomplete obstruction of the aqueduct radiologically at initial examination.

The 14 male and 13 female initial patients presented at age 5 weeks to 43 years. No etiologic factors were apparent. There were no clinical features permitting the condition to be recognized with certainty. Most patients had symptoms and signs of raised intracranial pressure without focal signs. Evidence of elevated intracranial pressure was a consistent finding on plain skull radiography. Angiography in 5 patients with focal neurologic signs showed only hydrocepha-

---

(1)   J. Neurol. Neurosurg. Psychiatry 40:521–532, June, 1977.

lus. In another 5 patients, pneumoencephalography after ventriculography allowed outlining of the 4th ventricle.

Six patients underwent 3d ventriculostomy initially; 4 of them required reoperation. In 8 patients given a Spitz-Holter valve, 4 valves required revision, and 1 valve was removed. Three of 11 patients who had ventriculocisternostomy by the Torkildsen technique initially required further operations. One patient had aqueduct cannulation initially.

Seventeen patients had satisfactory results at follow-up. Five patients died, 3 of meningitis. Three patients were retarded and 2 had poor vision; 1 patient was spastic, 1 was ataxic and 1 had chronic epilepsy.

Patients usually present some time after onset of pathologic changes of aqueduct stenosis. Before any form of internal shunting is carried out, the functional capacity of the subarachnoid space should be assessed and factors leading to its subsequent incapacity evaluated.

► [McMillan and Williams suggest that nontumorous aqueductal stenosis is more likely to be the cause of hydrocephalus than the initial cause of the dilated ventricles. They analyze their cases to indicate that they behave as if the aqueduct were being blocked by lateral compression of the midbrain between the enlarged lateral ventricles.

A Norwegian family with 8 cases of congenital hydrocephalus in male members is the subject of a report by Søvik, Van Der Hagen and Løken (Clin. Genet. 11:416, 1977). All but 1, who lived several weeks, died at or within 10 days of birth. Autopsy of a pair of affected twins showed marked stenosis of the aqueduct of Sylvius without signs of preceding inflammatory or neoplastic change. There were 4 cases of clubfoot in the family, but none of the 8 members (all in the same generation) showed that defect. The authors believe the stenosis of the aqueduct and hydrocephalus in this family was due to an X-linked gene.

A computerized tomographic, roentgenographic and psychometric study of 9 patients with achondroplastic dwarfism was carried out by Mueller et al. (Neurology (Minneap.) 27:430, 1977). All had ventricles ranging from normal to severely hydrocephalic, and 3 had enlarged sulci. Petrous ridges were asymmetric. Intelligence quotients were generally average, but performance deficits were found in all and presumed to be reflections of the hydrocephalic state or its secondary effects on the brain. Most data indicate that the hydrocephalus is of a communicating nature, usually ascribed to problems at the base of the skull. – Ed.] ◄

Hydrocephalus Drainage in Dandy-Walker Syndrome with Consideration of Morphology is discussed by B. Szepan[2] (Univ. of Bonn). According to available reports, the treatment of the Dandy-Walker syndrome (DWS)

(2) Z. Kinderchir. 22:99–110, October, 1977.

is determined by the morphological conditions as well as the cerebrospinal fluid (CSF) dynamics of the cerebrum and cerebellum. However, the author observed 4 patients with surprising morphological findings that oppose the general opinion that DWS represents a pathogenic entity in terms of a dysraphic disturbance. All 4 infants were admitted for excessive cranial size, presenting a high-degree internal hydrocephalus with a cyst in the posterior cranial cavity.

In 2 patients a primary ventriculoatrial drainage according to Pudenz was implanted in the right lateral ventricle, although with completely different subsequent courses. In 1 child the hydrocephalus persisted and repeated intermittent signs of cerebral pressure were registered. A CSF pressure crisis occurred at age 3. At age 4½ a large cyst was exposed in the posterior cranial cavity; the child died at age 5 after renewed cyst formation. The other child showed largely normal development after revision of the posterior cranial cavity. The ventriculoatrial CSF drainage led to diminution of the entire ventricular system and a significant augmentation of the cerebral coating thickness.

In another child, death was most likely attributable to a decompensation of CSF dynamics before ventriculoatrial drainage could be carried out. In another child, primary total extirpation of the posterior cranial cyst was accomplished, during which the radiologically suggested communication with the cerebrospinal canal could not be confirmed.

None of these children presented the pathogenically typical picture of DWS. In 2 patients a porencephaly of the cerebellum could be demonstrated. Morphological findings in another did not allow clear pathogenic evaluation; histologic examination showed a cystic wall reminiscent of either meningoencephalocystocele or porencephaly. In one child, exposure of the posterior cranial cavity at age 4 showed no cyst, although such had been clearly demonstrated at earlier age.

Although from the clinical standpoint DWS is considered treatable, a uniform pathogenesis in terms of a dysraphic disturbance was not confirmed in several cases. Observations to date allow the conclusion that a DWS associated with porencephaly is more likely to lead to decompensation of the CSF circulation than is the same syndrome associated with developmental disturbances, although these considerations must remain hypothetical for the present, pending further observations.

▶ [Salmon, Hajjar and Bada (Pediatrics 60:721, 1977) use the term "fontogram" to denote the recording of fontanelle pressures by use of an applanation transducer. This device flattens (applanes) the skin of the fontanelle, and a plunger within is displaced by the force within the membrane. Studies compared these results with those from direct measurements via a ventricular needle; correlation coefficients were 0.98 in 21 paired determinations. In 35 newborn infants, the mean pressure in mm Hg was 7.37±1.45 SD. Clinical cases demonstrate the use of the applanation transducer in determining patency of the shunt, determination of how much fluid to remove from the ventricle to keep pressure normal, how much mannitol to use to keep intracranial pressure normal and similar purposes.

Among the complications of ventriculoperitoneal shunts described by Adeloye and Olumide (Int. Surg. 62:525, 1977) were peritoneal fibrous pouch (4 cases), although the chief problem in these cases was mechanical plugging of the end of the tube. In 4 instances, the mother mistook the subcutaneous peritoneal tube for an *Ascaris* worm (in these undernourished children while the incision was not completely healed) and clawed the tube free. Two cases of accumulated fluid causing ascites were noted in these data on 154 cases. There was 1 case each of spontaneous extrusion of tube, bowel perforation and volvulus. — Ed.] ◀

Tension-Free Closure of Large Meningomyelocele Defects. Solid closure of meningomyelocele is necessary, but this can be difficult when a large skin defect is present. Mutaz B. Habal and John K. Vries[3] (Univ. of Florida) devised a technique for closing large meningomyelocele defects (Fig 16) without tension, which uses bilateral bipedicle flaps (Fig 17) developed from vertical flank incisions, advanced medially (Fig 18) and approximated in the midline (Fig 19). The lateral defects are closed transversely (Fig 20) and the outer margins of the bipedicle flaps are left free until the flaps adhere to underlying tissue. Children selected for repair are operated on as soon after birth as possible, under general endotracheal anesthesia. The residual gaps are closed after 10 days with sutures or skin clips (Fig 21). Occasionally the central part of the lateral defect requires a small split-thickness skin graft.

Twelve large meningomyeloceles, with an average width of 6 or 7 cm, were repaired by this technique. The width of each lesion exceeded half the width of the back; the largest lesion was 11 cm. Ten patients underwent repair within 12

(3) Surg. Neurol. 8:177–180, September, 1977.

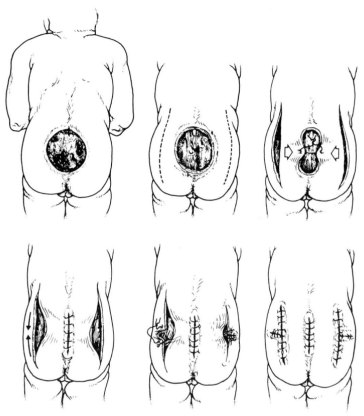

Fig 16 (top left). – Preoperative appearance.
Fig 17 (top center). – Position of lateral incisions for development of bipedicle flaps.
Fig 18 (top right). – Medial advancement of bipedicle flaps.
Fig 19 (bottom left). – Closure of medial margins of bipedicle flaps.
Fig 20 (bottom center). – Reduction of lateral defects by transverse closure.
Fig 21 (bottom right). – Final appearance of repair.
(Courtesy of Habal, M. B., and Vries, J. K.: Surg. Neurol. 8:177–180, September, 1977.)

hours of birth. A tension-free closure was obtained in each instance. The repair took only 5–10 minutes longer than closure by the undermining method, and no significant increase in blood loss resulted. There were no significant wound complications. Skin grafting was carried out in 4 patients. The children could be handled normally within 2 weeks of birth. Seven children followed for over 6 months have had no complications related to meningomyelocele. Six of the children have achieved normal milestones for intellectual development.

This technique provides tension-free closure of meningomyelocele defects, with minimal blood loss. The cosmetic result is better than with previous techniques for closure of large lesions. That children can be managed normally within 2 weeks of birth aids their psychosocial development.

▶ [Silon silicone sheeting is somewhat elastic and when used in closure of a large defect of the back, as described by Winston, Michle and Shuster (J. Neurosurg. 47:781, 1977) permits even tension on the lumbodorsal fascia and, through this, onto the skin. Within 10 days a defect 7×4.5 cm was reduced to 7×2 cm. The mesh (which had been tightened by sutures in the interim) was removed and the skin undermined and closed. – Ed.] ◀

Urinary Continence in Open Myelomeningocele. The chief handicaps of children with myelomeningocele are those related to hydrocephalus, lower limb function and the urinary tract. Urinary diversion has been recommended for all children before age 5. Roger J. Brereton, R. B. Zachary and James Lister[4] (Sheffield, England) analyzed bladder control in children born with open myelomeningocele 10 – 12 years after closure of the back lesion. Of the 200 consecutive cases operated on in 1962 – 64, 194 were treated in the first 36 hours of life. At follow-up in 1974 – 75, 106 children had survived for at least 10 years and had accurate information available.

Twenty-four children (23%) had normal continence and 82 were incontinent, but 46 of the latter were "socially dry," 26 with the aid of urinary diversion and 16 by using a penile appliance. Extremely few patients were kept socially dry by bladder expression. No patient was being managed by bladder catheterization at the time of review. Children with extensive lesions were less likely than the others to be continent. Only 1 of the children who were continent at age 5 lost control at a later time. Four children appeared to gain bladder control after age 5. Deterioration of the upper tracts was not seen on pyelography after age 5. No urinary tract infection has occurred in 21 of 24 continent children having repeated examinations; 12 of these 24 children required a shunt for hydrocephalus and 11 had considerable neurologic

(4) Arch. Dis. Child. 52:703 – 707, September, 1977.

involvement of the lower extremities. The rate of normal urinary control among patients with moderate or severe neurologic involvement was about 12%.

Early urinary diversion in children with myelomeningocele, even in the presence of neurologic deficit, is indicated only to prevent progressive deterioration of renal function. Urinary incontinence itself is not an indication for urinary diversion in the 1st decade of life.

Disk Problems

▶ For sheer numbers, I know of nothing to surpass the reports on lumbar disk surgery given at the proceedings of the meeting of the German Association for Neurosurgery in 1976 (Acta Neurochir. (Wien) 36:265, 1977). Series of 1,000 were commonplace; others had 2,000, 2,200 and 3,166 cases (e.g., Simon's series of patients operated on between 1970 and 1975). Analyses were made of differential diagnosis, complications, protrusions in childhood and in elderly people, recurrences and relationships with social and psychiatric situations. Three articles dealt with microsurgical approaches to the lumbar disk, some with incisions of only 2.5 – 3 cm. The articles involved have appeared now under the title *Lumbar Disc/Adult Hydrocephalus, Volume 4 of Advances in Neurosurgery*, edited by R. Wüllenweber et al. (New York: Springer-Verlag New York, Inc., 1977). The last 150 pages of the volume are a potpourri of "Free Communications" concerned with a variety of neurosurgical items, from head injury to reconstruction of spinal cord vessels.

Salibi (Wisc. Med. J. 76:82, 1977) has given the historical background, outline of modern concepts and analysis of 23 cases of neurogenic intermittent claudication. Disk hernias were removed in 8 cases; the standard operation, however, is wide laminectomy and facetectomy. How to do this with chisel and hammer instead of rongeurs is described by Verbiest, whose long experience with spinal stenosis is discussed below. – Ed. ◀

Results of Surgical Treatment of Idiopathic Developmental Stenosis of the Lumbar Vertebral Canal: A Review of 27 Years' Experience is presented by Henk Verbiest[5] (Univ. of Utrecht). In this study, diagnosis of developmental stenosis was limited to patients with midsagittal diameters of the vertebral canal measuring 12 mm or less. During 1948 – 75, 147 patients were treated surgically for developmental stenosis of the lumbar vertebral canal. The midsagittal canal diameters were measured in the entire stenotic area in 116 patients, 92 of whom were followed for 1 – 20 years.

In the presence of an obliterated interlaminar space, laminectomy was begun from the next normal space. Disk protrusions inside areas of absolute stenosis were not removed before resection of the related arches. Unroofing with a chis-

---

(5)   J. Bone Joint Surg. (Br.) 59-B:181 – 188, May, 1977.

el was preferred to use of a rongeur or punch to decompress an extremely narrow foramen.

There was 1 death and 1 case of coronary thrombosis after operation. Seven patients had a new radicular deficit or increased radicular symptoms, and 2 had a permanent deficit. No vertebral displacement was noted after extensive laminectomies, even when combined with excision of disk protrusions and clearance of the corresponding disk spaces. Combined laminectomy, bilateral foraminotomy and disk excision at the same level resulted in vertebral displacement in 1 case. Two patients had postoperative ossifying arachnoiditis, and 1 patient had annular nonossifying arachnoiditis. Three patients had recurrent symptomatic stenosis, and 2 had recurrent stenosis entirely due to scar formation in the area of previous decompression.

Sixty-two of 91 patients were completely relieved of symptoms and signs of stenosis. Two patients with paraplegia had no improvement in the paraplegia after decompression. Sciatica persisted in only 1 of 18 cases and intermittent claudication in only 4 of 74 cases. Symptoms were reduced in number in most patients who remained symptomatic after operation.

▶ [It seems to me that anyone interested in the problems of lumbar stenosis (and this should mean orthopedist, neurosurgeon and radiologist — the last with his new transverse computerized scans) must obtain and read and reread Verbiest's book, *Neurogenic Intermittent Claudication: With Special Reference to Stenosis of the Lumbar Vertebral Canal* (New York: Elsevier-North Holland Publ. Co., 1976). — Ed.] ◀

Indications, Technique and Results of Caudal Epidural Injection for Lumbar Disk Retropulsion. R. K. Sharma[6] (Royal Infirm., Preston, England) reviewed the results of epidural injection for low back pain and sciatica in 201 patients. Epidural injection can confirm the diagnosis. Therapeutic indications include acute "lumbago," intractable sciatic pain, chronic backache with sciatica, symptoms of disk prolapse complicating pregnancy, nocturnal cramps and coccydynia and failure of laminectomy or other treatment. Contraindications include local sepsis, a history of sepsis, and obliteration of the sacral hiatus by a bony mass. The needle should enter the sacral canal through its hiatus; puncture of the dural sac should be avoided. The solution

(6) Postgrad. Med. J. 53:1–6, January, 1977.

should reach the desired level within the vertebral canal. A volume of 40 ml of 0.5% lidocaine is used for the epidural injection. Diazepam is useful for sedation in some cases. The injection is made as a slow, stop-and-go procedure. If the first injection is ineffective, further injections can be given at 2-week intervals.

A total of 201 patients with disk degeneration and retropulsion had epidural injections of about 80 mg methylprednisolone. Most patients were aged 25–50. Thirty-six patients received more than one injection. Results, based mainly on pain relief, were extremely good in 59 patients, good in 54 and fair in 48, whereas 40 patients had no improvement. The average time lost was 14.8 weeks; just over half the patients lost 8 weeks only.

Epidural injection by the caudal approach is preferred to injection by the lumbar route because it is simple and relatively free from complications. In addition to the presumed anti-inflammatory effect of steroids that reduces edema and relieves pain, it is assumed that the anticollagenic activity of methylprednisolone minimizes nerve traction and subsequent pain production through depression of adhesion formation.

▶ [Our anesthesiologists far prefer the lumbar direct route for epidural injections to the caudal approach described above. The injection is easier, uses less local anesthetic and does not depend on an opening (sacral hiatus) that sometimes is quite variable.

I find it difficult to understand the presumption that corticosteroids act on adhesions; as Sharma points out, their role (if any) in this regard is related to inhibition of new adhesions. Once collagen has formed, the steroids do not dissolve it. For an even more controversial opinion, see the following article. – Ed.] ◀

Lumbosacral Arachnoepiduritides: Clinical and Etiologic Aspects. J. Pourel, R. David, L. Picard, J. Roland, J. Montaut and A. Gaucher[7] (Univ. of Nancy) state that after disk surgery or a first myelographic contrast examination, arachnoid or epidural alterations are often observed, which are grouped together under such disputable terms as lumbar arachnoepiduritis or chronic adhesive spinal arachnoiditis or are described simply as cicatricial aspects. The present study included 120 cases classified on the basis of radiographic criteria. Three forms were distinguished: arach-

(7) Sem. Hop. Paris 53:2109–2115, Nov. 9, 1977.

noid-type lesions limited to the region beneath L5–S1 (A1) or more extensive in height (A2) and epidural or arachno-epidural-type lesions (AE). The discovery of these lesions often poses diagnostic and therapeutic difficulties, as well as etiopathologic problems.

Clinical symptoms are varied; they are generally benign and nonspecific and without correlation with radiologic type. Evolution is marked by progression to chronicity and variation in distribution of symptoms (greater frequency of lumbalgia, diminution of sciatic radiculalgia). Cerebrospinal fluid abnormalities are variable and nonspecific. Among 3 cases of apparently primary arachnoiditis (without prior myelography or surgery), a herniated disk was the suspected cause in 2. In the 9 cases (A1 and A2) discovered after a first myelography, the effect of this examination could not be clarified. Most AE cases were observed after one or several interventions for herniated disk with laminectomy.

The role of operation seems to be established by the frequency (90%) of postoperative cases. As for arachnoiditis that follows myelography, clinical and experimental findings point to the nature of the contrast material as a possible influence. The recent introduction of metrizamide may represent some progress in this regard. The quantity injected may also play a role, and a volume of 5 ml Dimer-X should preferably not be exceeded. The noxious effect of water-soluble contrast mediums depends on the hyperosmolarity provoked by their subarachnoid injection, which suggests their use in diluted form. The results of Dullerud and Morland (1976) seem to show that simultaneous administration of corticoids favors development of arachnoiditis, although the role of corticoid infiltration is uncertain. Contamination of injected products with detergents, glass fragments or plastic particles is also a consideration.

Postlaminectomy Arteriovenous Fistula. The symptoms of postlaminectomy arteriovenous (AV) fistula can be vague, and delayed diagnosis is distressing. Usually patients present at a young age with congestive heart failure. Douglas H. Hildreth and Donald A. Turcke[8] (Univ. of Oregon) reviewed the records in 47 reported occurrences of postlaminectomy AV fistula and 2 recent personal experiences.

(8) Surgery 81:512–520, May, 1977.

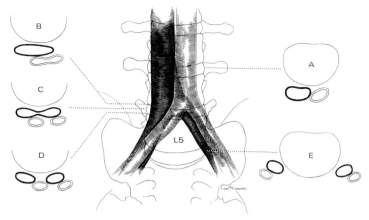

Fig 22. – Diagrammatic representation of the cross-sectional relationships between intervertebral disk, artery and vein at **A,** disk levels L3–L4; **B,** upper L4–L5; **C,** middle L4–L5; and **D,** lower L4–L5 (reflecting low, intermediate or high aortocaval bifurcations) and **E,** L5–S1. (Courtesy of Hildreth, D. H., and Turcke, D. A.: Surgery 81:512–520, May, 1977.)

The relevant anatomical relationships are shown in Figure 22. Although some AV fistulas are associated with pseudo-aneurysms and carry a risk of rupture, the major danger is high-output congestive heart failure. Symptoms are unusual with fistulas less than 10 mm in size. Nine patients had symptoms early in the postoperative period, including abdominal or groin pain, ascites, ileus and "failure to thrive." Forty patients presented months to years after surgery with fatigue, malaise, shortness of breath and other symptoms of congestive failure. Sixteen patients had lower extremity edema and venous engorgement. Ascites was uncommon in chronic cases.

Angiography delineates the precise anatomy of the AV fistula and defines any local vascular anomalies. Standard treatment to control heart failure is mandatory preoperatively. Closure of the venous side of the fistula alone may not be adequate. The four vessels supplying the fistula should be mobilized far enough away to prevent premature entry into the fistula. The artery may be divided completely if necessary and reapproximated after repair, either directly or with a Dacron prosthetic segment. The vein is preserved. Arterial ligation alone is unacceptable. If a large pseudoaneurysm is present, the ligation technique may be useful. Intravascular balloon catheter tamponade may also be extremely helpful. If thrombophlebitis is present, partial inferior caval interruption should be considered. Only 4 of 47 previously described patients died, 1 preoperatively.

By selection of the appropriate procedure for the individual patient with a postlaminectomy AV fistula, a successful outcome may be expected.

▶ [Here, in a nutshell, is a dilemma that typifies current surgical practice—and malpractice! If the operator desires to remove the entire disk (which includes the annulus and hence implies going deep inside the disk space), he takes a considerable risk of injury to anterior structures. He may not recognize the injury, for, as Hildreth and Turcke show, the symptoms may not bring the patient to the doctor for months or years after the operation. (Obviously, if there is an immediate gush of blood from inside the disk space, something better be done about it right away.) How responsible is such a physician for the injury he has (presumably unwittingly) produced? A total of 49 reported instances undoubtedly does not nearly represent all the times such fistulas have been formed, but when one considers the thousands of disk operations, certainly the incidence of this injury must be no more than 1 in 1,000. Its disastrous nature necessitates its inclusion among those complications of which current malpractice suits make it obligatory to inform the patient. As these authors put it, "Most of these complications have befallen excellent technicians, occasionally while a discussion of the very complication was taking place."

On the other hand, "Fear of recurrence has resulted in aggressive fragment removal." This is envisaged by the long-time practitioner who warns the patient that no attempt to remove the entire disk is to be made, and recurrence may take place. Of the two alternatives, it seems to me more sensible to take the risk of the recurrence. Furthermore, another argument in favor of not taking out the entire disk (or as much as possible) is the collapse of the disk space, which inevitably results in changes in the zygapophyseal joints, including their ligaments, which in turn may lead to persisting back pain. The shift of the vertebral bodies also may cause compression of the nerve roots at the top of the foramina (these holes are extremely large, to be sure, but the nerve roots stay near the top and get pulled on with disk narrowing). I believe that this disappearance of the disk space and body shifts are responsible for recurrence of back and radicular pain after chymopapain injections that function too well—that is, all the disk disappears!

So it appears that there is no one best way to deal with the herniated disk problem, nor with the possible complications. Not all of the patients are helped by epidural steroids; disk protrusions may cause acute neurologic deficit (including flaccid paraplegia), and operations will, I am sure, continue to give satisfying relief to a large number of patients.—Ed.] ◀

Jackson-Pratt Drain in Anterior Cervical Spinal Operations. Ralph B. Cloward[9] (Honolulu) describes the

(9) Surg. Neurol. 7:205–208, April, 1977.

Jackson-Pratt drain as a soft, flexible, perforated silicone tube with a gentle bulb suction, which he has used for the past year in all his anterior cervical spine operations, with gratifying results. It has markedly reduced morbidity by eliminating many objectionable postoperative symptoms and complications. A pliable, perforated, flat drain 10 cm long is placed in the wound, attached to a round, noncollapsible tube and hermetically sealed. The reservoir is a collapsible bulb 12 cm long and 5 cm in diameter at the meridian; it is marked with measuring lines. The drain can be doubled or kinked in the wound without obstructing flow. It is placed in all recesses of the operative field and secured tightly with inverted absorbable subcutaneous sutures. It is removed when less than 10 cc is recovered in 24 hours.

Esophageal and tissue "edema" was a constant finding 3 days after operation when rubber Penrose drains were used, and this often lasted 1 or 2 weeks or longer. The Jackson-Pratt drain has yielded 30–60 cc drainage in the first 24 hours, and a total averaging 48 cc in single-level cases. Marked clinical improvement occurred with removal of this fluid and blood. There was little or no fever and little difficulty swallowing. Patients took a regular diet the day after surgery. Postoperative interscapular pain was not reported. Postoperative x-rays have shown little or no increase in the vertebral-tracheal interval.

Only 1 patient has required reoperation for evacuation of a hematoma since the Jackson-Pratt drain has been used. This drain finds wide use in all operations in which large areas of raw tissue are exposed, including mastectomy, mammary augmentation and reconstruction, radical neck surgery and orthopedic procedures.

▶ [We have also found this drain to be useful in cervical operations. Cloward does not tell us if there have been any infections; these, after all, have been the reason for hesitation in the use of drains, which are said (in several reports on postoperative infections in neurosurgery) to increase the frequency of infection. – Ed.] ◀

Tumors

"Failure to Thrive" due to Pontine Glioma. Rarely the diencephalic syndrome may be caused by tumors of the posterior fossa that involve the cerebellar vermis, floor of the 4th ventricle or cervicomedullary junction. Joseph C. Maroon and Leland Albright[1] (Univ. of Pittsburgh) present a case illustrating the protracted course and minimal clinical findings that may be associated with brain stem gliomas.

Boy, 14, seen for large size at age 6, was noted to perspire excessively and had a height and weight above the 98th percentile. Weight loss was first noted at about age 10 and ascribed to an "adjustment reaction of childhood." Dizziness and vomiting led to admission at about age 13, when anorexia nervosa was diagnosed. Suboccipital "tightness" was reported 4 months later, when examination showed minimal left dysdiadochokinesia. A glucose tolerance test again gave abnormal results. The cerebrospinal fluid protein level was 260 mg/100 ml. A pneumoencephalogram showed only slight panventricular dilation, and posterior fossa angiography was reported as normal. A year later, a computerized tomographic scan showed a posterior fossa mass with ventriculomegaly. Symptoms were worse on hyperextension of the neck. Slight ptosis and palatal weakness were noted and a pneumoencephalogram showed a brain stem mass at the pontomedullary junction, with a component in the 4th ventricle. A brain stem astrocytoma was confirmed at suboccipital craniectomy. Radiotherapy was given postoperatively and substantial weight gain ensued.

Five previous patients with diencephalic syndrome due to posterior fossa tumor have been described. Five of the 6 children have been boys. All but 1 had symptoms in the 1st year of life. The average time to diagnosis was 30 months after the onset of symptoms. The symptoms were identical to those in patients with anterior tumors and diencephalic syndrome. Neurologic abnormalities are minimal in both groups. The cause of the syndrome in patients with posterior

(1) Arch. Neurol. 34:295–297, May, 1977.

fossa tumors is not known, but involvement of locus ceruleus-hypothalamic pathways has been postulated.

► ↓ Another cause of the "diencephalic syndrome" or failure to thrive can be optic glioma, as mentioned in the following article by Oxenhandler and Sayers. Incidentally, the diagnosis of anorexia nervosa in a male child or adolescent must be looked at with great suspicion. — Ed. ◄

Dilemma of Childhood Optic Gliomas. The management of childhood optic gliomas is controversial. Donald C. Oxenhandler and Martin P. Sayers[2] (Ohio State Univ. Hosp.) reviewed the records of 12 male and 16 female patients seen in 1954–75 with childhood optic glioma. Twenty-three patients were seen at age 10 or less. The chief initial complaints were loss of vision, headaches and proptosis. Strabismus occurred in most younger children with significant visual loss. Four patients presented with clinical hypothalamic involvement, manifested as diabetes insipidus or diencephalic syndrome. There was no surgical mortality. Four patients have died during follow-up for 1–20 years and 2 were lost to follow-up. Neurofibromatosis was present in 36% of patients. Two of 7 patients with chiasmal glioma and neurofibromatosis died; 7 patients without neurofibromatosis were followed after resection of unilateral optic nerve gliomas and all have stable normal vision in the remaining eye. Two of 6 patients who were irradiated for chiasmal glioma without phakomatosis have had progressive visual loss. Among 8 patients with hydrocephalus, 2 of 5 with hydrocephalus due to 3d ventricular tumor have died.

Presently patients with chiasmal gliomas are followed closely by neuro-ophthalmologic studies. Any evidence of field loss or a decrease in acuity might be an indication for radiotherapy. Hypothalamic involvement also calls for radiotherapy. Hydrocephalus is managed by shunting if increased intracranial pressure supervenes. Individualization of patient care is necessary in this condition. Optic gliomas appear to be a potentially progressive neoplastic entity, at best one of slow subclinical progression and at worse one of relentless hypothalamic infiltration or, rarely, malignant degeneration.

► [Nowhere is this controversy about optic gliomas more explicitly stated than in the masterful multivolume work *Neuro-Ophthalmology: Clinical Signs and Symptoms* (Philadelphia: Lea & Febiger, 1978). The section on the treatment of these gliomas is separately presented by Drs. Walsh and Hoyt — who differ on the treatment. Hoyt is unhappy with the results of biopsy of the optic glioma, for decline in vision may occur thereafter. Walsh is in favor of operation for confirmation and resection of unilateral optic nerve glioma, which is the procedure supported by Oxenhandler and Sayers in the young patient in whom follow-up examination is unreliable, unilateral visual loss is profound or proptosis is excessive. If there is any question as to the origin of an anterior hypothalamic tumor, exploration should be undertaken to rule out the presence of meningioma, teratoma, craniopharyngioma, ectopic pinealoma or dermoid cyst, all of which have mimicked optic glioma. With the advent of computerized tomographic scanning and fractional polytome pneumoencephalography, explorations and resections should become necessary less often.

Meningeal tumors that encase the optic nerves at the inner end of the optic canal, or at its orbital entrance, are associated with exophthalmos, loss of vision, optic atrophy and opticociliary shunts. Hollenhorst, Hollenhorst and MacCarty (Mayo Clin. Proc. 53:84, 1978), report data on 9 patients with meningioma of the optic nerve sheath, bilateral in 2, right-sided in 6 and left-sided in 1. In 10 of the 11 affected eyes, opticociliary shunts developed. Indentation and flattening of the globe (and hypermetropia) were noted in 5. Nine eyes progressed to blindness; 1 was worse after operation. Surgical treatment has not been effective in these cases or similar ones reported in the literature. The presumptions are that the tumor interferes with the pial blood supply to the optic nerve and that operation only causes more vascular interference. However, it is also true that when eyes have nerves that are severely atrophied, anything that can be done may be followed by blindness. I have seen the same happen with severe atrophy after papilledema from posterior fossa tumor; despite prompt and adequate decompression, vision continues to deteriorate. The obvious answer seems to be either to do nothing unless exophthalmos makes it imperative — or operate early. — Ed.] ◀

Immediate Visual Deterioration after Attempts at Radical Excision of Pituitary Adenomas. Debate continues about whether or not to attempt radical removal of pituitary adenomas. Technical problems in removal of large tumors have been simplified by use of the operating microscope and bipolar coagulation. J. Sanchis and M. Bordes[3] (Valencia, Spain) have, since 1970, attempted total removal of the tumor mass and as much as possible of the suprasellar capsule adherent to the inferior aspect of the optic nerves and chiasm. In the past 5 years 30 cases have been managed in this way by means of a transfrontal intracranial approach. Five patients had postoperative visual loss. Two had an insignificant reduction of the visual fields, but 3 were totally blind immediately after surgery.

(3) Acta Neurochir. (Wien) 38:251–258, 1977.

All totally blind patients had long histories, advanced loss of acuity, bilateral optic atrophy and large tumors. No relationship with age, sex, diabetes or hypertension was apparent. Surgical manipulations were difficult in all cases because of the large tumor or because of adhesions after previous surgery. No accidental hypotension occurred. The blindness does not seem to have been related to intrasellar hematoma, a secondary empty sella or direct trauma to the optic pathways. Local disturbances of blood supply from surgical manipulations are believed responsible for most of the early visual damage. Recovery may begin after an interval of several weeks. Patients were given high doses of dexamethasone, dextran and vasodilators.

Radical tumor excision does not necessarily require removal of the suprasellar capsule, and this does not appear to reduce the risk of tumor recurrence. Traction on and manipulation of the suprasellar capsule involves a risk of damaging the chiasm, probably through interference with its blood supply from below. The capsule should not be disturbed. If the main goal of surgery is to improve vision, this can best be achieved by as complete a simple internal decompression as is possible.

► [Ciric (J. Neurosurg. 46:596, 1977) is convinced that there is a single common membranous layer that invests the anterior and neural lobes of the hypophysis and the pituitary stalk. Because of this capsule, it is necessary to section deliberately and sharply the pituitary stalk early in hypophysectomy to prevent postoperative diabetes mellitus. He proposes that the capsule is a derivative of the primitive pia mater that develops from the mesoderm separating the cerebral vesicle from the stomodeum.

In a 3-year period at the Mayo Clinic, 203 transsphenoidal procedures were carried out. Of 129 patients with normal vision preoperatively, none had visual impairment postoperatively although 3 had transient diplopia. Of 62 patients with preoperative visual impairment, 45 had pituitary adenoma, 10 had craniopharyngioma, 3 had chordoma and single patients had ectopic pinealoma, fibrous dysplasia, arachnoidal cyst and cholesteatoma. Laws, Trautmann and Hollenhorst (ibid. 46:717, 1977). Two patients died; the others had postoperative visual studies indicating 81% had improvement, 11% were unchanged and 5% were worse. The authors consider the results for vision to be comparable to those with other surgical techniques, and hence the transsphenoid hypophyseal approach should be continued and expanded.

Analysis of 70 cases of pituitary adenoma by Mohanty, Tandon, Banerji and Prakash (J. Neurol. Neurosurg. Psychiatry 40:987, 1977) showed 18 with hemorrhage. Three patients had acute apoplexy, 3 had an acute episode of deterioration in a known adenoma, 11 had chronic bleeding, found only at operation, and 1 had had an acute episode 4 years before progressive visual loss, diabetes and other symptoms caused his hospitalization. Subarachnoid hemorrhage was found in 2 of the 3 with acute apoplexy. Such patients should have emergency surgical decompression. Diagnosis of hemorrhage into a known tumor (acute or chronic) is important in providing impetus to operation that may quickly reverse visual loss. Small hemorrhages in chronic tumors are of incidental interest and represent the largest group. The authors believe their high incidence of overall hemorrhage may be due to the large size of the tumors that they see. – Ed.]

Prolactin-Secreting Pituitary Tumors. J. Lobo Antunes, Edgar M. Housepian, Andrew G. Frantz, Donald A. Holub, Robert M. Hui, Peter W. Carmel and Donald O. Quest[4] (New York) reviewed data on 69 patients with pituitary tumors, seen in 1971 – 75, in whom prolactin secretion was evaluated. The 41 women and 28 men had a mean age of 40.6. Visual field defects were present in 33 patients and 5 had compromise of the 3d or 6th cranial nerves, or both, as well. Galactorrhea was documented in 21 women, 19 of whom also had amenorrhea; 7 women had amenorrhea without galactorrhea. Two men had galactorrhea and decreased libido. Ten patients had evidence of acromegaly. Pituitary tumor was confirmed histologically in 50 patients.

Prolactin was elevated in 37 (79%) of 47 patients before treatment. Eight of 22 previously treated patients were hyperprolactinemic. All but 2 of 21 women with galactorrhea and all but 2 of 26 with amenorrhea had hyperprolactinemia. Four of 6 acromegalic patients were hyperprolactinemic. Serum prolactin levels were usually not elevated by chlorpromazine or thyrotropin-releasing hormone, but L-dopa reduced the levels in the 3 patients evaluated. Six of 36 patients with hypersecretion of prolactin had reduced adrenal function and 7 had reductions in both adrenal and thyroid function. All tumors in hyperprolactinemic patients were of the chromophobe type. Prolactin levels usually declined substantially shortly after removal of the adenoma and in 7 patients returned to normal.

Little correlation was found between the serum prolactin level and tumor size in this series. Both transsphenoidal surgery and radiotherapy greatly reduced the hyperprolactinemia, but a more rapid reduction was achieved with microsurgical removal of the secreting adenoma. Normal pituitary function was preserved in most patients. It is not clear

(4)   Ann. Neurol. 2:148 – 153, August, 1977.

whether serial prolactin determinations are a reliable index of tumor recurrence.

► [In the series of 34 patients with galactorrhea or amenorrhea studied by Chang et al. (Am. J. Obstet. Gynecol. 128:356, 1977), 18 had microadenomas of less than 1 cm diameter, 7 had lesions over this size and 5 had unidentified lesions. One patient explored by the transsphenoidal route had a normal pituitary gland, and 3 had cryosurgery without biopsy. Menses resumed in 16 of 17 women with microadenomas and in 2 of 7 with macroadenomas who presented with amenorrhea. Galactorrhea disappeared in 15 of 17 with microadenomas and in 4 of 7 with macroadenomas who presented with galactorrhea. Sellar polytomography in women with hyperprolactinemia is a useful technique for diagnosis of pituitary tumors, and microresection by the transsphenoidal route is safe and effective.

Galactorrhea in men and boys is very rare, and in most cases is due to drug ingestion. Van Meter, Gareis, Hayes and Wilson (J. Pediatr. 90:756, 1977) report a case in a boy, aged 12, in whom pituitary functions were normal except for persisting hyperprolactinemia. X-rays showed an asymmetrically enlarged sella turcica, without suprasellar extension on air study. Lactation ceased and hyperprolactinemia disappeared after transsphenoidal hypophyseal resection of a microadenoma.

The meeting of the Society of Neurological Surgeons in Philadelphia in 1978 contained a symposium on pituitary microadenomas. The panelists were endocrinologists, presenting new statistics and reinforcement of the concept of surgical treatment of microadenomas, while admitting the utility of treatment with bromocriptine. Snyder from the University of Pennsylvania reported that special stains reveal that 25% of 300 pituitary glands contained lactotrope hyperplasia and 8% had adenomas. Mikhail, from the same university, reported on newly released figures from French and Swedish investigators of the amenorrhea-galactorrhea syndrome. Tolis, from McGill University, said the amenorrhea may be due to tumor in 16% cases, but if galactorrhea is also seen, tumor is present in 70% cases. Bromocriptine lowers the prolactin level, but there is usually a rebound after it is discontinued. In male patients, the usual presenting symptoms for prolactin-secreting tumors are decreased libido and impotence; 43% had visual impairment and 30% had headaches, compared to about 3% with women with prolactin adenomas. Tolis believes that operation is the treatment of choice, with bromocriptine to be used only if remission is incomplete.

Zervas, speaking at the Interurban Neurosurgical Society in February, 1978, gave a figure of 6% adenomas in 838 cases of amenorrhea, usually with asymmetric sella. He felt that if a patient has a high prolactin level with a normal sella, one should observe the patient, and if the sella is enlarged with high prolactin levels, one should operate for tumor. He thinks transsphenoidal operations (method of choice) should be followed by radiotherapy. — Ed.] ◄

Division of Hypophyseal Stalk (Mischotomy) for Malignant Exophthalmos after Treatment of Graves' Disease with ^{131}**I** was performed by J. Le Beau and A.

Corlcos[5] (Paris) in a case in which the condition had proved resistant to corticosteroids, thyroxine in large doses and reserpine.

Woman, 54, was seen in November, 1958, for bilateral retraction of the upper lids and unilateral right-sided exophthalmos. Ocular difficulties had progressively increased during 2 months, but neither goiter nor tachycardia had been present. A discrete tremor had been attributed to emotionalism. She had been widowed 1 year earlier. Weight loss of 25 kg and cessation of menstrual periods thereafter had been reported.

Basal metabolism was +71%; cholesterol, 2.16 gm/L, protein-bound iodine, 6.5γ. Exophthalmometry showed 18 mm protrusion on the left and 20-21 on the right. After treatment with 10 drops of thyroxine and 60 drops of chlorpromazine daily for 2 months, conjunctival hypervascularization was present on the right, weight was 63 kg and pulse rate was 90. The thyroid gland was nonpalpable, and thermophobia and gross sweating of the extremities were noted. Four months later, treatment with reserpine, thyroxine, phenobarbital and local hydrocortisone was started, without improvement of protrusion (22 mm on the right and 18 mm on the left). Ten months after treatment was begun, the edema of the lids was distinct bilaterally, the thyroid was palpable and somewhat firm, pulse rate was 90 and the exophthalmometric result was 25½-21 mm.

In October, 1959, she was hospitalized and received 7 mCi [131]I. One month later, she had gained 3.5 kg, pulse rate was 68 and exophthalmos, 25-22 mm in front of the lateral rim of the orbit. She was discharged on a regimen of 3 tablets of reserpine and 2 of thyroxine daily. Six months later, she had gained 9 kg and resumed work on a half-time basis.

In May, 1960, the exophthalmos was increased — 26 mm on right and 24 on left. After retrobulbar injections of hyaluronidase and cortisone, photophobia and significant ocular disturbance were noted.

The patient was not seen again until December, 1962. Ocular protrusion had increased — 30 mm on the right and 28 on the left. Appearance was slightly hypothyroid, with somewhat puffy face and sparse eyebrows. A large myxedematous subdermal plaque (5 × 3 cm) on the left tibial crest and hippocratic fingers were noted. Cholesterol and lipids were augmented. Basal metabolism was −19%. Low iodine and protein-bound iodine of 1.5γ confirmed the impression of hypothyroidism. Trials with dexamethazone, thyrox-

(5)   Sem. Hop. Paris 53:2181-2184, Nov. 16, 1977.

ine and reserpine resulted in improvement of the general condition, but exophthalmos persisted (29 mm on the right, 27 on the left), and surgical intervention was decided on.

METHOD. – After difficult exposure of the stalk concealed under numerous suprasellar adhesions, it was isolated with an Oliver hook and sectioned with a short Adson's knife. Coagulation of the central point of the stalk was followed by placement of two folded polyethylene strips, pushed as far as possible back and downward so as to isolate the hypophyseal dura mater.

Long-term results were satisfactory, with marked progressive regression of exophthalmos and return to work and normal social life.

Treatment of Colloid Cysts of the Third Ventricle by Stereotactic Aspiration. D. A. Bosch, T. Rähn and E. O. Backlund[6] (Stockholm) performed stereotactic aspiration of colloid cyst in the anterior 3d ventricle, causing obstruction of the foramina of Monro, in 4 patients after exact neuroradiologic localization that included computerized tomographic (CT) scanning.

Man, 40, had had attacks of vertigo and progressive headache for 1 month and vomiting in recent days. The symptoms were provoked and worsened by tilting the head backward. A neurologic examination, EEG and echoencephalogram were negative, but plain skull films showed the pineal calcification displaced caudobasally. Air encephalography showed an expanding lesion in the anterior 3d ventricle that bulged into the widened lateral ventricles; the estimated cyst volume was 1.3 ml. The patient was bradycardic and drowsy after the air study, but was improved by ventricular drainage. Stereotactic cyst puncture was carried out 4 days later, with removal of a little more than 1 ml mucous fluid. The patient recovered rapidly and was free of symptoms a week postoperatively. He is in excellent health 7 years after surgery. A recent CT scan showed cyst remnants and slightly dilated lateral ventricles.

If late refilling of the cyst occurs, repeat cyst aspiration is indicated. Stereotactic biopsy for diagnosis should be the first step in the management of patients with intracerebral and intraventricular tumors. Needle puncture and aspiration biopsy are quite easily done stereotactically after exact localization of the lesion by ventriculography or CT scanning, or both. A carotid angiogram is necessary preoperatively to avoid injury to the internal cerebral vein by the

(6) Surg. Neurol. 9:15–18, January, 1978.

biopsy needle. Complications are essentially absent in cases of colloid cyst when careful attention is paid to the location of the internal cerebral venous angle.

▶ [As these authors point out, the "typical" story of paroxysmal headache related to change of position is uncommon, and many patients present with a clinical picture resembling normal-pressure hydrocephalus syndrome. Other methods of managing this condition include bilateral Torkildsen ventriculocisternostomies, and we have recently had the opportunity to do bilateral ventriculoperitoneal shunts for such a colloid cyst. Long-term observation is obviously necessary to determine the optimal treatment, which may well be cyst aspiration and follow-up with CT scans. — Ed.] ◀

Treatment of Tumors of the Posterior Part of the Third Ventricle and the Pineal Region: Long-Term Follow-up. M. B. Camins and E. B. Schlesinger[7] (Columbia Univ.) reviewed the records of 126 patients treated during the last 30 years for tumors of the posterior 3d ventricle and pineal region. The EMI scanner has provided objective information on the effects of irradiation. There were 43 histologically verified tumors of the posterior 3d ventricle and 21 proved tumors of the pineal region in the series. The treatment of these tumors without pathologic verification is advocated. If a posterior fossa mass distorting the posterior 3d ventricle is considered, a suboccipital exploration is indicated. If the area is free of pathology, a Torkildsen procedure can be done at the same time. Eight negative suboccipital explorations have been carried out to date.

Patients are now treated with a tumor dose of 5,000 rad over 6 weeks. The spinal axis is not treated unless cerebrospinal fluid cytology is positive. Five patients with pinealomas had cord metastases and 5 had evidence of intracranial spread. If signs and symptoms do not subside after a course of radiotherapy, direct operative treatment should be considered. Five patients, 2 with pineal lesions and 3 with para-3d ventricular lesions, have survived more than 30 years after direct surgery and radiotherapy. A total of 34 patients with pineal lesions and 21 with paraventricular tumors have lived over 5 years, with a 5-year survival rate of 43%. Thirty of 79 initial patients died within a year, many in the immediate postoperative period without steroid therapy. Correcting for this factor, the 5-year survival rate is 57%.

(7) Acta Neurochir. (Wien) 40:131–143, 1978.

These results confirm the conservative approach to these lesions. The goal is the surgical relief of elevated intracranial pressure, followed by postoperative irradiation to arrest tumor growth. The key to treatment is radiotherapy. Many long-term survivors have only radiotherapy and shunting.

Cranial Chordomas. B. E. Kendall and B. C. P. Lee[8] (London) review the features of 44 cranial chordomas in patients with definite histologic evidence of chordoma and adequate x-rays for analysis. The 28 male and 16 female patients had an average age of 37.9 years at onset of symptoms. Average duration of symptoms was 3.45 years. Seventeen patients presented with cranial nerve palsies alone. Twenty-one presented with cranial nerve palsies associated with facial pain in 1, conductive deafness in 1, paresis or ataxia of limbs in 13, paresis of limbs and epilepsy in 1 and facial pain with paresis of limbs in 2. Two patients had tetraparesis plus neck pain; 2, nasal blockage plus epistaxis, 1, amenorrhea with headache and dementia; and 1, headache alone.

Plain films and tomograms of the skull showed that about half of the patients had classic features of a partially calcified midline tumor, destroying the clivus and causing a soft tissue mass in the sphenoid sinus or nasopharynx. Erosion of the tip of the clivus was noted in 4 patients. Unilateral bone erosion was evident in nearly a third of the patients. Bone sclerosis was seen in 5. Twenty-six patients had bilateral roentgenographic abnormalities. Increased uptake of technetium was seen in the 5 patients having gamma encephalography. Computed transmission tomography was useful in showing intracranial extensions of the tumors and changes in the ventricular system and also in outlining extent of the mass within the skull base.

Chordomas tend to displace the dura before transgressing it, so that the subarachnoid space is usually patent adjacent to quite large tumors, permitting the margins of any intracranial or spinal extension to be outlined at encephalography or myelography. Displacements of basal vessels are useful in confirming the site and extent of the tumor. Narrowing of arteries by compression is not infrequent, but encasement is rare. Pathologic circulation was observed in 6 of the

---

(8)   Br. J. Radiol. 50:687–698, October, 1977.

present cases. Selective angiography now available may well show abnormal vessels in more of these tumors, especially now that subtraction is also available.

Ependymoma: Follow-up Study of 101 Cases. Sverre J. Mørk and Aagot C. Løken[9] (Oslo) reviewed 101 cases of histologically confirmed ependymoma, seen over a 22-year period in 1953–74 in Norway. Choroid plexus papilloma and subependymoma were excluded from the series. Ependymomas comprised 1.2% of all primary intracranial tumors and 32% of intraspinal glial tumors seen in the review period. Of the 48 intracranial tumors, 34 were infratentorial, all in close relation to the 4th ventricle. Of the 53 intraspinal ependymomas, 29 were in the spinal cord and 24 in the conus region, filum terminale or cauda equina. Headache or vomiting, or both, predominated in patients with intracranial tumors and back pain in those with intraspinal tumors. Over two thirds of the intracranial tumors occurred in children, whereas nearly all intraspinal tumors were in patients over age 15. Only 3 "pure" papillary tumors were encountered. A myxopapillary pattern was seen in 9 cauda ependymomas; 7 intracranial tumors were anaplastic.

Fourteen patients, 12 with intracranial tumors, had no operation. There were 8 operative deaths in the intracranial tumor group and 1 in the intraspinal tumor group. The postoperative prognosis for all intracranial lesions was poor, only 53% of patients living 1 year and about 13% for 10 years or longer. Survival was greater in patients having irradiation than in those having surgery alone. The prognosis of intraspinal lesions was far more favorable, 96% of patients living 1 year and 72% for 10 years or longer. Myxopapillary ependymomas appeared to have a better prognosis than the cellular type. Total extirpation was done in 15 intraspinal cases and improved the prognosis. No obvious advantage was seen in the use of combined treatment of surgery and irradiation.

Postoperative irradiation appears to extend survival after initial surgery in patients with intracranial ependymomas, but a long-term effect on survival has not been demonstrated. Further research is needed to clarify the basic properties of tumor cells in the central nervous system.

► [An excellent French monograph published as a supplement to the

(9)   Cancer 40:907–915, August, 1977.

May, 1977, issue of *Neuro-Chirurgie* deals with ependymomas. Coutelle, of Lyons, France, is responsible for the section on supratentorial ependymomas, Pierluca offers a chapter on posterior fossa ependymomas and G. Fischer, of the Alexis Carrel Institute, presents the section on spinal ependymomas. As Wertheimer points out in his preface, the total of identifiable observations numbers 332. Several collaborators have helped in chapters on neuroradiology, anatomy, pathology, diagnosis and treatment. A 3-page English summary should whet the interest of any neurosurgeon dipping into this paperbound book from Masson, of Paris. — Ed.] ◄

Use of High-Dose Corticosteroids in Patients with Inoperable Brain Tumors.

Abraham Lieberman, Yves Le Brun, Peter Glass, Albert Goodgold, Warren Lux, Arlene Wise and Joseph Ransohoff[1] (New York Univ. Med. Center, New York) reviewed experience with high-dose steroids (methylprednisolone, 200–2,000 mg daily) in 11 patients seen in 1 year with inoperable brain tumors. They represented 15% of all brain tumor patients seen in this period. All patients were treated for at least 3 weeks, the mean treatment time being 55 days. The steroid was given in increasing doses to control elevated intracranial pressure.

The mean patient age was 57 years. All patients were symptomatic when admitted. Six patients had primary and 5, metastatic tumors. Dominant hemispheric tumors were present in 6, multiple tumors in 3 and deep thalamic lesions in 2. Five patients had been treated previously, 4 by radiation. Seven patients were irradiated while on high-dose steroid therapy, and 6 received concurrent chemotherapy. Five patients received 1 gm steroid daily for up to 3 weeks, and 3 of these received up to 2 gm daily.

All 8 patients who had deteriorated on conventional doses of steroids and then continued on dosages of up to 1 gm daily improved. No additional improvement occurred with higher doses in these patients. Steroids could be discontinued for several months in 2 patients with primary brain tumors. Two of 3 previously untreated patients with uncal herniation and signs of rostral-caudal deterioration improved dramatically on high-dose steroid therapy.

Three patients had serious bacterial infections while on steroids and chemotherapy. No deaths were attributable to steroid therapy. All patients developed features of hyperadrenocorticalism, but no gastrointestinal bleeding occurred.

---

(1)   J. Neurol. Neurosurg. Psychiatry 40:678–682, July, 1977.

Two patients developed pulmonary emboli requiring anticoagulant therapy; both had metastatic tumors. Two patients developed myopathy.

High doses of steroids are an effective and relatively safe short-term treatment for patients with brain tumors who no longer respond to conventional doses. An arbitrary upper limit on dosage should not be applied. A large multi-institutional study has been undertaken to investigate the effects of steroids on inhibition of tumor growth and on oncolysis.

▶ [Methylprednisolone sodium succinate (Solu-Medrol) may help patients with brain tumors achieve clinical improvement and reduction in periventricular elastance before significant reduction in raised intracranial pressure, according to Miller et al. (Neurosurgery 1:114, 1977). It is possible that this corticosteroid has less of an adverse effect than dexamethasone on bacterial phagocytosis and microphage migration and it also may have less of an interaction with Dilantin and phenobarbital. The authors used intramuscular methylprednisolone in doses of 40 mg every 6 hours for the 72 or more hours until malignant tumor (glioblastoma, metastatic carcinoma) was removed. Periventricular elastance was estimated from the changes in intraventricular pressure after injection of 1 ml saline into the ventricle, followed by removal of cerebrospinal fluid.

The use of high-dose corticosteroids (dexamethasone) has been examined by Marshall, King and Langfitt (Ann. Neurol. 1:201, 1977) in a prospective manner in 121 neurosurgical patients, with a view to clarifying the incidence of complications. Patients with a history of gastrointestinal ulceration were not excluded and no special precautions were taken in their management. Doses of 16 mg/day were given to 36 patients, 40 mg to 43 patients and 80 mg to 42 patients, in 4 divided doses per day. Tapering of the dose was done according to the clinical course (and these details are not given). The dosage of 40 mg daily was given to 19 patients on a long-term basis (mean 206±56 days) without any steroid complication. Five patients developed hyperglycemia and 3 required insulin. One developed *Candida* esophagitis that resolved, 1 had gastric hemorrhage requiring transfusion of 2 units and 1 patient with duodenal perforation died. The disorders were not apparently dose related. Serum gastrin levels were not raised in any of 12 patients who were comatose at the time of study. Concurrent antacid therapy probably should be used, and although a history of gastrointestinal erosive disease suggests caution, the benefits of corticoid therapy should be assayed and subtle signs of complications looked for. — Ed.] ◀

Combined-Approach Surgery for Removal of Glomus Jugulare Tumors was used in 10 cases by Gale Gardner, Edwin W. Cocke, Jr., James T. Robertson, Merlin L. Trumbull and Robert E. Palmer[2] (Memphis, Tenn.). Five male and 5 female patients (average age, 42) with glomus

---

(2) Laryngoscope 87:665–688, May, 1977.

tumors of the temporal bone that originated in the jugular bulb had operations in which combined approach through the neck and skull base was used. Seven patients had had hearing loss for an average of 39 months and 6, tinnitus for an average of 31 months; 2 patients had dizziness as an initial symptom. In all cases retrograde jugularography showed an obstruction of the jugular bulb. Angiography gave positive results in 7 patients. Five patients had cranial nerve deficits preoperatively; 1 had bilateral carotid body tumors. Six patients had two-stage procedures. Total tumor removal was achieved in 7 patients. Five patients have been followed for 1–4 years. Six patients had preoperative radiotherapy. Skull base exposure preceded the otologic phase of tumor exposure. If possible, tumor and attached venous system are removed en bloc.

Tumor specimens appeared smaller and less extensive than the earlier appearances suggested. Specimens from 6 patients who received irradiation therapy showed swelling in blood vessel endothelium which reduced bleeding at surgery, but tumor tissue was present in 5. All patients are alive at present, all but 1 without central nervous system complications or long-term disability. One patient had a postauricular fistula postoperatively and has had severe pain, weakness and dizziness and impaired coordination. Two patients have had revision surgery. Five patients had reduction in tinnitus postoperatively and 4 reported reduction in dizziness. Only 1 patient has had persistent postoperative cranial nerve dysfunction. The semicircular canals had to be sacrificed in 1 instance but vertigo and nausea resolved in this case.

The problem of intracranial extension of glomus tumors may be solved, at least in many cases, by collaboration between the otolaryngologist and neurosurgeon. The problem of extensive bleeding has been largely solved by preoperative irradiation and wide surgical exposure. The authors have had no experience with tumor embolization.

► [The key to excision from a neurosurgeons's point of view is removal of the soft tissue at the base of the skull, removal of bone from around the tumor and preservation of the facial nerve. The otologist's concern is control of the sigmoid sinus and removal of posterior fossa extension. By working as a team, they can meet these interdisciplinary requirements to accomplish the total removal of these large tumors. Transposition of the facial nerve is necessary for controlled removal of the tumors. No mention is made of the possibility of reduced blood loss by operating under hypotensive therapies. The authors have not used embolization, but the merits of that technique are beautifully illustrated in the book *Superselective Angiography of the External Carotid Artery*, by the late R. Djindjian and his colleague, J. J. Merland (New York: Springer-Verlag New York, Inc., 1977). They also illustrate selective angiography in cases of nasopharyngeal angiofibroma, another bloody tumor, which is the subject of the following article. – Ed.] ◄

Surgical Management of Nasopharyngeal Angiofibroma with Intracranial Extension is discussed by Edmund A. Krekorian (Fitzsimons Army Med. Center, Denver) and Ronald H. Kato[3] (Freedom, Calif.). Surgery continues to be the mainstay of treatment of nasopharyngeal angiofibroma. An estimated 10 – 20% of these tumors have intracranial extension. Three of the authors' 11 patients were proved at craniotomy to have such extension. No well-defined technique can diagnose extension short of craniotomy. Stereo x-rays and polytomography can show bony changes that may or may not represent intracranial extension. Angiography with subtraction technique may show an intracranial blush compatible with intracranial tumor extension.

The intracranial part of a combined operation is done first, by means of a frontotemporal flap. If the intracranial extension is small it may be left to be removed during the extracranial procedure. The internal carotid artery can be ligated whenever indicated. The chief aspect of extracranial removal of angiofibroma is adequate exposure. Some form of the Weber-Ferguson incision is supplemented by a lateral rhinotomy, except for small localized tumors. Tumor in the sphenoid sinus is approached last and with caution. Tumor removal should be done with gentle finger dissection where possible, exploiting planes of separation. The sphenoid sinus was filled by tumor in all 11 of the authors' patients. In all cases the tumor could be dissected away from the dura without lacerating it. Four of 5 patients in whom the sphenoidal roof was eroded acquired diabetes insipidus postoperatively. No blindness or cavernous sinus injury resulted. The angiographic findings in 1 patient are shown in Figure 23.

A combined approach is feasible for treating nasopharyngeal angiofibroma with intracranial extension. Despite the great risk to vital structures, other treatment methods have

(3) Laryngoscope 87:154 – 164, February, 1977.

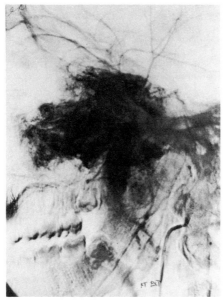

Fig 23. — Arteriogram of right external carotid artery showing magnitude of tumor. (Courtesy of Krekorian, E. A., and Kato, R. H.: Laryngoscope 87:154–164, February, 1977.)

been notably unsuccessful and the combined approach offers a chance of cure.

Clinical Differential Diagnostic and Radiologic Pictures of Primary Sarcomas of the Brain are reviewed by P. Distelmaier[4] (Univ. of Bonn), in an attempt to establish the particular properties of these lesions in terms of neurologic, neurosurgical and neuroradiologic consequences. During an 11-year period, 153 cases were investigated.

The general term sarcoma of the brain includes varied groups of tumors, differing significantly on biologic, clinical and radiologic levels, as well as in their amenability to certain types of treatment. The present classification, used at the author's institution, differentiates monstrocellular adventitial sarcoma; fibrosarcoma of the brain; supplement to the first two, gliosarcoma; diffuse adventitial sarcomatosis; hemangiopericytoma of the brain; nonclassifiable primary

(4) Nervenarzt 48:405–418, August, 1977.

undifferentiated sarcoma of the brain; sarcoma of the reticuloendothelial system; and medulloblastoma.

Clinically, the sarcomas of the brain possess important characteristic properties, clearly differentiating them from the gliomatous cerebral lesions. First, they tend to metastasize and there is a possible hereditary disposition. Second, there is the possibility of traumatic cicatrical or radiologic etiology or the occurrence as malignant degeneration of a primary benign lesion. Induction may occur by a gliomatous tumor or there may be simultaneous induction by a mutual oncogenic noxious agent. Last, they are seemingly more amenable to therapeutic intervention than are the malignant neuroectodermal lesions.

In terms of age distribution, the peak in youthful patients is formed by the medulloblastoma and its more mature variant, the circumscribed arachnoid sarcoma. The second peak corresponds with the peak onset of the differential diagnostically most important brain tumors, the gliomas and meningiomas. This second peak encompasses the 5th and 6th decades of life; the relative scarcity of brain sarcomas in the elderly is noteworthy. There are clear localizational predilection sites: the cerebellum (33%), with the reticuloendothelial system being favored, and the temporofrontobasal region (41%), this possibly attributable to the developmental history of the primitive meninx.

The monstrocellular sarcoma is an absolutely brain-specific lesion, without even approximate correspondence in other organs. The present group included 27 of these mostly round, grayish rose tumors of firm consistency. They are fibrous in the sectional plane and have a precise macroscopic circumscription, surrounded by a pseudocapsule of compressed cerebral tissue in 30% of the cases. In more than 80% of these tumors, extensive internal necrosis was found and even occasional extensive cyst formation. Meningeal infiltration was always more pronounced than is true for glioblastomas; sarcomas seem to possess a greater affinity for related tissue. Diagnosis was most frequently established by arteriography. The lesion was hypervascularized and well stained in 66% of the cases, typically without "tumor clouds," but showing a network of spiraled vessels with characteristic irregular aneurysmatic contrast pools or patchy staining. The average postoperative survival time is 9–12 months, although 2 patients had a 4-year symptom-free period; both patients had had intensive postoperative irradiation.

Among fibrosarcomas of the brain, Abbott and Kernohan differentiate three levels of malignancy: fibroma, fibroblastoma and the actual fibrosarcoma. In contrast to those found in other organs, intracerebral fibrosarcomas do not grow diffusely into the adjacent regions, but are usually round, coarse and of grayish rose color, with a pseudocapsule of compressed edematous cerebral tissue, seemingly preferring the frontotemporobasal localization. The angiographic picture partially resembles that of monstrocellular sarcomas, although with less dye retention. In the group of 18 seen in this series the average survival time was about 6 months.

Gliosarcomas represent an interesting form of mixed tumors composed of part glioblastoma, part fibrosarcoma or less frequently monstrocellular sarcoma. Recurrence after total excision often shows only a sarcomatous character, as is true for the metastases of this tumor. A clear predilection for female patients was noted (8:3). One notable clinical aspect is the decidedly short history of several weeks and the increased blood sedimentation rate of between 30/50 and 50/80 mm. All patients died in less than 6 months, with about 25% dying immediately after surgery.

The group of primary undifferentiated cerebral sarcomas includes all lesions not subject to clear classfication due to poor differentiation, usually small cellular lesions of a relatively homogenous structure. Distinct and progressive signs of increased cerebral pressure mark the clinical picture. Radiation treatment is of some benefit but a combination of surgery and irradiation result in survival times of 16 – 18 months.

Hemangiopericytomas of the brain are richly vascularized, relatively coarse, reddish brown lesions of usually clear macroscopic delineation. They originate from vascular pericytes, most likely developing in the meninges rather than primarily in the brain. The occurrence in two different locations and the clear tendency for recurrence are noteworthy.

According to Zülch, diffuse adventitial sarcomatosis consists of sarcomas originating from vascular perithelia without actual tumoral nodules. Two such patients were observed, presenting recurrent bouts of high temperature and rapidly progressing neurologic symptoms with increasing loss of consciousness.

Sarcomas of the reticuloendothelial system represent a class of sarcomas possibly composed of varied subgroups. Differentiation is difficult and was not attempted. The tumors are white and often round, particularly when localized in the cerebellum. Some showed a pseudocapsule, with cysts in 2 cases; others presented diffuse growth with multiple foci, without allowing recognition of a primary tumor with metastases. Most often they were not connected to the meninges but localized in the marrow.

The position of medulloblastomas has not yet been clarified. Gullotta assumes them to be mixed embryonal tumors with a neuroectodermal and a mesenchymal portion. Thirty-five such patients were seen, corresponding to 26% of all sarcomas. Diagnosis is usually achieved by ventriculography.

Presently available methods do not allow clear preoperative differentiation of cerebral sarcomas; no absolutely reliable characteristics have been demonstrated. Most important are meticulous observation of clinical data and angiographic investigation. Clinical characteristics include a rapidly progressive course and often a moderate increase in the blood sedimentation rate. Cerebral sarcomas differ from those found in other organs by their round shape and clear macroscopic delineation, being frequently surrounded by a pseudocapsule of edematous cerebral tissue, and their usually high degree of malignancy. Another significant aspect is the relatively frequent simultaneous occurrence of sarcomas and gliomatous tumors, which can greatly vary the clinical picture and suggests the overgrowth principle possibly being at work in their development. Generally prognosis seems somewhat better than for malignant gliomas.

► [This article demonstrates the necessity of reading more than an author's summary, for *that* in this instance speaks only of 153 sarcomas. Only in the text does one learn that Distelmaier includes hemangiopericytomas, and, even more confusing, also medulloblastomas, amounting to 35 cases in this series. His own figures for the distribution of sarcomas among brain tumors amount to 7% without medulloblastomas, but 9.1% including the medulloblastomas (in contrast to prior series of Zülch, for instance, with 4.1% in 1975, and Kernohan's figures for 1962 of 3%). — Ed.] ◄

Radiation Therapy of Brain Tumors. Glenn E. Sheline[5] (Univ. of California, San Francisco) reviewed the results of radiotherapy obtained over about 20 years in various histologic types of brain tumor. Treatment usually encompassed the suspected tumor volume plus a margin of several centimeters. The dose was carried to 5,000 or 5,500 rad at a rate of 180 rad per day in 5 fractions per week. Recently, treatment has been started with a full daily dose, and side effects suggesting brain edema from radiation have been rare or absent. Also in recent years, treatment of highly invasive lesions has included the entire intracranial contents, with a dose of 6,000 rad. In cases of tumor with a tendency to seed via the cerebrospinal fluid, such as medulloblastoma, the entire central nervous system is irradiated. Steroids have been used only when clinically indicated.

Of 147 patients with biopsy-proved astrocytoma, 25 died postoperatively. Fourteen patients had complete tumor resection without radiotherapy, and none had a recurrence. Of 71 patients with incomplete resection who received radiotherapy, 46% survived 5 years and 23%, 20 years, compared with 19 and 0%, respectively, without irradiation. One of 7 irradiated patients with gemistocytic astrocytoma survived. In patients with grade III malignant glioma, the 5-year survival rate without recurrence was 16% with irradiation and only 2% without irradiation. Radiotherapy also improved survival rates at 1 and 3 years in patients with grade IV gliomas, but by 5 years, there was no survivor in either treatment group.

Quality of survival of medulloblastoma patients has been improved by radiotherapy, but inhibition of spinal growth is a possible complication. In ependymoma, it is not clear whether or not to include the entire central nervous system in the radiation fields. Postoperative radiotherapy appears to improve survival of patients with oligodendroglioma. About 7% of patients with brain stem tumors have improved after radiotherapy. Meningioma has recurred in 74% of nonirradiated patients having subtotal resections, compared to only 30% of 34 irradiated patients. Radiotherapy may increase the recurrence-free interval significantly in patients with incompletely resected meningioma.

▶ [Brown, Gunderson and Plenk (Cancer 40:56, 1977) have followed

(5) Cancer 39 (Suppl.) :873–881, February, 1977.

13 patients with an initial diagnosis of medulloblastoma who were treated with radiation therapy to the posterior fossa and spinal canal. A 5-year survival rate of about 70% was achieved. The authors suggest that in the absence of evidence of spinal cord involvement, a dose to the spinal column of 2,500 rad is sufficient, which decreases the potential for spinal column arrest. A boost to the posterior fossa of 4,500–5,000 rad is given. The only patient with metastases had a ventriculoatrial shunt placed for control of intracranial pressure.

Spinal subarachnoid implants developed in 11 of 32 patients who received local irradiation for intracranial ependymoma in the series from the University of Michigan reported by Kim and Fayos (Radiology 124:805, 1977). Eleven had supratentorial and 21 had infratentorial tumors. Radiation therapy was applied to the local area of tumor, none received whole brain radiation, and spinal axis irradiation was not routinely given. Spinal implants developed mainly in those with infratentorial tumors and from poorly differentiated neoplasms. In view of this experience, the practice now is to give a whole brain dose of 4,500 rad; primary site radiation is 5,500–6,000 rad, and the entire spinal axis is now given 3,000–3,500 rad. The only exception is in well-differentiated supratentorial ependymoma.

Eight male and 12 female patients were studied by Shalet, et al. (Acta Endocrinol. (Kbh.) 84:673, 1977) 8–32 years after receiving radiotherapy for brain tumor. Eight had medulloblastoma, 5 had cerebellar glioma, 4 had brain stem or pontine glioma, and single patients had glioma of the basal ganglia or frontal lobe or reticulum sarcoma of the orbit. Nine patients had impaired growth hormone responses to hypoglycemia, and 7 of these were below the 3d percentile for standing height. These all received more than 2,950 rad to the hypothalamic-pituitary axis. Multiple pituitary hormone deficiencies do not develop with time if the radiation dose is below a critical level. – Ed.] ◄

Preliminary Results Using Superfractionation in Treatment of Glioblastoma Multiforme are reported by B. G. Douglas [6] (Vancouver, B. C.). With superfractionation radiation therapy, doses per fraction are smaller than with conventional fractional therapy, and smaller total doses can be given.

Use of superfractionation was evaluated in a randomized prospective trial at the British Columbia Cancer Institute in 33 consecutive new patients seen during 1974–76 with glioblastoma multiforme or astrocytoma of grade III or higher. Tumor histology was confirmed in 31 cases. Three patients first received conventional fractional therapy; 2 are living, 1 in good condition at 70 weeks. The other 30 patients received three 100-rad doses daily at 3- or 3½-hour intervals for the whole brain part of their treatment, followed by 1,000 rad in 5 daily treatments to the known tu-

(6)   J. Can. Assoc. Radiol. 28:106–110, June, 1977.

mor. In the parallel-pair part of the treatment, both fields were treated at each sitting, and all ports were treated daily for the restricted-volume part of treatment. A quadratic dose-effect relationship for human skin was used to select dosages. Initially, dose levels were selected cautiously. Most commonly, patients received 5,400 rad in 54 fractions in 3½ weeks, with 1,000 rad in 5 fractions as a booster dose to the primary site.

Results with superfractionation were significantly better than those obtained in 100 previous consecutive patients with the same type of lesions who had a 1-year survival rate of 27%. Nine patients treated with 4,500 rad in 45 fractions and 1,000-rad booster dose have a crude 1-year survival of 44%. None of 6 patients given 6,000 rad with a 1,000-rad booster are dead, but 3 of 5 patients who completed this treatment will probably die. The actuarial survival curve for the group as a whole coincided with the crude survival of the patients given 4,500 rad. Both curves yielded a survival of 44% at 1 year.

Superfractionation appears responsible for the improved results obtained in these cases. A controlled trial might now be undertaken to compare various radiation regimens using whole brain treatment with a booster dose to the known tumor.

Radiation Therapy for Pineal Tumors and Suprasellar Germinomas. William M. Wara, Carol F. Fellows, Glenn E. Sheline, Charles B. Wilson and Jeannette J. Townsend[7] (Univ. of California, San Francisco) reviewed the records of 19 patients seen in 1950–75 who were irradiated as a result of a diagnosis of pineal or suprasellar tumor. Biopsy was considered too risky in 13 cases. All 6 confirmed tumors were germinomas. Patients were irradiated with a 1-Mev x-ray unit, a cobalt-60 device or a 4-Mev linear accelerator. Radiation doses ranged from 4,000 to 5,500 rad and were delivered to the entire ventricular system, but not the spinal axis.

Fifteen patients (73%) were alive without disease on follow-up at 2–21 years; 9 of them have been followed for 5 years or longer. Two patients died of recurrent disease 2–3 years after treatment; both had massive tumor recurrence

(7) Radiology 124:221–223, July, 1977.

that had been partially excluded from the treatment portal; both had been treated with small portals. One of these patients had a pineoblastoma. One patient died 10 months after treatment with an infiltrative lesion characterized as reactive gliosis. Another patient had multiple brain stem and cortical infarcts with thrombosis of the major cerebral veins at autopsy. Treatment had been complicated by hydrocephalus and meningitis.

The total control rate in 53 patients reported in the literature was 64%; most of these patients did not have biopsies. Elective irradiation to the spinal axis is not recommended, but rather treatment of the entire ventricular system with a dose of 4,500 – 5,000 rad given over 5 – 6 weeks. It remains to be determined whether germinomas may be treated with the same therapeutic doses as testicular seminomas. A reduction in dose with no loss of therapeutic efficacy in a growing child would likely result in reduced long-term complications of irradiation to the pituitary region. Computed tomography may be of benefit in assessing early responses of germinomas, possibly permitting a dose reduction.

► [Review of 32 patients with craniopharyngioma made by Onoyama, Ono, Yabumoto and Takeuchi (Radiology 125:799, 1977) indicates that doses of 5,500 – 6,000 rad (approximately 1,700 rets) after the first surgical intervention definitely improve the prognosis. At 5 years, 69% of patients were still alive and at 10 years, 60%. Only 12 patients were younger than age 15, however, and the tables show appreciably higher survival for patients younger than age 25 as compared to older ones. At 10 years, 77% of those less than age 25 survived compared to only 33% of those older than age 26. – Ed.] ◄

Delayed Radiation Necrosis of the Brain. A small risk of disabling brain necrosis attends the use of even standard therapeutic doses of irradiation for intracranial neoplasia. Delayed radiation necrosis of the brain is often mistaken for recurrent tumor, and craniotomy and biopsy have usually been necessary for identification. Albert N. Martins, James S. Johnston, James M. Henry, Thomas J. Stoffel and Giovanni Di Chiro[8] report 6 cases; 5 were verified histologically.

Symptoms usually began 9 – 24 months after radiotherapy. Progressive visual impairment and dementia are common after perisellar irradiation, whereas hemispheric signs predominate after irradiation of the cerebrum. The cerebro-

(8) J. Neurosurg. 47:336 – 345, September, 1977.

spinal fluid protein level may be elevated. Focal delta slowing is usually present on EEG examination. Necrotic brain may appear as an area of abnormal uptake on nuclide brain scanning and may also act as an avascular space-occupying lesion. On computerized tomography scanning, radiation necrosis appears as an intracerebral area with reduced absorption coefficient, often enhanced by intravenous contrast injection. Exploration and biopsy may not be necessary in all cases.

Pathologic studies showed a continuum of changes characteristic of radiation necrosis. The cerebral white matter was selectively damaged, though small isolated areas of cortex were also necrotic. Damage in white matter primarily affected small arteries and arterioles; small pial vessels were often involved. Extensive areas of parenchymal necrosis were seen in most cases. Many necrotic and fragmented vessels were surrounded by hemorrhage and edema.

The pathogenesis of delayed radiation necrosis of the brain remains unclear. Both a direct effect on parenchyma and vascular mechanisms have been proposed. The risk-to-benefit ratio of radiotherapy appears to become increasingly unfavorable for most patients with benign intracranial neoplasms when the standard brain tumor dose of 5,000 – 7,000 rad is fractionated at over 200 rad daily. Dexamethasone often improves symptoms dramatically, but excision of necrotic tissue is necessary when there is intracranial spatial decompensation and impending tentorial herniation. When the risk of spatial decompensation is small, a trial of dexamethasone may carry the patient over the period of maximum swelling and make surgery unnecessary.

▶ [Most attention has been placed in the past on the adverse effects of radiation on the central nervous system. However, in 2 cases that are presented by Ashenhurst, Quartey and Starreveld (Can. J. Neurol. Sci. 4:259, 1977) lumbosacral radiculopathy developed after radiation therapy of cancer (of the bladder in a man and of the cervix in a woman). The clinical picture is one of progressive motor and sensory loss in the legs, with onset usually within 1 year but sometimes delayed up to several years after radiation. A similar clinical picture can be produced experimentally in the rat. Similar findings are noted in 20 other cases from the literature. However, "There was no pathologic examination of the spinal cord or nerve roots in these or other reported cases."

Six patients in 9 years were found at the Memorial Sloan-Kettering Cancer Center to have evidence of an intracerebral mass after irradiation of extracerebral cranial neoplasms and at operation were found to have pathologic changes associated with delayed radiation necrosis of the brain. Rottenberg et al. (Ann. Neurol. 1:339, 1977) give in detail the clinical, radiologic and pathologic findings in these cases. They involved osteogenic sarcoma of the maxillary antrum, rhabdomyosarcoma of the parotid gland, adenoid cystic carcinoma of the lacrimal gland, squamous cell carcinoma of the auditory canal, squamous cell carcinoma of the ethmoid sinus and nasopharyngeal carcinoma. All had some part of the brain included in the radiation portals, and symptoms occurred 4–31 months after therapy. Vascular injury rather than neuronal or glial damage is the most likely primary significant factor in pathogenesis. – Ed.] ◄

Indications for Nonoperative Treatment of Spinal Cord Compression due to Breast Cancer. Patients with cord compression due to epidural cancer have long been a problem in neurosurgical management. Cully A. Cobb, III, Milam E. Leavens and Nylene Eckles[9] adopted a primarily nonoperative approach to these patients about 8 years ago. Review was made of data on 12,478 patients with breast cancer, including 2,467 with spinal metastases. Local treatment was not necessary in 688 patients, whereas 1,735 patients were irradiated without acquiring neurologic deficits. Only 44 patients had myelopathy due to cord compression. Twenty-six had laminectomy initially and 18, radiotherapy. Both groups consisted of middle-aged women with a long history of breast cancer. About one third of the group having operations and half the radiotherapy group could walk before treatment. A myelographically complete block was present in 88% and 78% of the groups, respectively. Seven of 12 patients having operations and no postoperative radiotherapy had received radiotherapy previously.

Motor function deteriorated in 6 (23%) of patients initially operated on and in 4 (22%) of irradiated patients. Power improved in 12 (46%) and 9 (50%) of patients, respectively. Radicular pain was less after treatment in 12 (46%) of patients operated on and in 13 (72%) of irradiated patients. Pain increased in 2 patients having operations and 1 irradiated patient who had laminectomy subsequently. Two patients initially having operations lost the ability to walk after treatment, as did 2 of the 9 irradiated patients. Six patients who had surgery regained the ability to walk after laminectomy and 5 irradiated patients became able to walk by the end of the course of irradiation.

(9)   J. Neurosurg. 47:653–658, November, 1977.

Treatment of spinal metastases by radiotherapy without laminectomy is reasonable in patients without a rapidly developing myelopathy and with a radiosensitive tumor such as breast cancer. Strict bed rest should be observed until at least the 1st week of radiotherapy is completed or symptoms have subsided. High-dose steroids may be advisable during radiotherapy. Radiotherapy alone can give results as good as those of laminectomy and radiotherapy.

▶ [Review of 344 consecutive cases of brain metastasis from the Massachusetts General Hospital was carried out by Solis et al. (Comput. Tomogr. 1:135, 1977). Lung contributed 38% and breast 24% and 8% came from melanoma, 6% from the gastrointestinal tract and 5% from the genitourinary tract. The source was undetermined in 14%. The colon and rectum contributed 80% of the gastrointestinal sources and the kidney contributed 34%, uterus 23% and prostate 14% of the genitourinary sources. Analysis of the computerized tomography scans done in 14 of the 25 cases of metastatic melanoma indicates high absorption abnormality with hemorrhage range density values. Most of the tumors did not enhance with injection of contrast medium. Solitary masses were more common than multiple ones, but the latter masses were more often seen after contrast enhancement.

Small cell carcinoma of the lung may be complicated by relapses within the brain during treatment, so Jackson et al. (J.A.M.A. 237:2730, 1977) carried out a randomized study of 29 patients. All received irradiation of the primary lesion and chemotherapy and, in addition, 14 did and 15 did not receive prophylactic irradiation of the brain. None of the 14 with prophylactic brain irradiation had a brain metastasis, whereas 4 of 15 without such treatment did, during a medial survival period not significantly different in the two groups (9.8 and 7.2 months, respectively). Although brain irradiation did not improve response rate or survival, brain metastasis with its attendant complications was effectively prevented.

Electroencephalography, echoencephalography, radionuclide brain scan and carotid angiography were the objective tests used by Romodanov et al. (from Kiev) (Zentralbl. Neurochir. 37:161, 1976) in assaying possible benefits from endolumbar injections of methotrexate in cases of malignant brain tumor. Doses ranged from 0.25 to 0.6 mg/kg body weight repeated every 2nd day for 5−7 injections. Higher doses were usually followed by some temperature elevation, headache, dizziness, anorexia, vomiting and meningism. In 5 cases, there was a rapid onset of a syndrome of intracranial hypertension, intoxication, stomatitis and fever to 39−40C. In 52 patients so treated, there was an objective decrease in the size of the neoplasm, and repeated biopsies showed a destructive effect of the preparation on these malignant brain tumors (24 glioblastomas, 14 undifferentiated gliomas, 5 sarcomas, 3 chorionepitheliomas and single instances of ependymoma, medulloblastoma and metastatic carcinoma).

The attention of the reader is directed toward a two-part article on neurosurgical perspective of tumor immunology (Bull. Los Angeles Neurol. Soc. 41:168, 1976; and ibid., p. 196). The first part, by Apuzzo and Sheikh, deals with general concepts of tumor immunology. The second part, by

Apuzzo alone, has to do with the immunology of glial neoplasms. Certainly a glioma-associated antigen does exist, but there is depression of the cell-mediated vanguard of the immune response. Both active and passive immunotherapy have been used in a small number of patients with malignant gliomas. Evidence of benefit is fragmentary. Apuzzo writes, ". . . it is apparent that reductive therapy consisting of surgery, radiation and chemotherapy will be necessary before the immune system will be effective against the tumor burden."

At the Philadelphia meeting of the Society of Neurological Surgeons in 1978, Bruno reported on his experiences with 317 glioma patients in four hospitals. The 1973–78 survival figures were 8.4 months for patients with grade IV gliomas, 15 months with grade III and 38 months with grade II. Immunotherapy was tested in a mouse ependymoma module. It appeared to help control the tumor only if the number of cells was small enough, necessitating preliminary lowering of malignant cells by some other techniques: operation, radiation therapy and chemotherapy in succession followed by immune therapy seemed to be the therapy of choice. — Ed.] ◄

Vascular Problems

HEMORRHAGES

▶ Some patients who come to emergency rooms or offices with sudden severe headache have hypertension; others have infections of the nervous system. Some have aneurysms, and the problem has been how to identify the patient with unruptured aneurysm at this stage. Olinger and Wasserman have devised an electronic stethoscope for this purpose. The system consists of a two-track magnetic tape recorder, two acoustically shielded air microphones, an amplifier and filter network and a headset. Impulses are picked up from the closed eye and from the heart, filtered, passed through a computer for Fourier analysis and visually displayed. Spectral analysis shows a large spike when an aneurysm lurks behind an eye. Serial monitoring also permits differentiation of arterial stenosis from arterial spasm (Surg. Neurol. 8:298, 1977).

The practical importance of identifying the patient with an incipient aneurysm rupture lies in at least two spheres: (1) the desire to find this aneurysm and do something about it before it ruptures and (2) the recent rash of malpractice suits based on the failure properly to diagnose such an aneurysm, when a doctor has seen the patient in the emergency room or the office. Here is an example of a situation that is going to lead to "defensive medicine" with its attendant costs. The implication of the legal attack is that anyone who appears before a doctor complaining of sudden severe headache without neurologic findings will have a computerized tomographic scan or an angiogram, or both. Such increased utilization will in turn bring down the wrath of the cost-conscious minions of the Department of Health, Education and Welfare; the conflict will then certainly induce the formation of a committee to establish a set of rules to determine which patients shall be admitted and which shall be sent home. The era of cookbook medicine and of branched mandatory paradigms is upon us.

Morelli and Laubscher (J. Neurosurg. 46:532, 1977) add another report to the growing, but still small, number of cases of aneurysm in infancy. Their patient was 4 months old when the aneurysm bled, was discovered by angiography and was removed, with apparent cure. The child in the report by Mabe and Furose (ibid., p. 795) was of the same age and was found to have an arteriovenous malformation after the head enlarged. The posterior fossa anomaly caused hydrocephalus. Shunting was done and follow-up angiography at age 1 year disclosed no sign of the malformation.

Aneurysms distal to the circle of Willis are seldom congenital or arteriosclerotic in origin, according to Olmsted and McGee (Radiology 123:661, 1977). The chief exceptions to this rule are those found at the genu of the middle cerebral artery and the pericallosal aneurysm at the origin of the callosomarginal or frontopolar artery. Peripherally located aneurysms may be secondary to infection, tumor embolus, moyamoya or trauma.

According to West et al. (Neurology (Minneap.) 27:592, 1977) non-visualization of a cerebral aneurysm probably represents the most common explanation for a normal cerebral angiogram in a patient with spontaneous subarachnoid hemorrhage. Perhaps due to improved techniques of femoral catheterization, magnification, unusual projections and subtraction, normal angiograms were found in only 7% of 220 patients with subarachnoid bleeding. Under these circumstances, the authors advise bed rest for 10–14 days, control of hypertension, repeat cerebral angiography and supine myelogram for spinal vascular malformation only when indicated clinically. ϵ-Aminocaproic acid is not used.

Hayward (J. Neurol. Neurosurg. Psychiatry 40:926, 1977) lists aneurysms undergoing thrombosis at the time of hemorrhage and minute (2 mm) aneurysms that are destroyed by the bleeding as the most likely reasons for subarachnoid hemorrhage of unknown origin. The analysis included 592 cases of subarachnoid hemorrhage, from which 91 cases were culled for lack of cause of bleeding. Of these, full angiography and computerized tomographic scans were done in 51 without cause for the bleeding being disclosed. In this group, no patient died or had a further hemorrhage, and only 2 were rendered unfit for work by reason of the bleeding of unknown origin. – Ed. ◄

Significance of Fundal Hemorrhage in Predicting the State of the Patient with Ruptured Intracranial Aneurysm. Hemorrhages are often seen in the fundus after rupture of an intracranial aneurysm. P. Rácz, M. Bobest and I. Szilvássy[1] (Univ. Med. School, Pécs, Hungary) studied the relationship between the presence of fundal hemorrhage (FH) and the state of patients with ruptured aneurysm in 201 patients admitted with subarachnoid bleeding due to verified intracranial aneurysms. Fundal hemorrhage was found in 49 patients (24.6%). Hemorrhages were bilateral in 23 patients. Twenty-eight patients had pool-like retinal, preretinal and vitreous hemorrhages. About two thirds of patients with FH and less than half of those without FH were drowsy or confused on admission or were stuporous with severe hemiparesis or early decerebrate rigidity (Hunts' classes III and IV). Serious pathology such as intracranial hemorrhage, ischemic infarction or massive hematoma were found in 31 of 49 patients with FH and in 54 of 152 without FH. Mortality was 65.3% in the group with FH and subarachnoid hemorrhage and 46.8% in the others without FH, a significant difference.

(1) Ophthalmologica 175:61–66, 1977.

Fundal hemorrhage was not related to the site of aneurysm in this series, but patients with FH had a higher mortality than those without. In the presence of FH, subarachnoid hemorrhage is often accompanied by intracerebral bleeding, cerebral infarction, extended spasm of vessels and disturbed cerebrospinal fluid circulation. In the presence of FH, patients should be classed in a less favorable category, as recommended for severe arteriosclerosis and vasospasm.

▶ [The cause of the fundal hemorrhage is still not clear. The authors refer to some of the recent hypotheses, which include the idea that blood from the subarachnoid space passes up the optic sheath to the lamina cribrosa and then to the fundus. Others believe the sudden increase in intracranial pressure causes rupture of the central retinal vein. It has also been proposed that transmitted increased intracranial pressure dilates the optic sheath, compressing the central retinal vein and making it possible for bridging veins from the dura to the pia mater to rupture. Hemorrhage in the optic sheath does occur in patients with sudden raised intracranial pressure. This hemorrhage may compress retinochoroidal anastomosis, leading to the rupture of retinal veins. – Ed.] ◄

Ruptured Intracranial Aneurysms: Case Morbidity and Mortality. Kalmon D. Post, Eugene S. Flamm, Albert Goodgold and Joseph Ransohoff[2] (New York Univ. Med. Center) examined the outcome in 100 consecutive patients with ruptured intracranial aneurysms who were seen in 1972 – 74. The goal was to carry patients through the acute period to the point at which intracranial obliteration of the aneurysm could be carried out safely. Eighty-five patients were placed on a regimen for subarachnoid bleeding, including control of blood pressure, anticonvulsants and antifibrinolytic therapy. Sedation was with phenobarbital, and blood pressure control was with methyldopa or hydrochlorothiazide, alone or in combination. The dose of ϵ-aminocaproic acid was 36 gm daily intravenously for 3 days, followed by 24 gm daily until surgery, or for 6 weeks in unoperated patients. Fifteen patients were managed by bed rest and sedation only until surgery could be done. Twenty-eight patients had a total of 60 aneurysms.

Ten patients on the bleeding regimen (11.8%) had early rebleeding. ϵ-Aminocaproic acid and hypotension are now continued until the aneurysm had been obliterated. Three patients had nonfatal pulmonary emboli during treatment. Results were considerably poorer in patients with vaso-

(2) J. Neurosurg. 46:290 – 295, March, 1977.

spasm. Seven of 12 such patients improved clinically when given intravenous isoproterenol and aminophylline, and 5 had angiographic evidence of lysis of spasm. Intracranial surgery was done in 86 cases. Surgical mortality was 6.3% for patients in grades 1–3 and 47% for those in grades 4–5. None of 13 patients given long-term hypotensive therapy after occlusion of the bleeding aneurysm, in the presence of multiple aneurysms, have rebled to date. Four patients not operated on have had a good or excellent outcome.

The overall surgical mortality in this series was 8.1%. Sixty percent of the patients were able to return to their previous activities, and 25% were incapacitated with moderate deficits. The total case mortality was 15%. The risk of future rebleeding has been eliminated for these patients. A regimen of active medical treatment before neurosurgery has improved overall case morbidity and mortality as well as the chance for long-term survival.

► [Tranexamic acid has been used in reducing risk of rebleeding after subarachnoid hemorrhage, but, as with ε-aminocaproic acid, controlled studies have been scanty. A double-blind controlled clinical trial in 51 patients from three Dutch hospitals is reported by van Rossum et al. (Ann. Neurol. 2:238, 1977). The dose was 4 gm/day for 10 days. Neither mortality nor rebleeding rates were improved after a follow-up of 3 months.

Piracetam (2-oxo-1-pyrrolidineacetamine) is a cyclic derivative of γ-aminobutyric acid (GABA) that appears to facilitate learning and memory and the transfer of information from one hemisphere to another, to reinforce cortical control over subcortical structures, and to protect the cortex against hypoxia. Alan Richardson and F. J. Bereen (Lancet 2:1110, 1977) have tried this material in 50 patients undergoing craniotomy for ruptured aneurysm or brain tumor, whereas 50 others had placebo. Otherwise, operation and treatment were the same in both groups. Groups reasonably well matched for age, sex, blood pressure and general medical condition were available, but there were actually fewer patients with ruptured aneurysms in the piracetam group and a higher proportion of fully alert patients in the placebo group. A standard dose of 10 gm daily of this drug given for 10–21 days produced no adverse effects, and did not appear to interfere with antibiotics, anticonvulsants, corticosteroids and other drugs. There was an apparently significant improvement or maintenance of consciousness in the piracetam group, especially if consciousness was impaired before operation. Whether this benefit is due to protection against anoxia or not is unclear.

Randomization of a clinical trial including regulated bed rest was carried out between 1963 and 1970 in the United States. Henderson, Torner and Nibbelink (Stroke 8:579, 1977) used various actuarial and statistical analyses. The designated period (21 days) of bed rest was completed by 198 patients; 22 had middle cerebral artery aneurysm, 35 had internal carotid aneurysm and 130 had anterior cerebral-anterior communicating artery aneurysm. The 7 with vertebrobasilar artery aneurysms were excluded from statistical analyses because of the small sample size. In the 5-year follow-up, cumulative mortality was 50%, associated with 47% rebleeding; 30% of the patients rebled during the 1st month and 1–3% after the 1st year.

The poorest prognosis was for patients with middle cerebral artery aneurysm with poor initial medical and neurologic conditions, presenting soon after the ictus, especially for men of advanced age. High mean blood pressure, large aneurysm size, multiple bleedings in the past and evidence of diffuse vasospasm were other unfavorable factors. The mean blood pressures included those at the time of original bleed, but how hypertensive these patients were "normally" is unclear, especially in view of the findings of others that blood pressures found to be in the normal range before bleeding rise after the ictus.

The treatment regimen included subdued lighting and the head of bed elevated no more than 30 degrees; the patient does not sit up or feed himself although he may turn. Bowels are regulated with common stool softeners; a bedside commode was used after the 1st week. Airway and oxygen maintenance was insured; phenytoin, 300 mg/day was given for at least 4 weeks. Fluid intake was 1,800–2,000 ml/day, with 1,000 calories per day. Restlessness was treated with sedatives, and pain was controlled with salicylates, codeine or meperidine. Condom or catheter drainages was used for those with urinary incontinence. No corticosteroids or osmotic diuretics were used, and a high level of nursing care was required.

Treatment of patients who had bled and whose blood pressures were kept low constitutes a different modality whose results are to be reported separately.

Sixty-two patients with intracranial aneurysm had operation directly at the aneurysm, and the results are reviewed by Ballenger, Salcman, Ducker and Perot (J.A.M.A. 237:1845, 1977). Eight were in grade I of Hunt and Hess, 31 in grade II (moderate headache, stiff neck, cranial nerve palsy the only neurologic defect) and 23 in grade III (drowsiness, confusion or mild focal deficit). None was in a more critical state (grades IV and V). Overall mortality was 5%. Patients were kept at bed rest, blood pressures over 150 mm Hg were treated with diuretics, hydralazine and sedatives, and aminocaproic acid was used to hinder lysis of clots. Intraoperative osmotic agents, steroids, magnification and hypotension were used. In 95% of patients, the aneurysms were on the anterior part of the circle of Willis, and 11% had more than one aneurysm. Only 3 of 62 had aneurysms on the posterior circulation. The average time from hemorrhage to operation was 12.4 days for most favorable cases and 27 days for grade III patients (usually due to delayed referrals rather than waiting for improvement in grade). Operative treatment in experienced hands should be greatly preferred to conservative therapy of ruptured aneurysms.

Microsurgical techniques were used in treatment of 137 patients with intracranial aneurysm by the Russian neurosurgeons Zlotnick, Oleshkevich and Stolkarts (J. Neurosurg. 46:591, 1977). There were 45 aneurysms on the internal carotid artery, 62 at the anterior cerebral-communicating artery area and 30 of the middle cerebral artery. The approaches used were, respectively, subfrontal sphenoid wing, interhemispheric fissure and via separation of the sylvian fissure. Results were good in 117 cases, fair in

10 and poor in 3. Seven patients died (mortality, 5.8%). The preoperative status of the patients was given, but not the interval after bleeding or the incidence of spasm. — Ed.] ◄

Surgical Management of Unruptured Asymptomatic Aneurysms. Duke S. Samson, Richard M. Hodosh and W. Kemp Clark[3] (Univ. of Texas, Dallas) have encountered a significant number of patients who had subarachnoid hemorrhage with multiple aneurysms that were injudicious to approach at a single sitting, as well as an increasing proportion of patients with asymptomatic incidental aneurysms in addition to a variety of disease processes. A significantly more aggressive approach has been adopted. Elective surgery is recommended to obliterate the unruptured aneurysm in all patients considered stable enough to have general anesthesia.

Fifty-two patients were seen in a period of about 5 years; only 3 refused the proposed elective procedure. Forty-nine patients underwent 50 elective craniotomies. There were 33 women and 16 men in the series. In 19 patients, aneurysms were found incidentally at angiography being done to investigate other neurologic symptoms.

Internal carotid lesions predominated. Most aneurysms were 7 – 10 mm in size. All aneurysms visualized at angiography were attacked surgically. The mean interval from primary surgery to elective aneurysm surgery was 11 days in patients with multiple aneurysms and 9 days in those with incidental aneurysms. Three aneurysms were ruptured during dissection, but bleeding was easily controlled. Two aneurysms were coated with polymerizing adhesive rather than being clipped. All 42 intraoperative or postoperative angiograms have shown adequate clip placement. No operative deaths occurred. Three patients had permanent deficits attributable to surgery, and 7 had transient deficits. All permanent deficits were paralyses of the frontal branch of the facial nerve due to excessive traction on the small skin flap. Two patients had minor local wound complications. No patient has had bleeding on follow-up for 3 months to nearly 5 years.

Modern anesthetic and microsurgical techniques justify

(3)   J. Neurosurg. 46:731 – 734, June, 1977.

an aggressive approach to most unruptured asymptomatic intracranial aneurysms.

Diagnosis and Treatment of Postoperative Cerebral Vasospasm. Cerebral vasospasm is a leading cause of morbidity and mortality in patients with intracranial aneurysms. Steven L. Giannotta, John E. McGillicuddy and Glenn W. Kindt[4] (Univ. of Michigan) have for 6 years attempted to counteract the ischemic effects of postoperative vasospasm by increasing cerebral blood flow and cerebral tissue oxygenation. Review was made of the records of 86 patients having 92 craniotomies in 1973 – 75. Seventeen had neurologic features suggestive of vasospasm and arterial narrowing on angiography in the postoperative period. Elevated systolic blood pressure was reduced preoperatively with α-methyldopa or hydralazine to a level of 130 – 150 mm Hg. Most patients had topical lidocaine or papaverine applied intraoperatively. Whole blood or colloids were infused when vasospasm was demonstrated to raise the central venous pressure to 8 – 10 cm water. These measures were sufficient in 10 of 17 patients. In the later years, routine overtransfusion of whole blood was used; dexamethasone in 4-mg doses was given intravenously for up to 3 days and low molecular weight dextran for the 1st day, with decreasing doses over the next 2 days. If the deficit did not improve, intravenous phenylephrine or dopamine was used to maintain a systolic pressure over 150 mm Hg. If the deficit progressed the patient was intubated and mechanically hyperventilated. Two patients received mannitol and urea after instillation of a subdural pressure monitor.

Twelve patients had no neurologic deficit on follow-up and returned to their former work. One had no deficit but has not returned to his former way of living; 2 patients had fair results and 2 had poor results. One died postoperatively of a pulmonary embolus and 1 probably had cerebral infarction before adequate treatment was instituted.

Neurologic deficits caused by postoperative cerebral vasospasm in patients operated on for intracranial aneurysm can be promptly reversed by the rapid application of these treatment methods. Hyperventilation may be necessary in

---

(4) Surg. Neurol. 8:286 – 290, October, 1977.

patients who show continued deterioration or increased intracranial pressure. Where necessary, the intracranial pressure should be monitored and it should be controlled with dehydrating agents.

▶ [At the Philadelphia meeting of the Society of Neurological Surgeons in April, 1978, Simeone reported on the state of the art so far as vasospasm is concerned. Although numerous hypotheses have been offered, the actual cause (causes?) of vasospasm remains unclear. After presenting the long list of materials used for treatment, Simeone opined that there is no specific treatment, but that experienced neurosurgeons agree that the best current treatment is to maintain blood volume and pressure after operation. Transfusion is given after clipping of the aneurysm and the blood pressure is kept up with pressor agents thereafter.

Sweet reported that in Boston a randomized study was begun and then stopped when it became evident that operative results were superior when the regimen of Zervas was used; this includes reserpine, 0.2 mg four times a day, and kanamycin, 1 gm four times a day. Patients had much less trouble with spasm when they were so treated than when placebo was given. (See Zervas: Trans. Am. Neurol. Assoc. 102:25, 1977.)

Hunt suggested operating during the first 3 days after operation before spasm appears, and then keeping the blood pressure and volume up during the spasm, which usually begins after 3 days following hemorrhage. Doctor Pia, from Giessen, West Germany, suggested the return to an old treatment — bilateral sympathetic blocks.

Patients with subarachnoid hemorrhage who were hemiparetic but conscious were put in class II (Botterell) by Nilsson, who analyzed the outcome of operation for ruptured aneurysm in relation to cerebral blood flow as measured by intravenous injection of ^{131}I-Hippuran or ^{99}Tc-pertechnetate and two gamma detectors placed bilaterally over the skull. Depressed blood flow was found even in patients with no or slight neurologic symptoms. With normal or only slightly disturbed flow, morbidity and mortality were estimated at 8%. When blood flow was more than 40% reduced, the figure climbed to 30%. Twenty-five percent of patients with consciousness in grades I and II and minimal neurologic findings could still have reduced flow more than 2 weeks after bleeding. Although it is clear that surgery should be delayed when there is low flow, rebleeding may occur during the waiting period, as happened in 12 of the 160 cases in this series.

Endo and Suzuki (Stroke 8:702, 1977) show that vasospasm of the cat basilar artery induced by fresh blood is slight and short-lived. If blood (alone or mixed with cerebrospinal fluid) is incubated at 37 C for 5–10 days, the vasoconstriction is severe and prolonged; mixtures incubated for 7 days with clotted components give more constriction than those not incubated with clots. It appears that there is a vasospasmogenic substance in blood shed into cerebrospinal fluid; it becomes active about 3 days after bleeding, increases at 5–10 days and disappears after 15 days.

The exact mechanism for production of vasospasm is still unclear. Osaka (J. Neurosurg. 47:403, 1977) believes that the vasoconstrictors from lysis of erythrocytes are more important than platelets in induction of spasm. The responsible material may be iron pigment. The importance of vasospasm in treatment of ruptured aneurysms is emphasized by Saito, Ueda and Sano (ibid., p. 412). They note a lapse of at least 4 days between hemorrhage and vasospasm in their 96 cases. When operation was carried out more than 7 days after onset of spasm, preoperative vasospasm was not aggravated by surgery. There were no deaths in the group operated on in the first 3 days after bleeding, and postoperative spasm was usually mild, presumably because blood clot or bloody cerebrospinal fluid was removed at operation. The authors now routinely drain a lateral ventricle, the cisterns at the base (via optic chiasmatic cisterns) and the epidural space after operation for aneurysm. Direct surgery is not delayed more than 2 weeks after onset of vasospasm lest rebleeding occur. In cases of aneurysms of the vertical anterior cerebral artery or the middle cerebral artery, the presence of localized spasm should not hinder prompt operation, because these patients do well. There is no reasonable reason given as to why their patients operated on in the first 3 days did well, while Drake considers this to be a period of terrible results from operation. In the past 7 years, 388 patients with aneurysms underwent microsurgical attack at the University of Tokyo Hospitals. Mortality was 5.4% overall.

A definite correlation between vasospasm shown by angiography and clinical grade (Hunt) was not found in the 26 patients with subarachnoid hemorrhage studied by Hayashi et al. (ibid., p. 584). Their studies may indicate that patients in grades III and IV are in a condition of cerebral vasomotor instability and that patients in grade V have cerebral vasomotor paralysis. – Ed.] ◄

Reinforcement with Gauze Wrapping for Ruptured Aneurysms of the Middle Cerebral Artery.

Julien C. Taylor and Abdur R. Choudhury[5] (Derby, England) treated 35 patients having ruptured aneurysms of the middle cerebral artery (MCA) by gauze wrapping alone in 1961 – 74. The age range was 19 – 60; 10 patients were aged 51 – 60. Arterial hypertension was present in 15 patients. All patients had had subarachnoid bleeding and 10 had a history of multiple bleeds. Of 24 other patients seen in this period with ruptured MCA aneurysms, 10 high-risk patients deteriorated and died without surgery and 7 over age 60 had conservative management. Surgery was usually done 7 – 10 days after the last bleed in low-risk patients and later in higher-risk patients with significant vasospasm. Induced hypotension and hypothermia were not used but hypertonic urea was given routinely. A small temporofrontal craniotomy was used. The aneurysm was approached from above and laterally, dissected and wrapped with postage stamp-sized pieces of gauze. All survivors have been followed for 2 – 15 years.

Twenty-two patients eventually had a good outcome, re-

(5) J. Neurosurg. 47:828–832, December, 1977.

turning to their previous work with minimal or no neurologic deficit. Six patients had fair results and 3, poor results, with severe disability due to dementia. Three patients (8.6%) died shortly after surgery, only 1 in direct relation to surgery. There was 1 late death unrelated to aneurysm. Postoperative disorders were mostly direct sequelae of preoperative conditions. All 3 patients with disabling dementia presented with massive frontal hematomas. No patient had late recurrent hemorrhage.

All but 3 of 32 survivors in this series are working after gauze wrapping of a ruptured MCA aneurysm and over two-thirds have resumed their previous work and are leading normal family lives. No recurrent subarachnoid bleeding has been observed. This operation gives highly acceptable results. Its chief merit is its freedom from occlusive infarcts.

Carotid-Ophthalmic Aneurysms: Direct Microsurgical Approach. M. G. Yasargil, J. C. Gasser, R. M. Hodosh

Fig 24.—Operative findings. (Courtesy of Yasargil, M. G., et al.: Surg. Neurol. 8:155–165, September, 1977.)

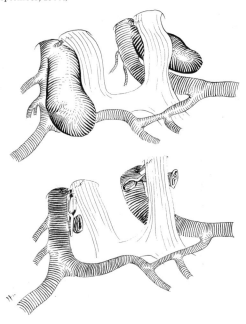

and T. V. Rankin[6] (Zurich) reviewed the results of operations on 30 carotid-ophthalmic aneurysms performed in 25 patients in 1967–76. The 23 women and 2 men had a mean age of 43.7 years. All 5 patients with bilateral aneurysms were treated at a single session by a unilateral frontolateral pterional approach (Fig 24). Eleven patients with aneurysms at other sites on the anterior circle of Willis were treated at the same time. Seventeen patients presented with subarachnoid hemorrhage and 4 had a second bleed before surgery. Six patients presented with visual signs. No patient had endocrine abnormalities preoperatively. The great majority of carotid-ophthalmic aneurysms arise from the medial or superomedial wall of the carotid just distal to the ophthalmic artery. Removal of the anterior clinoid process was necessary in 9 instances. Papaverine was routinely applied to the carotid artery and its branches early in the operation. Two ruptures occurred during dissection.

Twenty-six aneurysms were directly clipped. No deaths have occurred on follow-up for up to 8 years. All patients but 3 recovered completely. One patient had postoperative diabetes insipidus and amenorrhea, presumably due to compromise of the hypophyseal vasculature. One had transient oculomotor palsy. One patient with a large subchiasmatic adenoma had temporary visual deterioration postoperatively.

The microsurgical pterional approach appears to be indicated for intracranial carotid-ophthalmic aneurysms. There were no deaths in this series.

▶ [Direct attack on carotid ophthalmic and large internal carotid artery aneurysms has also been carried out by Benedetti and Curri (Surg. Neurol. 8:49, 1977). They emphasize the usefulness of manual compression of the common carotid artery in the neck during the direct operative approach. Tantalum clips, sometimes glued with acrylic, may be needed to occlude a large aneurysm neck; removal of adjacent bony parts, and even section of an optic nerve, may be necessary. In 6 cases, the aneurysm was completely excluded; in 1 case, closure was partial. Results were good in 3 patients and fair in 3; 1 patient died 15 days postoperatively of bronchopulmonary complications.

Sonntag, Yuan and Stein (ibid., p. 81) operated on 8 of 13 patients whose aneurysms ranged in size from 2 to 4.5 cm in diameter. In 31%, another aneurysm was also present and in 70%, presentation was via subarachnoid hemorrhage. Two of the anterior circulation sacs were at the bifurcation of the carotid artery, 1 was on the middle cerebral artery and the other 5 were "paraclinoid carotid." There were 4 at the basilar artery

(6)   Surg. Neurol. 8:155–165, September, 1977.

bifurcation and 1 at the trunk of the basilar artery. Of 5 patients with anterior giant aneurysms operated on directly, 2 died and 3 are working. One with carotid ligation in the neck is working. Two without operation died, 1 by suicide. Of those patients with posterior aneurysms,1 with wrapping is working, 1 with coating is institutionalized, 1 with negative exploration died, 1 with no treatment died and 1 with no treatment is working.—Ed.]

Aneurysms of the Posterior Cerebral Artery: Locations and Clinical Pictures. H. W. Pia and H. Fontana[7] (Univ. of Giessen) reviewed 34 reported and 8 personal cases

Fig 25.—Distribution and extension of posterior cerebral artery aneurysms. **A,** authors' cases. **B,** cases reported in the literature. (Courtesy of Pia, H. W., and Fontana, H.: Acta Neurochir. (Wien) 38:13–35, 1977; Berlin-Heidelberg-New York: Springer.)

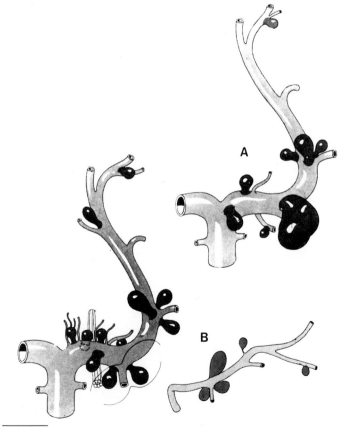

(7)   Acta Neurochir. (Wien) 38:13–35, 1977.

of posterior cerebral artery (PCA) aneurysm. Most adequately described aneurysms of the PCA arise from the main trunks of the vessel near the basilar bifurcation; the distribution is shown in Figure 25. Aneurysms of the PCA are not different in size and form from other aneurysms. The mean patient age was 37.4. There were 26 male and 16 female patients in the overall series. Subarachnoid bleeding was the first sign in 34 patients; 8 patients had more than one bleed. Hematomas were found in 10 patients, and 8 patients had ventricular bleeding. Coma or disturbed consciousness was noted in 13 patients. Two patients had signs of increased intracranial pressure. Twenty-two patients had local signs. Eight had oculomotor nerve paresis. Sensory disturbances were infrequent. Hemianopia was noted in 3 patients. One patient had speech disturbance.

Angiography in two projections is inadequate; oblique and tangential projections are necessary, and angiotomography and magnification angiography are useful. Preoperative magnification is of use in avoiding injuries to small central branches and to the midbrain and thalamus. The posterior communicating artery should be preserved if possible. Giant aneurysms and aneurysms of peripheral branches are particular surgical problems. The mortality of PCA aneurysms is low in reported series and in the present series. Direct 3d-nerve lesions are frequent, but the oculomotor paresis is usually reversible. Lesions of the central branches cause midbrain, peduncular and thalamic damage that is permanent despite a good collateral supply.

► [The surgical approach to the medial aneurysms (basilar-posterior cerebral anterior junction to posterior cerebral-posterior communicating artery junction) was via a frontal temporal approach. Anything distal to the posterior communicating artery was approached under the temporal lobe. Peripheral aneurysms were approached by occipital or similar craniotomy. – Ed.] ◄

Iron-Acrylic Compound for Stereotactic Aneurysm Thrombosis. The method is based on the attraction of intravascular iron to an extravascular magnet and was first described in 1965. In several cases of large aneurysms, part of the metallic thrombus fragmented to become an embolus and produced neurologic deficits. The magnet also had to be left in place for 5 days. John F. Alksne and Randall W. Smith[8] (Univ. of California, San Diego) have developed a

(8) J. Neurosurg. 47:137–141, August, 1977.

new iron-acrylic compound for stereotactic thrombosis of intracranial aneurysms. The material, carbonyl iron powder suspended in a liquid methylmethacrylate monomer, polymerizes rapidly, does not fragment and is nontoxic. After the magnetic properties of the mixture were shown to be adequate, it was injected into arteries of 20 animals. Boluses that were produced in the exposed carotid artery in the neck were left in place for 4 weeks to 4 months.

The optimal mixture was found to be 30 gm carbonyl iron in 12 cc monomer. The material had magnetic properties superior to those of iron-albumin. No changes in blood pressure, pulse, temperature or respiration resulted from intracarotid injections of the iron-acrylic compound. Loss of endothelium as well as subendothelial proliferation of granulation tissue were noted, but there was no inflammatory reaction, necrosis or alteration of the media. A patient with an anterior communicating artery aneurysm, who was a poor candidate for open craniotomy, had the aneurysm thrombosed stereotactically with iron-acrylic compounds and had no neurologic deficit.

Experimental and initial clinical studies of this iron-acrylic compound have given good results. The use of this material simplifies stereotactic aneurysm treatment and increases its safety. The injection system must be modified by a steel syringe that will create enough pressure to push the viscous material down a no. 20 needle.

► [Alksne has commented (Neurosurgery 1:29, 1977) on an article by Sheptak, Zanetti and Susen (ibid., p. 25) concerning injection of aneurysms with isobutyl-2-cyanoacrylate. It has been used for external coating of aneurysms in the past, as well as for repair of fluid fistulas and other disorders. He concurs with these authors on the difficulties in thrombosing aneurysms of the internal carotid artery as compared to those of the anterior communicating artery. The difficulties associated with operative treatment by craniotomy still encourage him to make more efforts at new methods of therapy. The authors had proposed the intra-aneurysmal injection especially for unclippable aneurysms and pointed out that only a small area of aneurysm need be exposed to permit the entry of a 25- to 30-gauge needle. — Ed.] ◄

Late Morbidity and Mortality of Common Carotid Ligation for Posterior Communicating Aneurysms: Comparison to Conservative Treatment.

H. Richard Winn (Univ. of Virginia), Alan E. Richardson and John A. Jane[9] (Wimbledon, England) report results of a long-term

(9)   J. Neurosurg. 47:727–736, November, 1977.

evaluation of 60 patients who survived 6 months after a subarachnoid hemorrhage. All were shown by carotid angiography to have a single aneurysm at the vicinity of the posterior communicating artery at its junction with the internal carotid artery. Forty-one patients had been assigned to conservative management and 37 to common carotid ligation; 26 conservatively treated patients and 34 having carotid ligation were alive at 6 months. The average follow-up of known survivors was 8 years, and over 60% of patients were followed for at least 5 years.

Morbidity was somewhat less in the surgical group at 6 months and during long-term follow-up. Three conservatively treated and 2 surgical patients had seizures during follow-up. Conservatively treated patients had significantly lower blood pressures on follow-up. Eight late rebleed episodes occurred in the conservatively treated group, three of them fatal. Five episodes occurred in the surgical group, four of them fatal. No protective effect of carotid ligation against late rebleeding was evident, considering either all types of rebleeding classifications (absolute, probable, possible) or absolute rebleeding only.

Late rebleeding occurred at similar rates in this series of patients with ruptured posterior communicating aneurysms, whether treatment was conservative or by carotid ligation. Morbidity is somewhat less after operative management, but little improvement in degree of morbidity occurred in either group many years after initial hemorrhage. Hypertension has been noted to develop in patients having carotid ligation.

▶ [Miller, Jawad and Jennett (J. Neurol. Neurosurg. Psychiatry 40:64, 1977) decided to evaluate the use of carotid ligation in management of intracranial aneurysms in view of the growing tendency to attack these directly. Of 72 patients treated by ligation of a carotid artery (internal or common was not clearly specified), overall incidence of temporary cerebral ischemia was 21%, and 5% had prolonged ischemia. Ischemic deficits were longer in patients rejected for ligation on the basis of cerebral blood flow measurements done at the time, almost always under general anesthesia. Of 28 rejected, 10 were later treated by direct clipping of the aneurysm and 6 died or were permanently severely disabled. Cerebral blood flow techniques should permit establishment of the degree of risk for carotid ligation in those patients in whom direct operation should not be done or in whom occlusion of the carotid artery will result (e.g., carotid-cavernous fistulas).

In a consecutive series of 500 patients with subarachnoid hemorrhage seen from 1967 to 1975, Blaauw and Braakman (Clin. Neurol. Neurosurg.

79:187, 1977) found 30 who had been treated by carotid ligation. Patients over age 60 were not treated surgically and hence angiography was not done, and this was also true of those over age 55 with hypertension. Other reasons for angiography not being done left only 315 patients with angiograms, of whom 159 had 1 aneurysm, 25 had multiple aneurysms, 45 had arteriovenous malformations, 84 had negative findings and 2 had both an aneurysm and an arteriovenous malformation. Carotid ligation was reserved for those whose aneurysms arose on the internal carotid artery; 62 had craniotomy for aneurysms elsewhere and 92 were treated conservatively. Common carotid ligation was done abruptly under EEG control, and only 1 patient developed EEG slowing, which decreased after the external carotid artery was also ligated. Ischemic complications developed in 7 patients within 24 hours, in 1 on the 2d day and in 1 on the 3d day after ligation. Two of the first 7 patients died; ischemic changes persisted in 3. One patient left the United States; of the other 27, none had recurrent hemorrhage in follow-up of up to 8 years (18 patients were followed more than 3 years). The authors consider their results to be no worse than those of direct attack, provided the patients are under age 60, have minimal angiographic spasm and are no worse than grade 3 so far as clinical condition is concerned.

We believe that carotid ligation is better than nothing at all, but should be reserved for those in whom direct attack is not to be done. With increasing development of technology, even these may well be attacked directly—but from the inside, via the catheter technique. — Ed.] ◄

Management of Ruptured Intracranial Aneurysm in Sickle Cell Anemia: Case Report is presented by Richard A. Close and William A. Buchheit[1] (Temple Univ.). Subarachnoid hemorrhage is not a common complication of sickle cell disease. When it occurs, it should be evaluated and treated in the usual manner.

Woman, 49, had sudden occipital headache and neck stiffness. She had a history of sickle cell disease with chronic pulmonary changes and a tendency to congestive heart failure, a history of leg ulcers, aseptic necrosis of both hips and shoulders and functional asplenia. Examination showed a stiff neck, a weak left leg, a Babinski sign and grossly bloody cerebrospinal fluid. A computerized tomography study was normal. Angiography showed an anterior communicating artery aneurysm, and ε-aminocaproic acid was given. A scan showed no evidence of cerebral ischemia. The cerebrospinal fluid cleared and the neurologic findings resolved. After a second partial exchange transfusion, surgery was done under enflurane-induced hypotension, urea and spinal drainage, with the use of the gyrus rectus approach. Left hemiparesis resolved after surgery, but right 3d nerve palsy persisted. An angiogram done 8 days postoperatively showed clipping of the aneurysm and vaso-

(1) J. Neurosurg. 47:761–765, November, 1977.

spasm. A repeat scintiscan showed no change in perfusion over the preoperative scan.

Angiography and hypotensive anesthesia can safely be carried out in these patients after the hemoglobin A level is raised to 60% by partial exchange transfusion. Hypoxemia, hypothermia and acidosis must be scrupulously avoided, and the blood volume must be maintained postoperatively. Urea has been used safely in the attempted treatment of sickle cell crisis. Postoperative angiography should be done whenever feasible, preferably within several days after surgery while the hemoglobin A is still at an acceptable level. All patients suspected of having sickle cell trait should be given a sickle cell screen and after diagnosis should be treated in the same manner, without an exchange transfusion.

▶ [Gendelman (Mt. Sinai J. Med. N.Y. 44:402, 1977) has reviewed the charts of 201 patients with hemophilia from either factor VIII or factor IX deficiency. Some central nervous system involvement was present in 14.9%, and peripheral nervous involvement was present in 12.9%. Of the central problems, subarachnoid hemorrhage occurred in 22 and intracerebral hemorrhage in 14. Involvement of the femoral nerve accounted for 16 of the peripheral nerve occurrences; 5 involved the median nerve. The former usually occurred with iliac muscle hemorrhage. Prompt recognition of the involvement, rapid adequate administration of the deficient factor, and invasive studies as indicated helped with resolution of the problems. Removal of further trauma and appropriate physical restrictions may promote a more normal life with reduction of morbidity. — Ed.]

Surgical Treatment of Arteriovenous Angiomas Localized in the Corpus Callosum, Basal Ganglia and Near the Brain Stem. J. Juhász[2] (Budapest) operated on 7 patients having deep angiomas in regions near the midline, including 4 in whom the malformation was not so circumscribed that it could be localized in one structure alone; 2 of these involved the corpus callosum and neighboring hemispheral substance. One involved the head of the caudate nucleus and the lateral ventricle. Two intraventricular angiomas, supplied by the choroidal arteries, involved the corpus striatum and the thalamus. Three juxtapeduncular angiomas were situated in the deep medial part of the temporal lobe, closely adherent to the peduncle, and were supplied by branches of the posterior cerebral and lateral choroidal arteries. All the lesions were true arteriovenous angiomas

(2) Acta Neurochir. (Wien) 40:83–101, 1978.

not of the cirsoid type and most involved more than one structure. Angiography and pneumoencephalography were done simultaneously in 2 patients to show the relation of a lesion to the ventricle.

All patients presented in the 2d or 3d decade of life with typical subarachnoid hemorrhage; 4 had repeated bleeding. Three patients were confused at the time of surgery and 1 of them had aphasia and hemiparesis. Two juxtapeduncular cases had intracerebral hematoma at operation. One malformation could only be partly removed, but 6 patients had total extirpation. The hemiplegic patient later improved satisfactorily after operation. Six patients are presently free of symptoms and working; 2 have had postoperative epilepsy at rare intervals. Postoperative cerebrospinal fluid obstruction occurred in 3 patients in which the ventricular system was opened. One patient had to have reoperation for evacuation of a high-pressure cerebrospinal fluid-containing cyst. Two had obstruction of the foramen of Monro and 1 required a ventriculocisternostomy.

Surgery should be attempted to remove arteriovenous malformations in the corpus callosum, head of the caudate nucleus, choroidal distribution area or a juxtapeduncular position. Striate and thalamic localizations are unfavorable, but attempts at radical intervention are justified where neurologic symptoms are present, especially in youth. If the patient deteriorates postoperatively with increasing intracranial pressure without rebleeding, an obstruction to cerebrospinal fluid circulation must be considered.

▶ [The descriptions of the operations are quite brief, but there is enough information to indicate that a bold approach to the vessels feeding the angiomatous malformations is required. Resections of frontal and temporobasal cortex may be required for access. The author emphasizes the need for simultaneous pneumography and angiography to delineate the relationship between the angioma and the ventricle. In several cases, operation was made easier by evacuation of intracerebral hematoma. Not all such intracerebral clots are due to bleeding from malformations. Thus, Kaneko, Koba and Yokoyama (J. Neurosurg. 46:579, 1977) assumed that if an intracerebral hematoma were operated on promptly, edema and other changes might be aborted and the amount of brain damage might be diminished. Lateral (?) hematomas were found in 40 patients admitted within 7 hours of attack, and all but 2 who had decerebrate rigidity were operated on in the acute stage. Access to the hematoma was gained by a 10-mm incision in the anterior upper temporal gyrus; a similar corticotomy was made after the insular cortex was reached through this approach. The hematoma was evacuated, and bleeding from a branch or trunk of the lenticulostriate group was controlled via microsurgical technique. At 6-month follow-up, 34 patients could walk unaided or with a cane, 1 was confined to bed and 3 had died. Right hemiplegia and aphasia had developed in 20 patients, 10 could communicate in society. Of 38 patients, hand movement was functionally complete in 12, and 4 had minimal movement, with the rest having intermediate movement (note that Table 5 in the original article adds up to 35 patients, since 3 died). What is obviously needed before we all rush to do similar emergency craniotomy is a valid comparison with similar patients not operated on. I presume that the term "lateral" with regard to these clots implies lateral in the basal ganglia; in the table of incidence, only 5 were said to be "medial" and 3 "subcortical." These were all called hypertensive hemorrhages and were differentiated from 6 "spontaneous intracerebral hematomas" on an unknown basis.

Luessenhop and Gennarelli (Neurosurgery 1:30, 1977) have put together a number of illustrations of varieties of supratentorial arteriovenous malformation as determined by their major vessels of supply. These have been used as a method of anatomical grading for determining operability. Assessment of operability also must include the clinical status of the patient and the anatomical-functional location of the malformation. — Ed.]

Angiographic Contribution to the Problem of Enlargement of Cerebral Arteriovenous Malformations.

H. A. Krayenbühl[3] (Zurich) reviewed 325 cases of cerebral arteriovenous malformation (AVM) and found 7 with a change in size of the malformation over several years. Increasing enlargement of the malformation resulted from progressive dilatation of preexisting abnormal vessels or from actual growth, especially in childhood. Knowledge of this is important for adequate diagnostic and surgical procedures.

Boy, 12, had had subarachnoid bleeding at age 3, and right carotid angiography had been negative a few days after the onset of bleeding (Fig 26). The boy had received a blow on the head a day before the onset. At age 12 he had progressive headache and suddenly became unconscious for 30 minutes, with vomiting and neck stiffness following. Blood-stained cerebrospinal fluid was found. Signs of severe meningeal irritation were present, with hyposmia on the right side. Four-vessel angiography showed a right frontal AVM (Fig 27) and a right frontal intracerebral hematoma, with shift of the right anterior cerebral artery to the left. The AVM was completely excised, along with a huge subcortical frontal hematoma. Angiography done 5 months postoperatively showed complete absence of the malformation. The patient was in excellent health.

Many cases of progressive enlargement of AVMs with clinical progression have been reported. Resistance to blood

(3) Acta Neurochir. (Wien) 36:215–242, 1977.

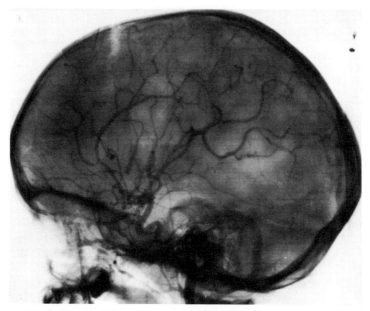

Fig 26. – Normal right carotid angiogram a few days after the first subarachnoid hemorrhage in boy, aged 3. (Courtesy of Krayenbühl, H. A.: Acta Neurochir. (Wien) 36:215–242, 1977; Berlin-Heidelberg-New York: Springer.)

flow through the malformation is reduced and arterial pressure is transmitted directly to the veins, leading to widening of the vessels and, in the course of years, enlargement of the malformation. The initial size of the AVM appears to be the crucial factor in change in size; small malformations have a marked tendency to grow. Autonomous growth of the AVM may also be a factor. A congenital arteriovenous shunt may lead to abnormal growth of pathologic vessels, or abnormalities in vessel structure may lead to the growth, with shunting being only incidental.

Only serial four-vessel angiography will show the actual size of the AVM, and this study is necessary because microsurgery permits radical removal of the lesions.

► [Szepan (Acta Neurochir. (Wien) 36:243, 1977) adds another case of growth of a small arteriovenous malformation over a period of almost 18 years. The lesion described by Szepan was in the left occipitotemporal junction in a pregnant woman, aged 20. She had mild right hemiparesis and hemianopia as a result of hemorrhage; no therapy was undertaken

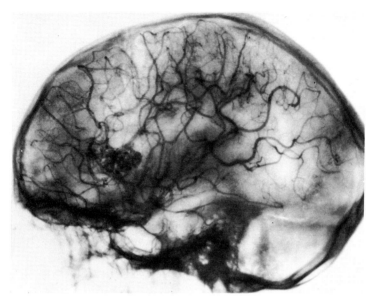

Fig 27. — Angiogram 9 years later, after second hemorrhage, in same boy as in Figure 26 shows AVM in the depth of the right frontal lobe. (Courtesy of Krayenbühl, H. A.: Acta Neurochir. (Wien) 36:215–242, 1977; Berlin-Heidelberg-New York: Springer.)

because of the pregnancy. She did well thereafter until recurrent bleeding at age 37+. No additional neurologic deficit resulted from total removal of the malformation, which had grown considerably in size and collaterals in the interim. — Ed.] ◄

Spinal Cord Arteriovenous Malformations and the Klippel-Trenaunay-Weber Syndrome. M. Djindjian, R. Djindjian, M. Hurth, A. Rey and R. Houdart[4] (Paris) reviewed 150 cases of arteriovenous malformation of the spinal cord and encountered 5 associated with the Klippel-Trenauney-Weber syndrome. Hypertrophic lesions, dilated arteries and varicose veins were present in each case, but only 2 patients had cutaneous angiomatosis. Each patient had an intramedullary arteriovenous malformation. Forty associated malformations were encountered in 35 cases, or 23% of 150 cases of arteriovenous malformations of the cord. Twelve of the 17 cutaneous angiomas were segmental. There were 5 segmental vertebral hemangiomas, 2 cases of

(4) Surg. Neurol. 8:229–237, October, 1977.

the cutaneous-vertebral-medullary angioma of Cobb's syndrome, 8 cases of Weber-Rendu-Osler disease, 2 visceral angiomatoses and 1 lymphatic dysplasia.

The Klippel-Trenaunay-Weber syndrome is characterized by segmental cutaneous angioma, the early development of unilateral varices and partial gigantism of the involved extremity. Trophic or nervous lesions may also be present. Most authors have included the Parkes Weber syndrome, which has as its basis an arteriovenous ectasia, with the Klippel-Trenaunay-Weber syndrome. Arteriovenous malformations of the cord have been encountered in several of the systemic angiodysplasias, including both diffuse angiomatous and predominantly regional phakomatoses, nonangiomatous phakomatoses and neurofibromatosis. These associations lead to the concept of a common neural pathogenesis, the result of an early embryonic abnormality, which depends on a unique factor, focal teratogenesis with a metameric expression.

► [A case of Cobb's syndrome is reported by Jessen, Thompson and Smith (Arch. Dermatol. 113:1587, 1977). This is the combination of a vascular skin nevus and an angioma in the spinal cord corresponding within a segment or two of the dermatome involved. This is the 28th case thus far reported and involved a boy, aged 15, with multiple hemaniomas when first seen. At age 19 he complained of weakness of the right leg and bladder difficulties. Despite a negative spinal angiogram, exploration was eventually done and it disclosed a nodular enlargement of the spinal cord with two mulberry-shaped hemangiomas on one side. No attempt at excision was made. Follow-up apparently consisted only of a 9-day postoperative period. — Ed.] ◄

Intradural Extramedullary Spinal Arteriovenous Malformations Fed by the Anterior Spinal Artery. M. Djindjian, R. Djindjian, A. Rey, M. Hurth and R. Houdart[5] (Paris) report 6 extramedullary arteriovenous malformations that derived their blood supply from the anterior spinal artery or the artery of Adamkiewicz. Their extramedullary site distinguished them from the more common malformations fed by the anterior spinal artery. Extramedullary malformations are clinically distinct from intramedullary malformations fed by the anterior spinal artery, alone or with the posterior spinal arteries, and they can be successfully extirpated.

All 6 malformations lay outside the pia and were supplied

(5) Surg. Neurol. 8:85–93, August, 1977.

exclusively or in part by the anterior spinal artery. Four were at the level of the conus medullaris. Anatomically they were characterized by arteriovenous shunting. Three lesions were simple arteriovenous fistulas arising from the artery of Adamkiewicz. Two patients had early onset of symptoms; 1 had a subarachnoid hemorrhage and the other had numerous sudden episodes of disability. The 4 older patients had progressive symptoms. All patients had symptoms probably resulting from cord ischemia due to a vascular steal by the malformation. This occurred acutely and repeatedly in 1 patient and was apparently precipitated by pregnancy.

Extramedullary arteriovenous malformations of the spinal cord supplied by the anterior spinal artery occurred only 6 times (7%) in 90 cases of malformation supplied by this vessel. It has been possible to excise the malformations completely without damage to the cord, with 1 exception. Results of operation on intramedullary arteriovenous malformations have been less satisfactory. Because extramedullary arteriovenous malformations have only a hemodynamic effect on the cord, symptoms appear later and the surgical prognosis is better than for intramedullary malformations.

► [I regret that we cannot reproduce the color illustrations of schematic representations of these lesions. Although the intramedullary malformations are quite distinct, even they can be operated on, and the authors stated they have been able to extirpate completely (controlled by postoperative angiography) 18 of 26 intramedullary malformations. – Ed.] ◄

OCCLUSIVE DISEASE

Noninvasive Evaluation and Management of the "Asymptomatic" Carotid Bruit are discussed by Mark M. Kartchner and Lorin P. McRae[6] (Tucson, Ariz.). Carotid phonoangiography (CPA) provides visualization of carotid bruits, and oculoplethysmography (OPG) is a reliable noninvasive screening test applicable to patients with asymptomatic bruits. Carotid phonoangiography consists of stethoscopic auscultation, direct visualization and photographic recording of carotid bruits. Oculoplethysmography consists of the comparative timing of simultaneously recorded ocular pulse wave forms that represent changes in volume of the

(6) Surgery 82:840–847, December, 1977.

globe with pulsatile arterial flow. The pulses are obtained from corneal suction cups.

Of 4,000 patients evaluated noninvasively for carotid occlusive disease, 1,287 presented with "asymptomatic" bruits; of these, 697 had nonhemispheric neurologic symptoms and 590 were clinically asymptomatic. With CPA, subbifurcation bruits were diagnosed in 619 patients and insignificant bifurcation bruits in 426; in 242 patients CPA demonstrated significant carotid bruits that persisted throughout systole, indicating a greater than 40% carotid stenosis. Oculoplethysmography detected 273 patients with significant internal carotid flow reduction and indicated that 5% of bifurcation bruits were of external carotid origin. The accuracy of 89% in determining over 40% stenosis by OPG-CPA in 295 patients having angiography was increased to 97% when both OPG and CPA were positive. Follow-up of patients for 6–70 months documented 156 carotid endarterectomies and 38 strokes. Analysis of the strokes favored angiography and operation only for patients with appropriately positive or progressive OPG-CPA findings or focal transient ischemic attacks.

Oculoplethysmography and CPA provide objective evaluations of asymptomatic carotid bruits and permit the noninvasive follow-up of patients with a high degree of safety. They lend objectivity to the long-term management of these patients, and can improve the selection of patients for carotid angiography and endarterectomy. The onset of focal transient ischemic attacks or progression to grade 4 stenosis is a strong indication for proceeding to angiography and carotid endarterectomy.

▶ [I find it difficult to understand the logic behind the decision to call "asymptomatic" those bruits that occur in patients who have dizziness, lightheadedness, blackouts or bilateral visual symptoms, which the authors term "nonhemispheric transient ischemic attacks." These are as typical for vertebrobasilar insufficiency as amaurosis fugax is for carotid disorders, a point touched on by A. L. Carney in the discussion in the original articles. The article does not give in detail how one is sure that the bruit does not come from the vertebral artery nor, indeed, that it does not come from the external carotid artery in the presence of a normal internal carotid artery. Nonetheless, it is an interesting exercise in how to approach the problem of cervical carotid circulation without invasive angiography.

See also the article by Sundt et al. in this chapter for a description of the variety of symptoms due to ischemic disease in the posterior circulation. H. Javid and his colleagues at Rush-Presbyterian-St. Luke's Medical Center in Chicago have long emphasized the utility of operating on carotid lesions when the symptoms are those of basilar insufficiency, for the connections of the circle of Willis are sufficient to explain how carotid occlusive disease can interfere with already compromised vertebral flow and can precipitate dizziness and other symptoms.

In a series of 144 patients who had carotid endarterectomies done at Oklahoma Health Science Center over a 6-year period, Kanaly et al. (Am. J. Surg. 134:821, 1977) found 14 who had had prophylactic operation prior to some other elective surgery, based on the finding of carotid bruits in the midcervical region. None of these patients had neurologic sequelae and none died from operation, although 5 died later from noncerebral causes. The authors believe that carefully selected patients with asymptomatic bruits may well undergo carotid endarterectomy to prevent future neurologic complications (all had had angiograms showing stenosis—5 unilaterally and 9 bilaterally).—Ed.] ◄

Thromboendarterectomy for Total Occlusion of the Internal Carotid Artery: Reappraisal of Risks, Success Rate and Potential Benefits. T. Kusunoki, D. W. Rowed, C. H. Tator and W. M. Lougheed[7] (Univ. of Toronto) reexamined the results of thromboendarterectomy for total occlusion of the internal carotid artery (ICA) in 40 consecutive patients with angiographically documented total occlusion. The 30 men and 10 women had a mean age of 58. Of 5 who had bilateral internal carotid occlusion, 2 had bilateral operations. A total of 42 thromboendarterectomies were attempted for complete ICA occlusion. Sixteen patients presented with major cerebral infarction with an established neurologic deficit and 5 presented with a minor cerebral infarction. Thirteen patients presented with transient ischemic attacks, 3 with progressing infarction and 3 with intellectual impairment or features of brain stem ischemia. Virtually all patients had anticoagulation therapy preoperatively.

Blood flow was restored in 52% of procedures. The ICA was patent in only 7 of 12 patients having angiography 3–6 months postoperatively. All 6 patients having endarterectomy without thrombectomy had total ICA occlusion. Flow was restored in 6 of 7 operations done within 72 hours of the presumed time of occlusion. Two of 26 patients with risk factors died of myocardial infarction and 4 died of intracerebral hemorrhage or massive cerebral edema secondary to cerebral infarction. None of 14 patients without risk factors

(7) Stroke 9:34–38, Jan.-Feb., 1978.

died, but 1 had a postoperative cerebral infarction resulting in a major neurologic deficit. Six patients with risk factors had cerebral infarctions after surgery and 2 had nonfatal myocardial infarctions. There was no long-term mortality or morbidity in patients with persistent patency.

The 52% overall success rate for restoration of patency of the totally occluded ICA in this series is comparable to that achieved in other series. The success rate of procedures done within 72 hours of occlusion was 86%. Risk assessment permits the selection of low-risk patients for early operation. Most patients with neurologic, medical or angiographic risk factors should probably not have thromboendarterectomy.

▶ [The authors discuss use of the Fogarty catheter when backflow does not occur spontaneously. The higher patency rate achieved with its use commends it, even considering the risks of distal embolization and possible carotid-cavernous fistula. The risk factors that tend to separate patients into those with and those without good prognosis include: major neurologic deficit of less than 2 weeks' duration; progressing deficit; deficits secondary to multiple infarctions; angina pectoris or myocardial infarctions; blood pressure greater than 180/110; congestive heart failure; chronic obstructive pulmonary disease; age more than 70 years and severe obesity; extensive atherosclerotic lesions in the aorta and its branches; and lesions of the opposite carotid artery, the vertebrobasilar system or the intracranial arteries. Some difficulty in evaluation of the results arises because of the postoperative use of anticoagulants for 6 weeks to 6 months after operation. – Ed.] ◀

Extracranial-to-Intracranial Vascular Anastomosis for Occlusive Cerebrovascular Disease: Experience in 110 Patients. A. John Popp (Albany Med. College) and Norman Chater[8] (Univ. of California, San Francisco) reviewed the results of extracranial-to-intracranial arterial bypass for occlusive cerebrovascular disease in 110 patients. The superficial temporal artery was anastomosed to a cortical branch of the middle cerebral artery on the brain surface with the use of microsurgical technique. A small craniectomy about 4 cm in diameter was used to expose a suitable cortical artery at least 1 mm in diameter in the region of the angular gyrus. Then an end-to-side anastomosis was performed. After surgery, patency was assessed by a Doppler flowmeter and by palpation of the superficial temporal artery. The average patient age was 59; the male-female ratio was about 5:1. Transient ischemia was present clinically in 64% of patients and a mild completed stroke in 18%.

(8) Surgery 82:648–654, November, 1977.

Patients with transient ischemia, progressive stroke or mild completed stroke were most consistently improved after surgery. Only 4 of 14 patients with moderate or severe completed strokes showed significant improvement. One patient had a permanent increase in deficit immediately after surgery. Three patients died within 30 days of surgery. Seven patients had strokes more than a month after surgery, 3 in the cerebral hemisphere supplied by the bypass. The anastomosis was not patent in 1 of the latter patients. Late stroke in the vertebrobasilar system caused 1 of 11 late deaths. The patency rate was high. Two postoperative thromboses of the anastomosis were attributed to technical problems where the cortical vessels were less than 1 mm in size. No difficulty has been found in locating a suitable recipient vessel in the last 100 cases, with exclusive use of the posterior temporal-angular artery complex.

This study showed a high patency rate of extracranial-to-intracranial arterial bypasses, with low permanent morbidity and operative mortality rates. Lesions producing transient ischemic attacks that were previously considered inoperable or inaccessible can be bypassed by this procedure.

► [Extracranial-to-intracranial bypass should have a low morbidity and mortality and it appears to have a prophylactic role in preventing further catastrophic cerebral ischemia, according to Yaşargil and Yonekawa (Neurosurgery 1:22, 1977). A graft patency rate of 87% has been achieved in the 34 cases operated on by Yaşargil and the 52 operated on by Yonekawa. It has been 100% in the last 20 cases. Complications included death (3), "morbidity" (2), infection (5), subdural hematoma (3), skin flap necrosis (5) and epilepsy (5). The authors believe that the donor and the recipient arteries should be at least 1 mm in diameter to insure patency. Infections have been diminished by a reduction in operating time to 3.5– 4.5 hours. The obvious implication is specifically stated: "The laboratory training of the surgeon in microvascular anastomosis techniques is a prerequisite of a high patency rate."

A new experimental model for extracranial-to-intracranial anastomosis is presented by Nishikawa et al. (Surg. Neurol. 8:249, 1977). A 100% patency rate was achieved 10 days after operation in which the canine external ethmoidal artery was anastomosed to the middle cerebral artery. Study of gas pressures and histology indicates that remarkable improvement of neurologic deficit should not be expected in the chronic stage of occlusive disease, even if blood flow is increased through an anastomotic procedure.

Anatomical details of exposure of the carotid artery in its petrous portion are expounded by Paullus, Pait and Rhoton (J. Neurosurg. 47:713, 1977). This area lateral to the trigeminal nerve can be readily approached and permits a 1-cm segment of artery to be uncovered, which might be used for bypassing cervical occlusion of the internal carotid artery.— Ed.] ◄

Staged Intracranial and Extracranial Revascularization. John M. Moran, O. Howard Reichman and William H. Baker[9] (Loyola Univ.) found 20 patients with a combination of intracranial and extracranial cerebrovascular lesions among 118 candidates for superficial temporal artery-to-middle cerebral artery (STA-MCA) bypass surgery. Two had an extracranial procedure in preparation for intracranial revascularization, whereas 18 had an additional extracranial procedure. The 14 men and 6 women had an average age of 59. Nine had a completed stroke but a relatively mild deficit. Ten patients had internal carotid artery (ICA) occlusion and contralateral ICA stenosis; 7 had combinations of ipsilateral lesions, usually ICA occlusion and external carotid artery (ECA) stenosis. Three patients had multiple lesions.

Of 18 patients having a STA-MCA bypass, 11 had contralateral reconstruction for ICA stenosis and 7 had ECA stenosis corrected. Two patients became asymptomatic after ECA endarterectomy only, and their proposed STA-MCA bypass has been postponed. Two deaths occurred, for an overall mortality of 10%. One patient with a progressive neurologic deficit had occlusion of the ICA siphon stenosis and died within 30 days of surgery. A neurologically asymptomatic patient died a year postoperatively of a presumed myocardial infarction. Ten of 11 patients with transient ischemic attacks are asymptomatic but 1 had a neurologic deficit related to a contralateral prophylactic endarterectomy. Seven of the 8 surviving stroke patients are improved and 1 is unchanged.

Repair of both lesions at the same operation would require reversal of heparinization before the neurosurgical stage, and prolonged anesthesia would be necessary. Patients with bilateral lesions should have the symptomatic lesion repaired primarily. The use of prophylactic STA-MCA bypass is entirely analogous to prophylactic carotid endarterectomy. Two of the present patients had fibromuscular hyperplasia of the ICA and bilateral symptoms due to occlusion and dissection, suggesting that this disease is not benign but may cause severe neurologic sequelae.

(9) Arch. Surg. 112:1424–1428, December, 1977.

► [Analysis of 28 patients with unilateral internal carotid occlusion and contralateral significant (greater than 50%) internal carotid stenosis has been made by Andersen et al. (Stroke 8:669, 1977). Indications for operation included transient ischemic attacks (TIAs) in 54% of the group, fixed neurologic deficits with TIAs in 21%, fixed defects without TIAs in 21% and operation as prophylaxis for major surgery in 4%. All 28 had endarterectomy on the stenotic side only, and none had endarterectomy during the acute phase of stroke. One patient had superficial temporal artery-to-middle cerebral artery bypass on the occluded side prior to endarterectomy on the other side, and 1 other patient had such an anastomosis done on the occluded side after endarterectomy on the stenotic side, because of persistent symptoms. Neither of these patients had neurologic complication, but 3 of the group (11%) developed fixed neurologic deficits lasting over 24 hours. Two of these cases were referable to the stenotic side, 1 to the side of occlusion. Review of the literature and observation of their own cases indicate to these authors that anastomosis is not justifiable on the side of an occluded internal carotid artery in an asymptomatic patient but it may be worthwhile if symptoms persist after endarterectomy, and a prospective study might show if such anastomosis is worthwhile on the occluded side prior to endarterectomy. – Ed.] ◄

Intracranial Bypass Grafts for Vertebral-Basilar Ischemia. Thoralf M. Sundt, Jr., Jack P. Whisnant, David G. Piepgras, J. Keith Campbell and Colin B. Holman[1] (Mayo Clinic and Found.) performed 14 operations in which an occipital branch of the external carotid artery was joined to the posterior inferior cerebellar artery (PICA) for occlusions or inaccessible stenotic lesions of the vertebral arteries proximal to the site of origin of the PICA. Eight patients had no major focal neurologic deficit but were considered at high risk for a posterior circulation infarct; 6 patients had been severely or moderately disabled before surgery. The chief ischemic symptoms were vertigo or nausea, or both, light-headedness and postural syncope.

Six patients at risk had had a trial of anticoagulant therapy without apparent benefit. Five of the 8 returned to normal activities postoperatively, essentially free of neurologic complaints; 3 were normal at neurologic examination but did not feel capable of resuming their previous work; 1 did not have a patent graft. All 6 disabled patients had had a trial of anticoagulant therapy. All 3 with increasing deficits had progression stopped after operation and 5 of the 6 patients gradually improved neurologically. Only 2 were able to achieve activities of daily living. Orthostatic symptoms were relieved. All but 1 of the 14 patients having oper-

(1) Mayo Clin. Proc. 53:12–18, January, 1978.

ations had a patent graft on postoperative angiography. The graft carried the major portion of flow to the posterior circulation in 9 of 10 cases in which the recipient vessel was the parent trunk of the PICA. One patient had a fixed hearing loss after surgery. One case each of pneumonia, subdural air and epidural hematoma did not lead to long-term morbidity.

This operation might be considered for patients with symptoms of bilateral occlusions or severe stenoses of the intracranial vertebral arteries proximal to the origin of the PICA, or unilateral occlusion or severe stenosis associated with a congenitally small vertebral artery that terminates in a PICA and does not communicate with the basilar artery. It is not indicated for extracranial vertebral artery stenosis or asymptomatic extracranial vertebral artery occlusion and should not be considered for patients with minimal symptoms. Anastomosis of the occipital artery with the superior cerebellar artery might be useful for cases of basilar artery stenosis or occlusion. Anticoagulant therapy should be tried in most patients before angiography and possible surgery.

► [From the symposium at the 1978 meeting of the Society of Neurological Surgeons in Philadelphia comes the report by Austin of monitoring blood flow for bypass operations; the flow can be increased by 12–18%, relieving transient ischemic attacks and preventing strokes. Austin still is not sure that the incidence of stroke is really decreased, but he is convinced that the quality of life is improved. He is also concerned (as are the aneurysm surgeons) with maintaining cerebral autoregulation and flow, and hence he uses a 1% Neo-Synephrine drip to maintain and increase blood pressure. Hypotension from halothane is avoided by shifting to nitrous-oxide-oxygen mixtures. Bypass should not be done in patients with severe neurologic deficit, according to Reimuth, who also disputes the published data of 50–90% for improvement in progressive stroke.

Peerless pointed out the various complications of operations, including subdural hygroma in 14 of 150 cases operated on. His group has been active in use of bypass before operation on giant aneurysms and tumors that can compromise the major vessels in the vicinity. On occasion, Peerless has used a saphenous vein graft from the carotid artery to the middle cerebral artery in such cases. He believes there is no firm evidence that the external carotid artery-middle cerebral artery bypass is effective in preventing progression of transient ischemic attack to stroke. Current medical therapy consists of aspirin and control of risk factors. A Fourth International Symposium of those interested in these operations was held in London, Ontario, September 6–8, 1978. — Ed.] ◄

Pain

Comparison of Percutaneous Radiofrequency Trigeminal Neurolysis and Microvascular Decompression of the Trigeminal Nerve for Treatment of Tic Douloureux. Ronald I. Apfelbaum[2] (Montefiore Hosp. and Med. Center, New York) compared the microvascular decompressive technique of Jannetta with radiofrequency trigeminal neurolysis in 103 consecutive patients treated for classic trigeminal neuralgia in 1974–77. All were refractory to or intolerant of medications. Forty-eight patients had percutaneous radiofrequency trigeminal neurolysis and 55, microvascular decompression via a suboccipital craniectomy. Five in the former group had multiple sclerosis. The respective average ages were 63 and 51. The microvascular decompression technique has been used for about 14 months.

Percutaneous trigeminal neurolysis was done under neurolept anesthesia. All but 6 patients were rendered free of pain, although 3 required two procedures. Two failures were due to anatomical abnormalities. Moderate morbidity occurred in a number of patients but there was no mortality. Seven patients had corneal anesthesia and 6 had anesthesia dolorosa or severe dysesthesia. One patient had an intracerebral hematoma during the procedure.

Forty-eight of 55 patients had complete pain relief after microvascular decompression and 4 others were improved. A number of initially relieved patients have had some recurrent pain and 2 had a moderate return of pain. One patient had hearing loss and facial palsy and 2 had mild hearing loss alone. No dysesthesia or corneal anesthesia occurred. There were no deaths in either group.

Both percutaneous radiofrequency trigeminal neurolysis and microvascular decompression are effective procedures for initially relieving symptoms of trigeminal neuralgia. The potential risks are greater with microvascular decom-

(2) Neurosurgery 1:16–21, July–Aug., 1977.

411

pression, but altered facial sensation, corneal anesthesia and dysesthetic complications do not occur after this procedure. Unsuspected tumors in the posterior fossa can be discovered early and cured with this approach. Follow-up is too short to conclude that microvascular decompression is curative, but the early results are extremely encouraging.

▶ [In a talk at the Interurban Neurosurgical Society in February, 1978, Jannetta gave details of his entire series of posterior fossa operations for nerve decompression, now amounting to 275, with 237 patients free of face pain after 1 operation and 19 free of pain after 2 operations. There were 20 benign tumors and malformations found by posterior fossa exploration. Jannetta finds that a third of tic patients have significant sensory abnormality on careful testing, and some of these disappeared after the decompressive operation. Snout and eye areas are said to be the only ones with exclusively trigeminal innervation; all the rest of the face gets some supply from cervical and other nerves. A single wisp of cotton may be needed to detect the sensory change in some patients (Jannetta tests from abnormal to normal areas), and early abnormal changes are found in sensory evoked potentials in some 86% of tic patients. – Ed.] ◀

Operative Approach to Persistent Trigeminal Artery Producing Facial Pain and Diplopia: Case Report.
Glen S. Merry and Kenneth G. Jamieson[3] (Queensland, Australia) report a case of persistent trigeminal artery producing intermittent facial pain and diplopia, in which the trigeminal and abducens nerves were attached to the trigeminal artery by a congenital membrane and the blood supply to the vertebrobasilar system was via the persistent vessel.

Woman, 31, presented with low back pain and left sciatica from a fall 4 days before and later had severe pain in the left side of the face in the trigeminal nerve area. There was also pain and some decrease in power in the left upper extremity. The facial pain was throbbing in nature and made worse by lying on the left and by stress. Similar episodes had occurred 11 and 4 years previously. There was hyperesthesia in the left side of the face and left extremities. Myelography showed a prolapsed disk at L4 – L5. The left trigeminal pain recurred after discharge and carotid angiography showed a persistent trigeminal artery supplying the vertebrobasilar system with retrograde flow in the vertebral artery to the level of the arch of the atlas. There was a reasonable response to carbamazepine but the pain subsequently recurred, with episodes of facial numbness, and diplopia developed for the first time. Aortic arch injection showed a grossly hypoplastic left vertebral artery

(3) J. Neurosurg. 47: 613 – 618, October, 1977.

arising directly from the arch and a patent, hypoplastic right vertebral artery.

Exploration through a curved incision behind the ear and an osteoplastic flap showed a thick congenital membrane enveloping the 5th and 6th cranial nerves, which were attached to the persistent trigeminal artery. The membrane was divided and a piece of Gelfoam was placed between the two structures. No facial pain was present at discharge, and the diplopia improved over the next 4 months. Numbness was noted inside the left cheek and on the left side of the tongue for several months. No further diplopia was reported 20 months after discharge.

Facial pain and diplopia were abolished by division of the congenital membrane present in this patient and facial sensation was preserved.

► [The operation in this patient was done June 26, 1974. The authors state, "In February, 1976, she had pain above the left eyebrow and was tender over the supraorbital notch. She responded to local injections of hydrocortisone acetate" (page 615 of original article). "The facial pain and diplopia remain absent and facial sensation is preserved" (page 617). — Ed.] ◄

Glossopharyngeal and Vagal Neuralgia Secondary to Vascular Compression of the Nerves. Glossopharyngeal neuralgia is uncommon and its association with syncopal attacks rarer still. F. Morales, P. Albert, R. Alberca, B. de Valle and A. Narros[4] (Seville, Spain) explored the condition of a patient with a glossopharyngeal and vagal neuralgia in whom the findings explained the etiology of these associated neuralgias.

Woman, 56, with severe intermittent pain at the angle of the jaw on the left side for 6 months, usually precipitated by swallowing, reported having lost consciousness for a few seconds after the pain began. Carbamazepine did not relieve the pain or episodes of lost consciousness. Cocainization of the throat abolished the pain for some minutes. Taste sensation was reduced in the posterior third of the tongue. X-rays showed minor basilar impression and an air study showed an extremely slight tonsillar herniation. Attacks of radiating pain were produced by touching the left posterior part of the tongue. The pulse slowed and the patient lost consciousness and had a tonic seizure of the four extremities. Unconsciousness lasted about 20 seconds. An EEG showed slow bilateral waves and a nearly flat period of 9 seconds during an attack. The heart rate and blood pressure both fell at the same time.

A left retromastoid craniectomy was performed, and the 9th and

(4)   Surg. Neurol. 8:431–433, December, 1977.

10th nerves were found to be severely compressed and distorted by a loop of the left vertebral artery. The artery and nerves were separated under the microscope and pieces of sponge were interposed. Decreased taste perception on the left posterior third of the tongue was noted immediately after surgery, but soon disappeared. No pain or syncope has occurred for over a year of follow-up, and neurologic examination was entirely normal. Touching the posterior part of the tongue and throat caused no pain or syncope.

The symptoms of this patient presumably involved the areas of sensory supply of the glossopharyngeal and vagus nerves and were due to compression of the nerves by a vertebral artery loop. In cases of glossopharyngeal neuralgia, the nerves responsible should be carefully explored to evaluate the possibility of neurovascular compression. When evidence of such compression is found, symptoms of glossopharyngeal and vagal neuralgia may be relieved by appropriate treatment of the compression, rather than by cutting the nerves.

▶ [Microvascular decompression was carried out in 4 patients with typical glossopharyngeal neuralgia at the University of Pittsburgh. Laha and Jannetta (J. Neurosurg. 47:316, 1977) have analyzed these patients and 2 others in whom part of the nerve was cut. One of the decompressed patients continues to have some pain, and 1 died in the postoperative period, presumably due to trauma at the operative site. If a proper means can be found for keeping the compressing vessel away from the 9th and 10th nerves, long-term results of this operation may be worthwhile. — Ed.] ◀

Treatment of Diffuse Metastatic Cancer Pain by Instillation of Alcohol into the Sella Turcica. The management of pain in patients with diffuse metastatic cancer is generally extremely difficult. Jordan Katz and Allan B. Levin[5] (Univ. of Wisconsin) evaluated a technique of "chemical hypophysectomy," involving instillation of alcohol into the sella turcica, in 13 patients having diffuse metastatic cancer. Seven had primary prostatic carcinoma. All had diffuse metastases and uncontrollable pain. The procedure was done under general endotracheal anesthesia. The target was the posterosuperior aspect of the sella in the midline. A hole was made in the floor of the sphenoid sinus and a 20-gauge spinal needle was inserted through the sellar floor to deposit up to 2 ml alcohol per injection at various depths within the sella. A total of 5–6 ml was usually used. In 10 patients α-ethyl cyanoacrylate was injected as the needle

(5) Anesthesiology 46:115–121, February, 1977.

was withdrawn to prevent cerebrospinal fluid leakage. The sphenoid sinus was irrigated with bacitracin solution.

On follow-up for up to 7 months, 11 patients have had good to excellent pain relief, which occurred almost immediately after the procedure. Five of 10 bedridden patients became ambulatory within several days after the procedure. The only significant complication was a cerebrospinal fluid leak complicated by bacterial meningitis. The patient died and the leak was attributed to widespread bony invasion by tumor tissue. One patient responded to a second alcohol instillation. Ten patients required treatment for diabetes insipidus. Before cyanoacrylate was used, 2 other patients had cerebrospinal fluid leaks. One patient had temporary cranial nerve palsies and 1 had a transient visual field defect.

This method of hypophysectomy is a technically simple one and should be considered for other related conditions where pituitary ablation is necessary. There is no neurophysiologic explanation for the immediate, profound pain relief obtained.

▶ [Just why the injection of alcohol into the sella turcica relieves pain even when the tumor involved is not hormone sensitive is quite unclear. Moricca introduced this treatment in 1963 when he found that the pain relief with endocrine-sensitive tumors was so immediate as to be incomprehensible on the basis of hormonal changes alone. And in fact, the technique does work for metastatic tumor pain from a number of causes. He has published pictures showing one to ten needles in the sella; why the current authors can do as well with using only one needle is not clear. Whether their stereotactic technique is better or easier than the freehand one of Moricca is also unclear. — Ed.] ◀

Pain Reduction by Electric Brain Stimulation in Man: Part 2. Chronic Self-Administration in Periventricular Gray Matter. Donald E. Richardson and Huda Akil[6] reviewed long-term effects of intermittent stimulation of the periventricular gray matter for relief from intractable pain in 8 patients with pain of known cause. All reasonable conventional methods had been tried or were refused. No patient was psychotic or severely disturbed. With 1 exception, narcotics and analgesics were discontinued before surgery. Electrode placement was carried out under local anesthesia, with a target site medial to the parafascicularis nucleus. After 1–2 weeks the electrode was connected to an induc-

(6)   J. Neurosurg. 47:184–194, August, 1977.

tion receiver and rectifying unit under general anesthesia. The receiver was placed subcutaneously over the pectoralis muscle. A Medtronics stimulator was utilized.

Stimulation relieved several types of pain over a long period, often bilaterally. With judicious use the effect did not appear subject to adaptation, but sustained uninterrupted stimulation for several hours did lead to a reversible reduction in efficacy. Side effects were minimal and caused little or no untoward emotional changes. Two patients who died about 2 months after electrode insertion exhibited no significant gliosis or tissue destruction.

Brain stimulation in the periventricular area can apparently effectively replace lesioning as a neurosurgical means of reducing pain. The present results are quite encouraging; 6 of 8 patients had good results and 1, a fair result. The longest follow-up exceeds 42 months. Pain throughout the body is controlled by this method, and the technique is not dependent on paresthesias for effectiveness. Apart from the electrode track, no irreversible brain damage occurs. It appears that the localized, intermittent nature of focal electric stimulation in the periventricular gray matter activates the pain inhibitory mechanisms harnessed by opiates while avoiding some of the side effects, including extreme tolerance with chronic use.

Pain Relief by Electric Stimulation of the Central Gray Matter in Humans and Its Reversal by Naloxone. Yoshio Hosobuchi, John E. Adams and Rita Linchitz[7] (Univ. of California, San Francisco) relieved intractable pain in 6 patients by stimulation of electrodes implanted permanently in the periventricular and periaqueductal gray matter. Narcotic analgesics in reasonable doses had not suppressed constant, diffuse pain in these patients. The target for stimulation was at the level of the posterior commissure and 2 or 3 mm lateral from the medial wall of the posterior 3d ventricle. The electrodes were implanted stereotactically. Initially the electrodes were externalized for trial stimulation over 1 or 2 weeks. Self-mediated stimulation began a few days after implantation; short bipolar square pulses of 10–20 Hz were used. After successful trial stimulation the electrodes

(7) Science 197:183–186, July 8, 1977.

were internalized and connected to a radiofrequency-coupled receiver. A ramp current was produced.

Five patients had total and 1 had partial relief from pain over a range of 3 – 6 v, with a latent period of 5 – 10 minutes. All patients noticed marked enhancement of well-being, increased appetite and better ability to sleep without sleep medication. Greater ease in general activities was possible than before electrode implantation. No change in neurologic or autonomic function was evident. Three patients who used stimulation almost continually noticed a rapid reduction in efficacy of pain control within 4 or 5 weeks. They also developed considerable tolerance for narcotic medication. After stimulation was stopped for a few weeks the demand for narcotics fell precipitously and stimulation again relieved pain. Patients then used stimulation not more than 1 or 2 hours at a time, at intervals of at least 3 or 4 hours. Only 1 patient had reduced sensitivity to pinprick. All patients but 1 reported total reversal of pain relief on intravenous naloxone administration. Naloxone alone had no effect on pain, except for exacerbation in 1 case. Two surviving patients have used the stimulator as their sole means of pain control for over 1 year.

These findings may support the view that a neural system that utilizes endogenous substances for pain relief may exist in the brain. Brain stimulation is potentially useful as a nondestructive means of controlling intractable persistent pain in human beings.

► [Naloxone can also be used to reverse the effects of narcotics used to relieve pain in persons with multiple injuries when there is doubt if drowsiness is due to narcosis or to rising intracranial pressure. It may also be used to determine if a patient is addicted to opiates, for if naloxone is given and the patient has immediate withdrawal symptoms, one can be sure that the patient is indeed addicted. – Ed.] ◄

Pain and Spinal Root Compression. M. L. Friis, G. C. Gulliksen, P. Rasmussen and J. Husby[8] attempted to obtain precise knowledge of the distribution of pain after compression of a spinal nerve root in 249 patients with herniated intervertebral disk or spondylotic nerve root involvement (Table 1). More than one nerve root was affected in 10 patients (Table 2). Most patients with monoradicular involve-

---

(8)   Acta Neurochir. (Wien) 39:241 – 249, 1977.

TABLE 1. – Diagnosis and Sex Distribution in 239 Patients with One Spinal Root Affected

		Prolapse				Spondylosis			
	♀	♂	♀ + ♂	♀/♂	♀	♂	♀ + ♂	♀/♂
C4 – C5	–	1	1	⎫	1	1	2	⎫
C5 – C6	2	–	2	⎬ 1,00	3	7	10	⎬ 0,85
C6 – C7	4	5	9	⎭	7	5	12	⎭
L1 – L2	–	1	1	⎫	–	–	–	⎫
L3 – L4	1	3	4	⎬ 0,71	–	1	1	⎬ 0,53
L4 – L5	34	45	79		7	20	27	
L5 – S1	30	43	73	⎭	9	9	18	⎭
All	71	98	169	0,72	27	43	70	0,63

ment had disk herniation. The average age of patients with disk herniation was 43 years and of those with spondylosis, 49.

The distribution of pain is shown in Figures 28 and 29 in patients with involvement of the 6th and 7th cervical roots. Neck and shoulder pain was present in about three fourths of patients. Lateral-radial pain predominated in cases involving the 6th root, and pain in the posterolateral aspect of the upper arm and medial aspect of the hand predominated in those involving the 7th root. Over two thirds of patients had shooting-lancinating pains in the arms. The distribution of pain in patients with lesions of the 5th lumbar nerve root is shown in Figure 30. Pain in the lumbar and gluteal regions occurred in three fourths of these patients and in

TABLE 2. – Diagnosis and Sex Distribution in Nine Patients with Two Spinal Roots Affected and One Patient with Two Main Diagnoses at Same Level

		Prolapse		Spondylosis		Prolapse + spondylosis	
		♀	♂	♀	♂	♀	♂
C4 – C5	C5 – C6				2		
C5 – C6	C6 – C7		1		1		
L3 – L4	L4 – L5				1		
L4 – L5	L5 – S1	1		2	1		
L4 – L5							1

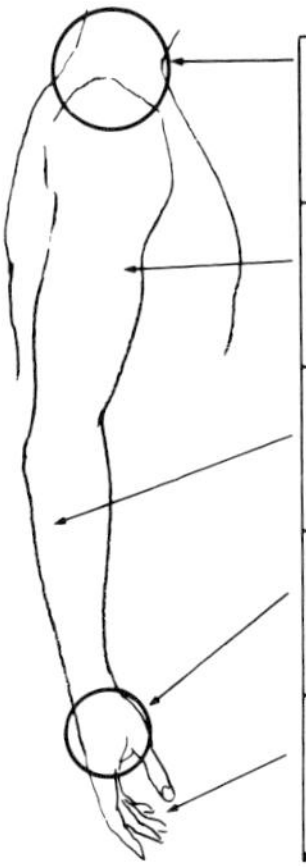

Region					
Neck-shoulder Prolapse spondylosis All:			+ Pain 2/6 8	O Pain -/4 4	
Upper arm		Posterior 1/2 3	Lateral -/6 6	O Pain 1/1 2	Other -/1 1
Lower arm		Ulnar 1/- 1	Radial 1/7 8	O Pain -/3 3	Other -/- 0
Hand		Ulnar -/1 1	Radial 2/3 5	O Pain -/4 4	Other -/2 2
Fingers	4th-5th -/1 1	2nd-4th -/2 2	1-(2) 2/3 5	O Pain -/4 4	Other -/- 0

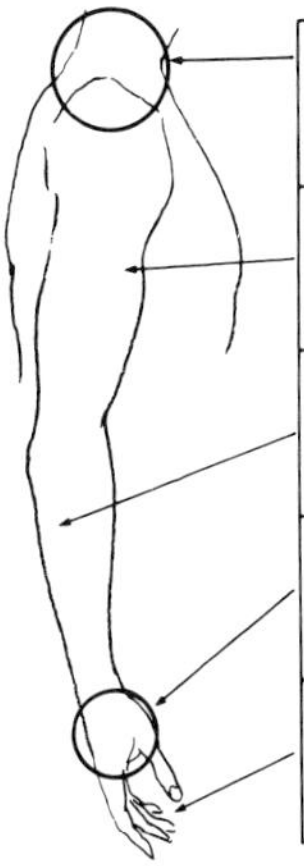

Region					
Neck-shoulder Prolapse spondylosis All:			+ pain 6/12 18	O pain 3/- 3	
Upper arm		Posterior 3/2 5	Lateral 4/7 11	O Pain 1/3 4	Other 1/- 1
Lower arm	Posterior 2/1 3	Ulnar 2/6 8	Radial 2/3 5	O Pain 2/2 4	Other 1/- 1
Hand	Posterior 1/- 1	Ulnar 1/5 6	Radial 2/1 3	O Pain 3/5 8	Other 2/1 3
Fingers	4th-5th -/6 6	2nd-4th 2/3 5	1-(2) 3/1 4	O Pain 3/2 5	Other 1/- 1

Fig 28 (top). — Pain distribution in 12 patients with prolapse-spondylosis affecting the 6th cervical root (C5 – C6 affection).

Fig 29 (bottom). — Pain distribution in 21 patients with prolapse-spondylosis affecting the 7th cervical root (C6 – C7 affection).

(Courtesy of Friis, M. L., et al.: Acta Neurochir. (Wien) 39:214 – 249, 1977; Berlin-Heidelberg-New York: Springer.)

two thirds of those with lesions of the 1st sacral root. Pain in the lateral aspect of the hip was more frequent in the cases involving the 5th root. Lower extremity pains were comparable in these two groups of patients. One third of patients had no pain in the foot or toes. Over two thirds of patients

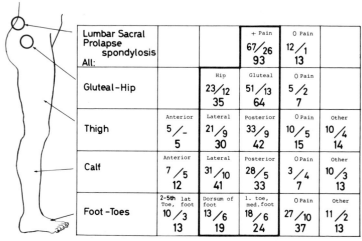

Fig 30.—Pain distribution in 106 patients with prolapse-spondylosis affecting the 5th lumbar root (L4–L5 affection). (Courtesy of Friis, M. L., et al.: Acta Neurochir. (Wien) 39:241–249, 1977; Berlin-Heidelberg-New York: Springer.)

had shooting-lancinating pains in the legs, though not necessarily extending into the toes.

These findings suggest that classic sciatic pain is rather infrequent and that it is not possible to determine with any certainty the site of nerve root involvement from the peripheral localization of the pain.

Commissural Myelotomy. Albert W. Cook and Yasuto Kawakami[9] (New York) describe commissural myelotomy and its effectiveness in 24 patients with intractable pain due to a variety of causes.

TECHNIQUE.—Under general anesthesia, an incision that starts a few segments higher than the level of pain is made over the spine. After a laminectomy is completed, a dural incision is made. Under microscopy or with the use of magnifying glasses, the posterior spinal vein is displaced from the sulcus, the pia is sharply incised in the midline, and the commissurotomy is made by using a special myelotome, with a blunt spatula 5.5 mm long, starting caudally. Every effort is made not to deviate from the midline. The dura and wound are closed in a routine manner.

No operative deaths occurred. Twelve patients had

---

(9) J. Neurosurg. 47:1–6, July, 1977.

marked hyperalgesia and dysesthesia immediately after the operation. These sensations began to abate the next day, and they resolved over 10–14 days. Methylprednisone was given for 10 days after surgery. Proprioception was sometimes disordered after surgery, but this defect resolved almost completely in most patients. No changes occurred in the motor system or in deep tendon reflexes. Pain disappeared promptly in 17 cases. Pain recurred after 2–5 years in patients with lumbar arachnoiditis. Patients with diffuse bilateral metastases from carcinoma showed the most dramatic pain relief after commissural myelotomy. They eventually died of carcinoma, but their pain was relieved while they survived.

There is no mortality from commissural myelotomy. Bilateral pain, especially due to metastasis, is effectively relieved. No permanent disturbance of urination, bowel function or motor function results. An open procedure is necessary, however, and proprioceptive sensation is modified. Pain relief has not been satisfactory in patients with pelvic metastases, and pain relief is only temporary in patients with lumbar arachnoiditis. The operation is not indicated in this nonmalignant situation.

► [Nine patients form the basis for King's article on anterior commissurotomy for intractable pain (J. Neurosurg. 47:7, 1977). Rostral cord segments were counted upward from the last dentate ligament insertion at T12. Myelotomy was planned from caudal S1 to at least two segments above the level of reported pain. The midline vein was not coagulated, the midline was incised with a no. 15 blade, and a 2-mm dissector was inserted to separate the dorsal columns. When the dorsal extension of the anterior fissure was entered, internal arcuate branches of the anterior spinal artery were seen but never the artery itself, which lies at the anterior aspect of the cord. The patterns of postoperative sensory loss could not be used to explain why patients were relieved of pain. Return to the use of narcotics was not necessary in 7 patients, except for 2 during the last 3–4 days of their illness. All 6 patients with cancer were relieved; all died within 6 months. Postlaminectomy pain recurred at 10 and 12 months in 2 patients, and 1 patient with a gunshot wound at L1 was relieved until he died, 26 months postoperatively. — Ed.] ◄

Miscellaneous

Genitofemoral Neuralgia. Entrapment neuropathy of the genitofemoral nerve is an uncommon syndrome characterized by neuralgic pain and paresthesias in the distribution of the nerve. Patients with the syndrome are not infrequently considered malingerers. Ranjit K. Laha, Sarojini Rao, Christopher N. Pidgeon and Manuel Dujovny[1] (Univ. of Pittsburgh) report data on a patient with bilateral genitofemoral neuralgia that responded to neurectomies of the genitofemoral nerve.

Man, 46, had had pain in the lower abdomen, radiating to the groins and testes, for 6 years and denied urinary symptoms and genital discharge. Pain had begun on the right 2 weeks after repair of a recurrent right indirect inguinal hernia. A small neuroma had apparently been excised from the right inguinal region without effect on the pain. Left groin pain developed shortly after a left indirect inguinal herniorrhaphy. Several local anesthetic injections on the right had given no relief and recently the pain had become refractory to stronger analgesics. The pain was considered psychogenic in origin. Hip extension produced the pain and hyperalgesia of the scrotal skin was noted. The right genitofemoral nerve was stimulated before being resected; endoneurial fibrosis was diagnosed. The neuralgic pain disappeared postoperatively and did not recur in the next 8 months. A left neurectomy was then performed, with disappearance of pain postoperatively. There was no sensory deficit on either side, but the left cremasteric reflex was absent.

Genitofemoral neuralgia consists of intermittent or constant inguinal pain radiating to the genitalia and upper thigh and aggravated by walking, stooping or hyperextension of the hip. The neuralgia is presumably caused by entrapment of the nerve in adhesions after herniotomy, appendectomy or inguinal trauma. The present patient had had an appendectomy. Neurectomy of the genitofemoral nerve is the treatment of choice for genitofemoral neuralgia. An extraperitoneal approach is indicated unless there is a reason

---

(1) Surg. Neurol. 8:280–282, October, 1977.

for a transperitoneal procedure. The incision and approach are similar to the transverse paraumbilical approach for lumbar sympathectomy. Differentiation is necessary between entrapments of the genitofemoral nerves and those of the ilioinguinal nerves; the latter may be treated with nerve block and neurolysis, in contrast to the necessary neurectomy with involvement of the genitofemoral nerve, betrayed by hyperalgesia in its distribution (scrotal skin), normal hip x-ray and increase in pain with hyperextension of the hip.

Peripheral Nerve Entrapments are discussed by Andrea Cracchiolo III, Norman S. Namerow, David S. Campion and Rodney Bluestone[2] (Univ. of California, Los Angeles). A peripheral entrapment neuropathy refers to injury to a peripheral nerve at a specific site, due to either an aberration of anatomy or mechanical irritation. Entrapment neuropathy is due to pressure or irritation from some anatomical structures next to the nerve and occurs frequently when the nerve passes through a fibro-osseous canal and is relatively fixed. Pain is the most common clinical feature; it can occur at the site of injury or along the distribution of the involved nerve. Muscle weakness and atrophy and paresthesias may also occur. Specific nerves that may be affected include the median, ulnar, radial, suprascapular, axillary, lateral femoral cutaneous, femoral, obturator and sciatic. Prolonged pressure results in a severely damaged fiber with partial or complete rupture of the myelin lamellae in the invaginated area. In chronic entrapment such as a carpal tunnel syndrome, the internodes of the myelinated fiber are swollen at the end away from the entrapment.

The pathophysiology and electrodiagnosis of entrapments are discussed. The sequence of events in a carpal tunnel syndrome, for instance, starts with mild compression that produces decreased amplitude of sensory potential and prolongation of latency (normal is 3.7 msec or less). As more compression occurs, the motor potential amplitude decreases and its latency is prolonged beyond normal (4.6 msec). As severity of involvement increases, conduction velocity decreases below the lowest normal, 49 m/sec, and finally needle examination shows denervation potentials in abductor pollicis and opponens pollicis.

(2)   West. J. Med. 127:299–313, October, 1977.

Entrapment within a confined space may be a local manifestation of a more generalized disease. Diseases of the bony components or of the interstitial tissue components may be responsible. Medical causes of nerve entrapment include the commonly recognized compression of nerve in a shallow groove or over an exposed area. Entrapment may occur in a confined space (e.g., median nerve at wrist) because of rheumatoid disease, edema of pregnancy, dependent edema with frozen shoulder, myxedema with hypothyroidism, tissue swelling with acromegaly, and mucopolysaccharide disorders. Nerves may themselves become enlarged or expanded, with amyloidosis, leprosy, idiopathic hypertrophic neuritis and other disorders. Management with diuretics, splinting and injection of corticosteroid in the tunnel space may be tried before operation.

Nonoperative treatment should usually be tried unless severe, unremitting symptoms or significantly abnormal nerve conduction are present, there is muscle atrophy or weakness or previous adequate nonoperative treatment has failed. If conservative care is not indicated, postponing surgery may be unwise. The exact site of entrapment must be determined preoperatively. Block anesthesia is satisfactory and preferable in some cases. A pneumatic tourniquet should be used proximally. The operation should thoroughly decompress the nerve and in certain cases the nerve may have to be transposed to a more favorable area to prevent recurrent entrapment. The success of a decompression operation depends on an absolutely accurate preoperative diagnosis and on thorough but gentle surgery.

▶ [The discussion by Cracchiolo of surgical treatment betrays his orthopedic orientation; most neurosurgeons would not use a longitudinal incision across the volar aspect of the wrist, nor would we use a tourniquet. Local anesthesia and bipolar coagulation make transection of the carpal ligament a virtually bloodless operation.

Another case of suprascapular entrapment neuropathy is reported by Gelmers and Buys (Acta Neurochir. (Wien) 38:121, 1977). The girl, aged 19, was a telephone operator who repetitively swung the left arm upward and to the right to reach a telephone clamp. Electromyography confirmed the localized involvement of the spinati muscles, and operation permitted section of the suprascapular ligament, with ultimate improvement.

Twenty-nine variations of the course of the median nerve were found in 246 hands by Lantz (J. Hand Surg. 2:44, 1977) during exploration of the carpal tunnel. There were variations in the thenar branch, accessory branches at the distal portion of the carpal tunnel, high divisions of the median nerve, and accessory branches proximal to the tunnel. These studies and those by Poisel in 100 cadaver hands emphasize the importance of approaching the median nerve from the ulnar side when opening the carpal tunnel. — Ed.] ◄

Ulnar Nerve Compression at the Elbow: Results of Surgery in 85 Cases. Per Hagström[3] (Stockholm) reviewed the results of surgery for ulnar nerve compression at the elbow in 49 male and 30 female evaluable patients having unilateral surgery 85 times in 1954–72 and followed for 1–18 years. All but 3 patients were right-handed and 52 patients had symptoms in the dominant hand. Over half the patients were aged 40–60 when symptoms began. Sixteen cases were attributable to direct trauma and 11 to indirect damage. Three cases with deformity of the ulnar sulcus occurred many years after an elbow fracture. Symptoms were present for over 3 years before operation in 18% of cases. The chief symptom was pain radiating from the elbow to the 2 ulnar fingers; numbness was less constant. About two thirds of patients had forearm and hand weakness. Reduced pain sensitivity was found in the ulnar fingers in 45% of patients, reduced power in the 1st dorsal interosseous in 55% and atrophy of the ulnar-innervated hand muscles in 42%. One fourth of patients had only a tender ulnar nerve in the sulcus.

Subcutaneous transposition of the nerve to the front of the medial epicondyle was done in 51 patients. In 8 others the transposition was accompanied by burying the nerve in the volar musculature. Neurolysis was done in 21 patients. Retransposition was necessary in 5 patients. Six patients had postoperative bleeding and 1 had infection. Complete cure was obtained in 31% of patients and radical improvement in 47%. Symptoms were unchanged in 13% of patients and worse in 9%. Men seemed to do better than women. Results were poorest in cases of direct elbow injury. The duration of symptoms had little influence on the outcome, and age was not an important factor. The best results were obtained by transposition, with and without nerve burial in the volar musculature. Associations with Dupuytren's contracture and hypertension were apparent in this series.

Surgical Management of Brachial Plexus Injuries is

(3) Scand. J. Plast. Reconstr. Surg. 11:59–62, 1977.

discussed by Hanno Millesi[4] (Vienna). Most brachial plexus injuries occurring in civilian practice are due to traffic accidents. The plexus may be compressed between the clavicle and 1st rib. The more the arm is elevated, the greater is the effect on the lower roots. If the shoulder is struck with the arm abducted, the upper roots are more vulnerable. Traction lesions can occur in the infraclavicular part of the plexus when the shoulder is dislocated or the humerus fractured. Until recently, physiotherapy has been advocated for patients without disorganization of the internal nerve structure, although compression can prevent spontaneous regeneration. A neurorrhaphy or a nerve grafting is possible if proximal stumps are available. Muscle and tendon transfers and stabilizing procedures are not adaptable to complete palsies.

Fifty-six patients with complete or partial brachial plexus lesions had operations in 1964–72. Of the 56, only 2 had avulsion of all five roots. Eighteen patients had both supraganglionic and infraganglionic lesions that led to complete palsy of the plexus and had nerve grafting. Grafts were united with the lateral and dorsal cords if two roots could be used. Eleven patients had root involvement that led to a partial lesion. Thirteen had a complete lesion due to damage to the supraclavicular or infraclavicular portion or both; continuity was preserved in 9 of them. Twelve patients with partial lesions of the infraclavicular portion had neurolysis or nerve grafting, or both. Intercostal nerve transfer was performed in 7 patients and useful function was obtained in 4 of them. Secondary procedures include resection of the distal suture site, tendon shortening and muscle transfers and restoration of protective sensibility.

Of 18 patients with complete palsy from lesions at root level, 15 gained protective sensibility and had improvement in trophy. Useful function was regained by 10 patients. Nine of 11 patients with partial palsy from lesions at root level gained useful function. Eight of 13 with complete palsy due to a peripheral lesion had useful function. All 5 failures were operated on more than a year after injury. Ten of 12 patients with partial palsies due to peripheral lesions acquired useful function. Pain disappeared in time in all pa-

(4) J. Hand Surg. 2:367–379, September, 1977.

tients but 1. In all, 38 of 54 (70%) patients had useful motor recovery in at least one important area and all but 1 of these were considerably improved. Complications included 2 cases of pseudarthrosis of the clavicle, 2 hematomas and 1 loss of function in a patient with a partial lesion. No pneumothorax occurred and no patient had any complication due to a lesion of a major vessel.

▶ [Sedel (Ann. Chir. Plast. 21:253, 1976) used Millesi's technique in replacing loss of neural substance by autograft. Although 19 brachial plexus lesions and 27 grafts for peripheral nerves were counted, the text of the article deals only with the latter. Most grafts were taken from the external saphenous nerve; some were from the internal brachial cutaneous or cubital nerve (when the latter was also damaged). Dissection of the injured nerve — as well as removal of the grafts — has been done with the use of a tourniquet. Each cable is sutured separately under magnification. Gaps of over 15 cm have been successfully grafted; included in this series were stretch lesions of the common peroneal nerve. Sedel believes results are better than those from conventional techniques of suturing injured nerves.

Repair of nerves with various suture material has been studied by De-Lee, Smith and Green (J. Hand Surg. 2:38, 1977). Wire, catgut, silk, polyglycolic acid (Dexon) and polypropylene (Prolene) were studied in rabbits. The synthetics available at the time were in size 6-0, so this size was used for all materials. Histologic study of nerves was carried out by a pathologist without knowledge of the material used for suture. Prolene was least reactive and silk was most reactive, with Dexon next. Plain catgut produced a minimal fibrous reaction, second only to Prolene. No consistent patterns of immediate cellular response could be found, indicating that technical variations in repair and possibly sterility factors may be important in an initial reaction. In this series, steel was not as innocuous as has been reported elsewhere, possibly due to trauma in manipulation of the suture.

Surgical indications for operating on the brachial plexus are also described by Valencak, Berger and Zaunbauer (Neurochirurgie 23:133, 1977). They also do not believe in section of the clavicle except in rare instances, lest new problems arise from the callus formed. Grafts may be obtained from the internal cutaneous nerves of the forearm and upper arm or the external saphenous nerve. Success has also followed grafts between the intercostal nerve and fascicles of the brachial plexus in instances of total lesions of the brachial plexus. The intercostal nerves (2d to 8th) are taken in the midaxillary line where there are large numbers of motor fibers available. One may also make an anastomosis between intercostal nerves and the peripheral nerves such as brachial radial or musculocutaneous. The basic technique is that of Millesi.

Nylon was the suture material used by Hudson and Dommisse (Can. Med. J. 117:1160,1977) for microneurosurgery of the musculocutaneous nerve after gunshot wound of the brachial plexus. The obviously separated elements were tagged with nonabsorbable suture and brought together loosely after the torn ends of the subclavian artery were sutured, and secondary repair was done about 9 weeks after injury. The central portion of the clavicle had been torn away in the original injury. Cervical myelogram was normal; intraoperative stimulation showed that the musculocutaneous nerve was the only one not in continuity, and this was repaired with sural autografts. Examination 18 months after injury showed considerable return of function. – Ed.] ◄

Method for Obtaining a Sural Nerve Graft. The sural nerve is preferred for nerve repair in the upper extremity if large gaps are present or several segments are needed. It is readily accessible, has several large fascicles, provides 30 – 40 cm usable graft and results in a minimal sensory deficit in the donor area. H. Louis Hill, Luis O. Vasconez and Maurice J. Jurkiewicz[5] (Emory Univ.) have used a Brand tendon stripper to obtain a long segment of sural nerve expediently, with little resultant morbidity or disability.

TECHNIQUE. – A 2-cm or 3-cm incision is made in the groove formed by the lateral edge of the Achilles tendon at the level of the lateral malleolus. The nerve is mobilized distally as far as possible and transected some 3 – 5 cm distal to the incision. It is then passed through the end of a tendon stripper, a clamp is placed on its tip and the stripper is passed proximally in a gentle rotary fashion until the tip is felt in the subcutaneous tissues near the popliteal fossa. The leg is wrapped with an elastic bandage.

This method has been used in 6 recent patients to obtain seven sural nerves for grafting of nerves in the upper extremity. A 30-cm to 35-cm segment of nerve can usually be obtained from each leg. No patient has had more than mild discomfort in the leg. Saphenous vein injury and excessive traction on the graft segment have not been problems. The communicating branch of the peroneal nerve is transected low with this technique, but this usually occurs also with the multiple-incision method of removal.

Etiology and Definitive Microsurgical Treatment of Hemifacial Spasm: Operative Techniques and Results in 47 Patients. Peter J. Jannetta, Munir Abbasy, Joseph C. Maroon, Francisco M. Ramos and Maurice S. Albin[6] (Univ. of Pittsburgh) treated 45 patients for classic hemifacial spasm and 2 with atypical features in 1966 – 74. Compression of the facial nerve root exit zone at the brain stem, usually by a crossing arterial loop, was present in all cases. The nerve was decompressed by microvascular manipulation of

(5)   Plast. Reconstr. Surg. 61:177 – 179, February, 1978.
(6)   J. Neurosurg. 47:321 – 328, September, 1977.

the vessel away from the nerve. The 32 women and 15 men, aged 20 – 75 years, had intractable, persistent hemifacial spasm, present for 1 – 14 years. All had disabling symptoms. Dexamethasone was given starting 12 hours preoperatively. A retromastoid craniectomy about 5 cm in diameter was made low and laterally to decompress the facial nerve root exit zone. The axis of the arterial loop was altered by interposing a small prosthesis of spongy material between the limbs of the loop and the brain stem. Muscle, Ivalon sponge or Teflon felt was utilized. A cholesteatoma was removed in 1 case.

Results were excellent in 38 of 45 patients with classic hemifacial spasm, good in 2, fair in 3 and poor in 2. Six patients had delayed temporary facial weakness; all but 1 regained fully normal function. Three patients had an ipsilateral hearing loss. The first 10 patients were treated with a gelatin foam prosthesis and have done well. Poor results were obtained in the 2 patients with atypical hemifacial spasm. Postoperative electromyography has shown progressive loss of spasm and a loss of preexisting denervation. Only 1 late recurrence has been noted on follow-up of all patients for up to 10 years.

Cross-compression at the brain stem is apparently truly causative of hemifacial spasm, and decompression is a definitive treatment. Operative trauma is not the cause of improvement. Experience with the surgical microscope is necessary if the procedure is to be carried out safely.

▶ [I do not understand why Gelfoam or muscle should work in this operation (or in decompression for trigeminal neuralgia); both should disappear within a few weeks.

Similar decompressive operations have, according to Jannetta, been useful in relief of selected cases of dizziness and atypical facial neuralgia. In spasmodic torticollis, the lesion possibly could be provoked by compression of the side of the medulla by an arterial loop (Interurban Neurosurgical Society, February, 1978). – Ed.] ◀

Results of Treatment in Peripheral Facial Paralysis: A 25-Year Study. C. B. Wynn Parry and P. F. King[7] (London) reviewed the records of 561 patients seen in the past 25 years with peripheral facial paralysis; 31 cases were due to trauma and 30 to herpes zoster, whereas 500 patients had idiopathic Bell's palsy. There was no suggestion of a

(7) J. Laryngol. Otol. 91:551 – 564, July, 1977.

predilection for one side. Taste was affected in 55 (18%) patients; 12 patients had subjective hyperacusis. There was no evidence that older patients did less well than younger ones. The end results were not related to the mode of onset of Bell's palsy, whether acute or gradual. Over two thirds of patients with partial lesions recovered fully by 3 months and 60% of patients with complete lesions had regained full function 3 months after the onset. Although 18% of those with complete lesions required a year to recover, only 9% of those with partial lesions took this long to recover. No particular benefit accrued from splinting during the stage of paralysis. Steroids were not used.

All but 1 of the 30 patients with zoster had complete paralysis when first seen. Recovery took longer than in Bell's palsy, 10 patients taking 1–3 years to gain their final degree of recovery. Since 1967, surgical decompression has been offered to all patients who had denervation on electrodiagnostic testing. Three fourths of 19 patients who were decompressed had a good outcome, compared with only 55% of 11 with denervation who were not decompressed. Recovery occurred in a shorter time after decompression. Fifteen of 27 patients who had complete facial paralysis as a result of traffic accidents regained normal function and 23 had extremely good functional results. None of 4 surgically damaged patients regained full function.

Facial palsy due to herpes zoster appears to carry a worse prognosis than idiopathic Bell's palsy. A complete palsy does not appear to carry a worse prognosis. Patients who have denervation may benefit from surgical decompression, but the presence of electric evidence of denervation does not necessarily imply a bad prognosis. The findings are not in accord with those of Taverner, who suggested the use of steroids in the early stages.

▶ [The authors found no evidence that electric stimulation of the face had any influence on recovery from peripheral facial paralysis. Decompression did — but exactly what is meant by "standard decompression" is unclear, especially because other workers have varied their operations considerably. For instance, it has been reported that decompression by bony removal is innocuous, but decompression by adding slitting of the nerve sheath is not.

It has been difficult to present convincing evidence of the utility of decompression of the facial nerve for Bell's palsy, because no controlled randomized series has been available. McCabe (Laryngoscope 87:246,

1977) has seen 7 patients who have regained partial but definite return of facial function detected on the evening of the day of operation. All were treated at least 4 months after onset. All lesions were infrageniculate, all nerves were completely without function and none responded to percutaneous electric testing. The odds of spontaneous return occurring immediately after a decompression operation for paralysis of 4–13 months "would stagger the imagination."

Trauma to the facial nerve in closed head injury is the third most common cause of facial paralysis. Adour, Boyajian, Kahn and Schneider (ibid., p. 380) found 12 patients with complete, 15 with incomplete and 3 with bilateral posttraumatic facial paralysis. Fracture could be identified in 80% of the 30 patients. Steroids were used to treat those who had incomplete paralysis, all of which cases were delayed in onset, and improvement was excellent. Of the 12 patients with complete paralysis, 10 had immediate onset and 2 had delayed onset. One had no treatment and no recovery; 1 was lost to follow-up. Seven of the 10 with immediate paralysis were operated on, with decompression in 4. Decompression was done on one side of the bilaterally paralyzed patients, and 1 was lost to follow-up. Decompression was found not to be of benefit in these cases, and substitution of facial nerve exploration for decompression seems warranted. Polytomography of the facial canal can help select patients for operation, such as removal of bone fragments that impinge on the nerve. Opening of the sheath is not of value to the patient and may, in fact, make the damage worse. – Ed.] ◄

Differentiation of Communicating Hydrocephalus and Presenile Dementia by Continuous Recording of Cerebrospinal Fluid Pressure. A. Hartmann and E. Alberti[8] (Univ. of Heidelberg) monitored the cerebrospinal fluid (CSF) pressure continuously and observed pressures during intrathecal infusions of normal saline at two rates in patients with communicating hydrocephalus and cerebral atrophy of other causes.

The CSF pressure was recorded for 24–36 hours. Then, with the patient lightly sedated with diazepam, saline was infused intrathecally for 60 seconds at a rate of 0.92 ml/minute, after which the CSF pressure was recorded for 15 seconds. Infusion and recording were repeated until headache or nausea developed or for 60 minutes or to a CSF pressure of 50 mm Hg. Some patients also received infusions at a rate of 1.84 ml/minute. The absolute infusion rates were 0.74 and 1.47 ml/minutes, respectively.

Twenty-seven consecutive patients were evaluated, 14 with communicating hydrocephalus and 13 with alteration

(8) J. Neurol. Neurosurg. Psychiatry 40:630–640, July, 1977.

of intellectual performance not due to communicating hydrocephalus (control subjects).

Eight of the 14 patients with communicating hydrocephalus had CSF pressures exceeding 15 mm Hg on occasion. No definite correlation was noted between the CSF pressure and occurrence of plateau waves. All 6 patients restudied after shunt surgery showed a fall in CSF pressure, and most showed clinical improvement. Control subjects never had pressure elevations that exceeded baseline pressure by more than 4 mm Hg. Lundberg's C waves were seen in both groups, but were higher in the group with communicating hydrocephalus. Seven patients with communicating hydrocephalus had normal responses to saline infusion. All with abnormal responses (type A or B) showed plateau waves on continuous monitoring, but the reverse was not true. No control showed an abnormal response with the low infusion rates. With the higher infusion rate, 6 of 8 subjects had such reactions: type A, steep rise in CSF pressure immediately after start of infusion and early headache and nausea; type B, slow continuous rise in CSF pressure and delayed headache and nausea.

The intrathecal infusion test can detect reduced absorption of CSF if more than one infusion rate is used. With use of both continuous CSF pressure monitoring and the infusion test, it is easier to determine which patients with communicating hydrocephalus should have shunt surgery. The proportion of patients who improve after shunt surgery can be increased with use of these tests.

► [Ventriculoatrial shunt produced tremendous improvement in a woman, aged 65, who had Paget's disease of the skull, dementia, parkinsonism, gait ataxia, urinary incontinence and a left hemicerebellar syndrome. Botez, Bertrand, Léveillé and Marchand (Can. J. Neurol. Sci. 4:139, 1977) could not do axial tomography because of the large head size, but hydrocephalus was diagnosed from a cisternogram with [111]In. They think it possible that the improvement in their patient was associated with the absence of pneumoencephalography, which can aggravate and decompensate a normal-pressure hydrocephalus syndrome.

A 3-year follow-up of 28 patients with idiopathic normal-pressure hydrocephalus is presented by Greenberg, Shenkin and Adam (J. Neurol. Neurosurg. Psychiatry 40:336, 1977), along with another 45 patients. Of the 64.3% who initially responded to treatment, 6 deteriorated, leaving a success rate of 42.8% at almost 3 years after shunting. In the second series, only 33% responded to treatment, but these patients generally had more dementia and less ataxia than the first group. The age of the patient and the duration of symptoms now appear to be unrelated to outcome. The presence of large sulci in computerized tomography scanning did not necessarily mean a poor result would occur. The authors still find that no single test or group of tests has predictive value, but gait disturbance and extremely large ventricles are apt to be related to good results.

Seventeen of 33 patients with normal-pressure hydrocephalus were found by Jacobs (ibid., p. 331) to have diabetes mellitus. This 51.5% incidence was in contrast to 12.1% in age-matched controls. It seems possible that the endocrine disturbance is due to disturbances in hypothalamic and brain stem autonomic functions produced by the expanding ventricles. – Ed.] ◄

Surgical Management of Hyperhidrosis. Excessive sweating often causes emotional and social problems, and treatment by psychotherapy, irradiation and drugs has proved ineffective in most cases. Only surgical removal of sympathetic paths or local excision of axillary sweat glands has given lasting relief. T. V. Keaveny, P. A. M. Fitzgerald, C. Donnelly and G. D. Shanik[9] (Dublin) reviewed experience with the surgical management of idiopathic hyperhidrosis in 42 female and 23 male patients with disabling hyperhidrosis, seen in 1971 – 76 and followed for 3 months to 6 years after surgery. Their mean age was 26.2. The operations included 42 bilateral supraclavicular cervical sympathectomies and 21 bilateral axillary skin excisions. Twenty-six patients had had the condition since childhood. The hands were primarily affected in most patients. Two patients had bilateral lumbar sympathectomies. Patients with axillary hyperhidrosis had removal of an ellipse of axillary skin.

Forty of 43 patients having cervical sympathectomy, 1 unilaterally, were totally satisfied with the results, whereas 3 were unimproved. Two patients were asymptomatic after lumbar sympathectomies. Horner's syndrome developed in 5 patients postoperatively, but was transient in 2. Two patients had a small pneumothorax and 2 a chylothorax; all resolved without treatment. Numbness near the wounds was transient in 1 of 2 patients. Fourteen of 21 patients were pleased with the results of axillary skin excision and another was improved after reexcision. Two patients obtained some relief, whereas 4 were unimproved. Four patients had wound disruption on suture removal. Two pa-

---

(9) Br. J. Surg. 64:570 – 571, August, 1977.

tients had transient numbness of the medial aspect of the upper arm; 1 had transient loss of power in the arm.

The results of axillary skin excision for idiopathic hyperhidrosis are encouraging, and this simple procedure is recommended for this most distressing condition.

▶ [Palmar hyperhidrosis can be mitigated by bilateral simultaneous upper thoracic sympathectomy by the supraclavicular approach, according to Kurchin, Zweig, Adar and Mozes (World J. Surg. 1:667, 1977). The preganglionic denervation is accomplished by removal of the T2 and T3 ganglia (with frozen sections fo confirm removal of neural tissue). Axillary sweating is best treated by removal of the axillary skin, so as not to extend the sympathectomy too far and thus induce more compensatory hyperhidrosis. The thoracic duct was injured in 4 of 308 operations in 155 patients, subclavian artery branches were torn in 3 cases and the pleura was torn in 68. Early Horner's syndrome appeared in 68 patients, and 10 failed to get a dry hand. Six needed chest drainage, and transient brachial plexus contusion occurred in 13. A posterior approach (Adson-Smithwick) and an anterior transthoracic approach (Palumbo) are considered too extensive; the transaxillary approach requires two separate operations and has a significant incidence of pulmonary complications, postoperative shoulder pain and intercostal neuralgia. – Ed.] ◀

Posterior Partial Rootlet Section in Treatment of Spasticity. Förster's method (1908) of treating spasticity has been criticized because of subsequent disorders of sensation, trophic changes and its effects on functional reeducation. Bernardo Fraioli and Beniamino Guidetti[1] (Univ. of Rome) used a modification of Förster's method in 26 patients aged 6– 16 years. The technique includes a partial section of the rootlets that constitute each posterior root.

TECHNIQUE. – A laminectomy limited to T11 – T12 is done under general anesthesia. After the dura is opened, the last 6 – 7 cm of the cord are exposed, usually over three laminae. The arachnoid is opened and removed and the rootlets of each root are separated as far as S1 at the junction with the cord. Under the operating microscope, half or two thirds of each rootlet is cut about 1 mm from its junction with the cord, from the dorsomedial to the ventrolateral site of each, starting with L1 and continuing down to S1, until the foot clonus disappears on reduction of anesthesia.

In the first 10 cases, one rootlet of each root was preserved. All patients were operated on bilaterally. The patients had the usual perinatal pathology and had had physiotherapy for many years. Ten had cerebral spastic diplegia and 14, cerebral spastic quadriplegia. Many patients were

(1)   J. Neurosurg. 46:618 – 626, May, 1977.

nearly independent when standing or walking. All had normal or only moderately reduced mental development. Seven of 13 patients who were not made worse by voluntary movements improved markedly, 2 moderately and 3 slightly. None of the 12 who were made worse by voluntary movements improved markedly, and only 2 improved moderately. Hyperextension and arching of the trunk were reduced, especially if the T12 level was treated. Increased stretch reflexes were markedly reduced or abolished in all cases. Exteroceptive sensations were normal clinically in all patients but 1. Proprioception was normal in all but 1 of the 21 patients so evaluated. No patient was ataxic. No general complications were observed.

This operation reduces or abolishes spastic disorders that are not made worse by voluntary movements. The afferent arcs of the stretch reflexes can be interrupted by partially cutting the posterior rootlets. Clinical disorder of exteroceptive sensations has not resulted from the procedure.

Physiologically Controlled Selective Thalamotomy for Treatment of Abnormal Movement by Leksell's Open System. The chief practical problem in stereotactic thalamotomy is identification of the critical point in each individual case. Ch. Ohye, A. Fukamachi, M. Miyazaki, I. Isobe, H. Nakajima and T. Shibazaki[2] (Gunma Univ., Maebashi, Japan) have used Leksell's open stereotactic instrument since 1972, and with semimicroelectrodes have attempted to obtain improved results with minimal lesions. Review was made of 20 cases, including 10 cases of Parkinson's disease. One-stage surgery was done in all but 2 cases. Simultaneous microrecordings were made while the electrodes were lowered in millimeter steps to delineate the deep subcortical structures, with the coagulating needle used as a guide tube. The neural noise level was estimated quantitatively, using audiomonitoring to indicate the approximate noise level. Repetitive high-frequency stimulation was applied through two electrodes alternately.

Typically, an extremely low noise level in white matter changed suddenly to a very high noise level at a high frequency, sometimes with spike discharges, when the electrode came close to the dorsolateral corner of the lateral

(2) Acta Neurochir. (Wien) 37:93–104, 1977.

ventricle in the posteroanterior view. This pattern was presumed to be due to activity of the caudate nucleus. Entry into the thalamus was easily recognized from an increase in neural noise with many spike discharges. A total of 182 points were stimulated in 18 cases, and responses were obtained from 123 points. The effects of stimulation between two parallel electrodes were often quite different. Operative effects on tremor and rigidity were satisfactory, completely abolishing them in 15 cases. Tremor recurred in 1 case. The initial effect has persisted at follow-up for up to 3 years. Transient weakness occurred in 5 cases and reduced mental activity in 4; these symptoms improved within a month.

Using this technique, the physiologic procedures needed to determine the final target are carried out under ideal conditions. The critical thalamic area presumably involves the lower border of the ventralis intermedius nucleus and a part of the caudal ventrolateral nucleus. The lesion avoids the internal capsule and specific sensory nucleus.

Long-Term Results of Surgery in Spasmodic Torticollis. Various intracerebral operations have been reported to be useful in this condition since the introduction of stereotactic neurosurgery. J. Hernesniemi and L. Laitinen[3] (Helsinki) reviewed data on 45 male and 35 female patients, aged 13 – 62 years, who were hospitalized in 1954 – 74. They had had torticollis for 1 – 33 years. Special attention was focused on patients' subjective opinions of short-term and long-term results of treatment.

Among the patients treated surgically, sternocleidomastoid myotomy was performed in 14, division of the accessory nerve in 4, a combination of sternocleidomastoid myotomy and accessory neurotomy in 4, a combination of multiple cervical and nuchal myotomies in 3, Foerster-Dandy cervical rhizotomy in 13, bilateral ventrolateral thalamotomy in 6, unilateral ventrolateral thalamotomy in 4 and unilateral internal ventral oral thalamotomy in 7. Follow-up for surgical patients averaged 7 years. Ten patients were treated conservatively. In these, the torticollis was only moderate or was accompanied by various psychologic symptoms. Only 2 patients in the latter group declared themselves to be satisfied with their condition 10 years later, clearly indi-

(3)   Neurochirurgie 23:123 – 131, 1977.

cating the seriousness of this condition and its poor "natural" prognosis.

Immediate results in the surgical patients were often good to satisfactory, but an average of 7 years later, their condition had again deteriorated. Half the group considered the benefit of surgery to be negligible. Only 6 patients (11%) declared themselves to be satisfied, though 37.5% were able to continue working. Thus, surgical treatment can be considered to be useful, because only 20% of those treated conservatively were able to keep their jobs. However, the high frequency of complications diminishes the value of surgical treatment. This is particularly true of thalamotomies. Peripheral operations such as myotomy and neurectomy are recommended as initial treatment for spasmodic torticollis, possibly to be followed by cervical rhizotomy under microscopic control. Unilateral thalamotomy might be attempted in patients in whom torticollis is accompanied by hyperkinesia, but the bilateral ventrolateral thalamotomy has been completely abandoned by the authors.

Modulation of Emotion with a Brain Pacemaker: Treatment for Intractable Psychiatric Illness. Robert G. Heath[4] (Tulane Univ.) has for 16 months used an implantable pacemaker for electric stimulation of specific sites on the cerebellar surface in patients with intractable mental illness. It is postulated that a stimulus that activates the physiologic system for pleasure in the septal region of the cerebellar cortex while inhibiting the system in the hippocampus and lateral amygdala for adversive emotion can be effective treatment for behavioral and seizural disorders. Psychosis is viewed as a result of disruption of the physiologic mechanism for emotional expression. Inappropriate emergency emotion consequent to faulty learning experiences is viewed as the principal pathognomonic factor in neurotic behavior. The receiver is implanted over the left side of the chest and a suboccipital craniectomy is then done to implant the electrodes subtentorially over the rostral vermal and paravermal regions. The external stimulator, usually carried in a pocket, delivers the stimulus through an antenna taped to the skin over the implanted receiver.

Eleven patients who had failed to respond to all other

(4)   J. Nerv. Ment. Dis. 165:300–317, November, 1977.

treatments were evaluated. Illness had been present without significant remission for 6–23 years. Four patients had uncontrollable violence-aggression, 2 with brain pathology, whereas 5 were chronic schizophrenics. Two had lifelong patterns of severe neurosis. Three patients had seizures in addition to behavioral pathology. Ten patients presently are functioning out of the hospital without medications or other treatment. Some are symptom free and others have improved significantly. The 1 patient who failed to respond had an organic lesion over the cerebellar site to be stimulated.

This procedure is noninvasive of the brain. The present results are not conclusive, but they are promising enough for the treatment to be considered for patients in whom adequate trials of conventional therapy have failed, especially those who have undesirable side effects from drugs. The time required for remission appears directly related to the time the patient has been psychotic, especially if he has been isolated in institutions.

▶ [All of the 1,830 Finnish veterans who survived a penetrating brain injury during World War II were studied by Virkkunen, Nuutila and Huusko (Dis. Nerv. Syst. 38:907, 1977) to elucidate the incidence of criminality over a follow-up of 32–37 years. Five hundred randomly selected noninjured veterans of the same war were used as controls. There was no statistically significant difference between the two groups for frequency of convictions of crimes punishable by imprisonment. Only 0.9% of the 1,830 patients and 0.6% of controls had committed crimes of violence. Criminal behavior was not recurrent; many convictions in both groups were for drunken driving or distilling of liquor. Follow-up was easy because all brain-injured veterans get a life annuity if they register with the Rehabilitation Institute; this appears to eliminate all except unusual economic pressures as a motive for crime. – Ed.] ◀

Safety and Efficacy of Chronic Stimulation. I. S. Cooper, I. Amin, A. Upton, M. Riklan, S. Watkins and L. Mc-Lellan[5] have used chronic cerebellar stimulation (CCS) to relieve spasticity and intractable seizures for 4½ years. Review was made of the records of 100 patients with cerebral palsy and 32 with epilepsy who had this procedure. Eighteen patients had investigative neurophysiologic procedures; 9 had intractable epilepsy and 9, cerebral palsy. Cortical somatosensory evoked potentials were recorded on median nerve stimulation in 14 patients.

Significant improvement was found in 68% of the 100 pa-

(5) Neurosurgery 1:203–205, Sept.–Oct., 1977.

tients with cerebral palsy. Spasticity was reduced after 30 days of CCS and was further improved at a mean follow-up of 13.2 months. Athetosis showed more improvement at follow-up than at 30 days. Younger patients had the best results, as did those with considerable muscular control. Nineteen patients reported improved vision after CCS. Eighteen epileptic patients showed a good response to CCS, with at least a 50% reduction in seizures. Half these patients had generalized seizures.

Virtually all patients reported increased alertness and better concentration after treatment. Depression was often reduced and the fluency of speech improved. No patient had adverse psychologic effects from CCS. Two patients died of postoperative hemorrhage. Seven cerebrospinal fluid leaks required surgical correction. No clinical neurologic sequelae of CCS were observed. Three autopsies showed cerebellar tissue damage confined to the area subjacent to the electrodes.

Chronic cerebellar stimulation inhibited H reflexes, V_1 and V_2 responses, blink reflexes, somatosensory evoked potentials and paroxysmal discharges in the EEG. No excitatory effects were observed during or immediately after CCS but a "rebound" of evoked potential amplitude and reflex responses was noted after cessation of stimulation. Thresholds for stimulation varied widely.

Chronic cerebellar stimulation is effective and safe in the treatment of selected neurologic disease. Each apparatus is presently calibrated at follow-up examination.

► [This abbreviated article appeared as a part of a symposium on neuroaugmentive devices, and the complete papers are being published in the journal *Applied Neurophysiology*. Davis et al. (Neurosurgery 1:205, 1977) report on chronic cerebellar stimulation to reduce spasticity and involuntary movements in 156 patients; they believe the patients are not transformed but are more independent, more ambulatory and more communicative. Sances et al. (ibid., p. 207) have studied the electrode configuration and current patterns with evoked potential change in the cerebellum. Applications in human beings are given by Larson et al. (ibid. p. 212). Other sessions of the symposium included discussions of deep cerebral stimulation, spinal cord stimulation and nerve and muscle stimulation. — Ed.] ◄

Cerebral Commissurotomy for Control of Intractable Seizures. Donald H. Wilson, Alexander Reeves, Michael Gazzaniga and Charles Culver[6] performed partial or

(6) Neurology (Minneap.) 27:708–715, August, 1977.

complete cerebral commissurotomy in 10 patients. "Frontal" commissurotomy consisted of division of the anterior commissure, one fornix and the anterior half of the corpus callosum. The complete operation included division of the entire corpus callosum with the underlying hippocampal commissure, one fornix and the anterior commissure. The operating microscope and microsurgical procedures were used. All patients had been incapacitated by seizures for at least 4 years despite vigorous anticonvulsant medication. None was considered a candidate for standard surgical methods. All had at least 4 daytime seizures per month and were unable to lead reasonably normal lives.

Three complete and 5 frontal commissurotomies were done, whereas 2 patients had total division of the corpus callosum and hippocampal commissure. With 1 possible exception, no patient had worse seizures postoperatively. Generalized seizures stopped or were converted to partial seizures. A good effect on complex partial seizures was also evident. Anticonvulsants were, however, necessary after the operation, because partial seizures continued to occur in some patients to a variable and unpredictable extent. The operation seemed most effective in patients with obvious unilateral brain damage. Invasion of the ventricular system was hazardous; ventriculitis and hydrocephalus were the most serious complications. The acute disconnection syndrome occurred to varying degrees in all patients.

Cerebral commissurotomy may eventually play a small but definitive role in the management of intractable epilepsy, but the procedure must be refined and criteria for patient selection clarified. Dexamethasone and prophylactic antibiotics are to be used in connection with the operation. Only the corpus callosum with the hippocampal commissure will be sectioned, with the ventricular ependyma spared. At present, patients without clear-cut unilateral brain damage will not be excluded solely for this reason, although the chance of seizure relief is greater if this can be proved.

Surgical Treatment of Epilepsy during Childhood and Adolescence. John R. Green[7] (St. Joseph's Hosp. and Med. Center, Phoenix, Ariz.) observes that the procedures most commonly used for neurosurgical treatment of epilepsy

(7) Surg. Neurol. 8:71–80, August, 1977.

in childhood and adolescence are temporal lobectomy, cortical excisions in extratemporal regions and hemicorticectomy. Less commonly used procedures include commissurotomy, stereotactic ablations and chronic cerebellar stimulation. Of 145 epileptics treated in 1948–76, 50 were aged 2–18 years; the rest were older. Temporal lobectomy was most commonly performed in both age groups, whereas hemicorticectomy was done only in younger patients. The seizure pattern should indicate a discharging lesion in a localized, accessible area of the brain, and serial EEGs and special studies should localize the epileptogenic area. Intensive anticonvulsant drug therapy should be shown to be inadequate to stop seizures before operation is performed. Major surgery must be possible without undue risk.

Thirty-two children and adolescents had temporal lobectomy, 10 had nontemporal cortical excision or lobectomy, 6 had hemicorticectomy or partial hemicorticectomy and 2 had no excision. Nine of 28 patients had permanent morbidity after temporal lobectomy. Nondisabling hemianopsia was most frequent. There was no mortality in this group. A highly satisfactory effect on seizures was obtained in all but 2 of the 28 patients. Five patients have had no seizures or aura while off medication and 12 have had none while on reduced amounts of medications. Effects on behavior have been generally satisfactory. The socioeconomic rehabilitation of these children has been gratifying. Two of 10 children were relieved from seizures by nontemporal cortical excisions and 4 were improved. Four patients were relieved by hemicorticectomy, whereas 1 died postoperatively. Partial hemicorticectomy resulted in improvement in 1 patient.

Children and adolescents with seizures, if unresponsive to medications, face more serious morbidity and mortality risks than normal subjects. Appropriate surgical treatment can result in excellent rehabilitation of about 80% of these patients who are disabled by seizures and frequently by behavior problems.

▶ [Jensen and Vaernet (Acta Neurochir. (Wien) 37:173, 1977) have followed 74 patients who had temporal lobe resection in 1960–69 for epilepsy. In the first 16, electrocorticography was done, but it is now considered proper to operate on the basis of a preoperative unilateral temporal lobe focus in a patient whose seizures are poorly controlled. Resection is done to 6 cm from the temporal pole in the dominant hemisphere and 7 cm in the nondominant hemisphere, with the tissue taken en bloc. At follow-up, 45 patients were free of seizures, 15 had reduction of seizures by at least 75% and 10 were not improved. There were 4 deaths. Paranoid and schizophrenic psychoses were not helped, but behavioral disturbances, especially aggression, were. Patients with anterior and medial foci did better than those with middle temporal or posterior temporal foci. The authors find a poorer prognosis with longer duration of epilepsy, so they advocate operation for temporal lobe seizures as early in life as possible and, in all events, as soon as the epilepsy has proved resistant to medication.

The experiences at the University of Washington Hospital from 1952 to 1976 with 45 epileptic patients subjected to operation have been reviewed by Rapport, Ojemann, Wyler and Ward (West. J. Med. 127:185, 1977). Ten were aged 10–20 and the others were aged up to 47 years. Nine had frontal and 31 had temporal lobe operations and 3 had partial and 1 had complete hemispherectomy; in single patients, the resections were temporoparietal and frontoparietal. One patient had no resection because no focus of abnormality was found at electrocorticography. Over an average follow-up period of 4.4 years, 36% were seizure free and another 40% were improved (i.e., either only an occasional seizure or such a reduction as to make a major beneficial impact on the life of the patient). Only 11% showed no improvement. Four tumors, 2 angiomas and 1 arteriovenous malformation were included in the series. The authors suggest earlier consideration of operation in epileptic patients with focal seizures in whom medical management fails or is complicated by drug reactions.

Zülch (Seara Med. Neurocirurg. 6:13, 1977) has used the phylogenic and ontogenic information available plus the results of studies on human beings with hemispherectomy to try to understand the organization of the functions of the central nervous system and the peculiarities of function after hemispherectomy. He emphasizes a chronological development of the three important functions—looking, grasping and walking. This orocaudal pattern is matched by the myelination of the appropriate segments of the pyramidal pathway. The uncoordinated motor pattern of the newborn is subserved by the already myelinated descending pathways from the extrapyramidal motor nuclei (globus, subthalamic nucleus and substantia reticularis). Synergistic movements in an anencephalic "midbrain being" are exactly like those of an early normal child. The archaic apparatus involved is later suppressed by the pyramidal pathway. In infantile hemiplegia or after total hemispherectomy including basal ganglia and thalamus, there still remains a compensatory motor system with synergies. Zülch believes this to be the parapyramidal motor system, which has descending fibers from the mesencephalon, reticular system and possibly part of the gamma systems, with bundles lying in the dorsal mesencephalon and medulla oblongata and later in the ventral half of the spinal cord. He does not believe there is an ipsilateral pyramidal pathway that can explain motor activities after hemispherectomy, in part because of the possibility of walking with synergistic movements in a patient with bilateral cortical destruction. (However, this does not take into account the supplementary motor pathways of the cortex.) There may be "triggering" of the mesencephalic apparatus either from ipsilateral or contralateral cortical areas. On the other hand, most of the sensory modalities perceived after hemispherectomy can be perceived entirely on an ipsilateral system, and evidence for this can come from evoked sensory potentials. – Ed.] ◄

Answers to Questions for Clinicians

The page references direct the reader to the articles containing the answers to the quiz.

Subject Index

ischemic attacks and, 201
Hypertensive vasculopathy: and
hydrocephalus, 218
Hypophyseal stalk division: for
exophthalmos after ^{131}I in
Graves' disease, 358
Hypothalamus: in Parkinson's
disease, 98

I

Ictal patterns: in epilepsy with
temporal lobe foci, 73
Ideation: motor, cerebral blood
flow in dominant
hemisphere during, 47
Ig (see Immunoglobulin)
Immunity: cell-mediated, of
lymphocytes to myelin
protein in demyelinating
diseases, 127
Immunodeficiency: and
poliomyelitis after
vaccination, in children, 59
Immunoglobulin
bands, CSF oligoclonal, 137
-containing cells in multiple
sclerosis plaques, 131
G
antibodies, oligoclonal virus-
specific, in CNS, 115
CSF, fluorometric assay, 236
deposition in immunologic
myopathy, 164
Immunologic
disorder, cerebral atrophy as, 21
myopathy, 164
Immunopathology: jejunal, in
sclerosis, 140
Immunosuppression: in
myasthenia gravis, 148
Infant: myasthenia gravis,
prednisone and thymectomy
in, 153
Infarction
cerebral, computed tomography
of, 230
myocardial, cardiac arrest in,
brain damage after, 213
Infection of wound: after
neurosurgery, 330

Injury (see Trauma)
Intensive care: neurosurgical, 261
Interictal behavior: in temporal
lobe epilepsy, 72
Intracranial pressure, 263 ff.
effect of bedside procedures on,
264
recordings in intracranial
hypertension, 263
Iodine-131 therapy: of Graves'
disease, exophthalmos after,
358
Iron-acrylic compound: for
stereotactic aneurysm
thrombosis, 393
Irradiation (see Radiation)
Ischemia: vertebral-basilar,
intracranial bypass grafts
in, 409
Ischemic attacks: carotid and
vertebral-basilar transient,
201
Isotope (see Radionuclide)

J

Jackson-Pratt drain: in cervical
spine surgery, 350
Jejunum, 138 ff.
immunopathology in sclerosis,
140
paramyxovirus from, in multiple
sclerosis, 138

K

Klippel-Trenaunay-Weber
syndrome: and spinal cord
arteriovenous malformation,
401

L

Lactate dehydrogenase isoenzyme
5: in Duchenne's muscular
dystrophy carriers, 162
Lactic acidosis: after grand mal
seizures, 71
Laminectomy: arteriovenous
fistula after, 348
Laminotomy: replacement, 308

Index to Authors